THERAPEUTIC PROGRESS IN OVARIAN CANCER, TESTICULAR CANCER AND THE SARCOMAS

BOERHAAVE SERIES
FOR POSTGRADUATE
MEDICAL EDUCATION
Vol. 16

PROCEEDINGS OF A BOERHAAVE COURSE
ORGANIZED BY
THE FACULTY OF MEDICINE, UNIVERSITY OF LEIDEN
THE NETHERLANDS
AND
THE PAGE AND WILLIAM BLACK POSTGRADUATE
SCHOOL OF MEDICINE OF THE
MOUNT SINAI SCHOOL OF MEDICINE (CUNY)
NEW YORK, U.S.A.
HELD DECEMBER 6-8, 1979

THERAPEUTIC PROGRESS IN OVARIAN CANCER, TESTICULAR CANCER AND THE SARCOMAS

edited by

A.T. VAN OOSTEROM, M.D.
State University Hospital
Leiden

F.M. MUGGIA, M.D.
New York University, Medical Center
New York

F.J. CLETON, M.D.
Netherlands Cancer Institute
Amsterdam

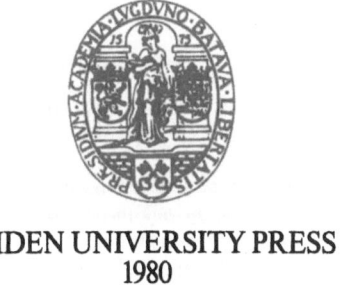

LEIDEN UNIVERSITY PRESS
1980

Distributors:

for the United States and Canada

Kluwer Boston, Inc.
160 Old Derby Street
Hingham, MA 02043
USA

for all other countries

Kluwer Academie Publishers Group
Distribution Centre
P.O. Box 322
3300 AH Dordrecht
The Netherlands

Library of Congress Cataloging in Publication Data

Main entry under title:

Therapeutic progress in ovarian cancer, testicular cancer, and the sarcomas.

(Boerhaave series for postgraduate medical education; v. 16)
"Proceedings of a Boerhaave course organized by the Faculty of
Medicine, University of Leiden, the Netherlands and the Page and William
Black Postgraduate School of Medicine of the Mount Sinai School of
Medicine (CUNY), New York, U.S.A."
Includes bibliographical references and index.
1. Ovaries - - Cancer - - Congresses, 2. Testis - - Cancer - -
Congresses. 3. Sarcoma - - Congresses. I. Oosterom, A. T. van. II.
Muggia, Franco M. III. Cleton, F. J. IV. Leyden. Rijksuniversiteit.
Faculteit der Geneeskunde. V. Page and William Black Postgraduate
School of Medicine. VI. Series. [DNLM: 1. Ovarian neoplasms - -
Therapy - -Congresses. 2. Testicular neoplasms - - Therapy - -Congres-
ses. 3. Sarcoma - - Therapy - - Congresses. W3 B0672 nr. 16 / QZ266
T398]
RC280.U8T47   616.99'46506   80-12670
ISBN-13: 978-94-009-9155-2   e-ISBN-13: 978-94-009-9153-8
DOI: 10.1007/978-94-009-9153-8

Cover design: Paul Burg

PREFACE

The Boerhaave Committee for postgraduate Medical Education
decided to organize a course on cancer treatment covering
selected solid tumors, in which they felt important changes were emerging in the basic biologic, diagnostic and
therapeutic concepts. Current management of cancer patients
is intimately dependent on precise morphologic diagnosis,
clinical staging and the proper application of all treatment modalities.

Many prominent investigators and clinicians of major cancer centers in the United States, Canada, and Europe con-
tributed by lecturing and during the panel discussions.
This book is the tangible outcome of the productive ex-
changes during the meeting held December 6-8, 1979.

In ovarian cancer the usefulness of histologic grading in
determining prognosis has become clear. The most important advance for the management of the patient is the -
careful staging procedure, based on new concepts of tumor
spread coupled with treatment tailored to the extent of
disease. Survival appears to be directly related to the
extent of the tumor mass. This has resulted in description
and application of optimal cyto-reductive surgery.
Radiotherapy and chemotherapy can both effectively eradicate small amounts of tumor.
In bulky disease treatment with new potent drug combination regimens may subsequently be complemented by reductive surgery. The complete remission rate in bulky disease has sharply increased with new therapeutic regimens

and gives hope that more patients will become longterm
survivors. The recently developed human tumor stem cell
assay and new methods for drug delivery and assessment
of response have the potential for identifying additional
systemic therapies.

In testicular cancer, a major problem lies in the equivalence of clinical versus pathological staging. In the
stage I non-seminomatous tumors, the results of surgery
and radiotherapy appear to be equal and consistent with
a 90-100 per cent cure rate. The problem, however, arises
with the presence of disease in retroperitoneal nodes and
how to reconcile the type of local treatment with the ur-
gent need for systemic therapy. Spectacular results have
been obtained with chemotherapy even in very late stages.
There are indications that application of chemotherapy in
all stages will be associated with dramatically improved
survival.
In fact the role of surgery has been changed from cytoreduction to adjuvant. This means that the best sequence
in the treatment of large tumor masses is chemotherapy
first, followed by surgery. With proper centralized treatment a 70 per cent cure rate is being obtained in advanced
disease.

In osteosarcoma major strides have been made in overall
survival results, however, the influence of histologic
type and grade on survival is often misjudged. Improvement of survival without adjuvant therapy has been reported and great variability exists in results from adjuvant
programs mostly in small series. The role of adjuvant
chemotherapy and radiotherapy on survival needs to be
clarified in larger prospective randomised controlled
studies with proper staging procedures.
Limb-salving procedures after pretreatment with chemotherapy also call for further exploration. The role of
surgery in minimal lung disease has been underestimated
and requires renewed attention.

In soft tissue sarcoma the histologic type and grading
are major discriminants for survival. This stresses the
need for adequate tissue sampling for histologic examination. The cornerstone of the treatment of the primary
is surgery; radiotherapy, however, must always be employed
if there is doubt about the margins. For chemotherapy the
role in the adjuvant situation is under study.
In advanced disease results are still disappointing by a
lack of drugs to build on the efficacy demonstrated by
Adriamycin. Further investigation in this field is actively being pursued and represents the hope for future improvements in survival.

This course was cosponsored by the Page and William Black
Postgraduate School of Medicine from the Mount Sinaï
School of Medicine, New York, N.Y., U.S.A.

We thank the authors for their splendid contributions,
Bristol Myers, the Netherlands, for financial support
and the personal support of Mrs. G. Boussauw-Weenink.
The secretarial work of Mrs. I. Blaschek-Lut is greatly
acknowledged.

A.T. van Oosterom, Leiden
F.M. Muggia, New York
F.J. Cleton, Amsterdam

30 December 1979

CONTENTS

CONTRIBUTORS

A. BARRETT, Division of Radiotherapy, The Royal Marsden
Hospital, Sutton, Surrey, London, England.

K. BREUR, Department of Radiotherapy, Netherlands Cancer
Institute, Amsterdam, The Netherlands.

D. CHASSAGNE, Department of Radiotherapy, Institut Gustave
Roussy, Villejuif, Paris, France.

F.J. CLETON, Department of Internal Medicine, Netherlands
Cancer Institute, Amsterdam, The Netherlands.

D. CROWTHER, Department of Medical Oncology, Christie
Hospital and Holt Radium Institute, University of
Manchester, Manchester, England.

A.J. DEMBO, Department of Radiotherapy, Ontario Cancer
Institute, Toronto, Canada.

R.B. GOLBEY, Department of Medical Oncology, Solid Tumor
Service, Memorial Sloan Kettering Cancer Center, New York,
New York, U.S.A.

C.TH. GRIFFITHS, Department of Gynecology and Obstetrics,
Harvard Medical School; Department of Gynecology and
Oncology, Sidney Farber Cancer Institute and Hospital for
Women, Boston, Massachusetts, U.S.A.

D.D. VON HOFF, Department of Medicine, Division of Oncology,
University of Texas Health Science Center, San Antonio,
Texas, U.S.A.

J.F. HOLLAND, Department of Neoplastic Diseases, Mount
Sinai School of Medicine, New York, New York, U.S.A.

C. MERRIN, Division of Urology, Loyola University Swedish
Convenant Hospital, Chicago, Illinois, U.S.A.

F.M. MUGGIA, Division of Oncology, New York University
Medical Center, New York, New York, U.S.A.

E.S. NEWLANDS, Department of Medical Oncology, Charing
Cross Hospital (Fulham), London, England.

A.T. VAN OOSTEROM, Department of Radiotherapy and Medical Oncology, State University Hospital, Leiden, The Netherlands.

H.M. PINEDO, Department of Medical Oncology, Free University Hospital and Department of Internal Medicine, Netherlands Cancer Institute, Amsterdam, The Netherlands.

CH.B. PRATT, St. Jude Children's Research Hospital, Memphis, Tennessee, U.S.A.

G. ROSEN, Departments of Pediatrics and Medicine, Memorial Sloan Kettering Cancer Center, New York, New York, U.S.A.

M. ROZENCWEIG, Investigational Drug Section, Department of Medicine, Division of Chemotherapy, Institut Jules Bordet, Brussels, Belgium.

TH.G. VAN RIJSSEL, Department of Pathology, State University, Leiden, The Netherlands.

S.E. SALMON, Section of Haematology and Oncology, Department of Internal Medicine, University of Arizona, Health Sciences Center, Tuczon, Arizona, U.S.A.

J. SESKI, Department of Gynecology, University of Texas System Cancer Center, M.D. Anderson Hospital and Tumor Institute, Houston, Texas, U.S.A.

W.F. SINDELAR, Surgery Branch, National Cancer Institute, National Institutes of Health, Bethesda, Maryland, U.S.A.

D.G. SKINNER, Division of Urology, Department of Surgery, University of California School of Medicine, Los Angeles, California, U.S.A.

J.P. SMITH, Department of Gynecology and Obstetrics, Wayne State University School of Medicine, Hutzel Hospital, Detroit, Michigan, U.S.A.

D.J. STEWART, Department of Developmental Therapeutics, University of Texas System Cancer Center, M.D. Anderson Hospital and Tumor Institute, Houston, Texas, U.S.A.

G. STOTER, Department of Medical Oncology, Free University Hospital, Amsterdam, The Netherlands.

P. THOMAS, Department of Radiotherapy, State University Hospital, Leiden, The Netherlands.

J.A.M. VAN UNNIK, Department of Pathology, State University Hospital,Utrecht, The Netherlands.

B.H.P. VAN DER WERF-MESSING, Department of Radiotherapy, Rotterdam Radiotherapeutic Institute, Rotterdam, The Netherlands.

S.D. WILLIAMS, Department of Haematology-Oncology, Indiana
University Medical Center, Indianapolis, Indiana, U.S.A.

E. WILTSHAW, Division of Medical Oncology, The Royal
Marsden Hospital, London, England.

R.C. YOUNG, Medicine Branch, National Cancer Institute,
National Institutes of Health, Bethesda, Maryland, U.S.A.

PART ONE

OVARIAN CANCER

1 CYTOREDUCTIVE SURGICAL TREATMENT IN THE MANAGEMENT OF ADVANCED OVARIAN CANCER

C. Th. Griffiths

Tumor resection without expectation of complete excision
violates the traditional tenets of surgical oncology and
obfuscates the concept of operability. Acquisition of
basic knowledge in tumor cell kinetics and the success of
chemotherapeutic adjuvants to presumably complete tumor
excision have led to a new concept often expressed as
"surgical debulking" or "reductive surgery." In this
sense an operation becomes a precedent adjuvant to chemotherapy which is employed with curative intent against a
known tumor residuum. Chemotherapy thus becomes the primary therapeutic modality in contrast to its secondary or
adjuvant role when residual tumor is only suspected.

For several decades surgeons have been admonished to
remove as much ovarian cancer tissue as possible, even
when disseminated intra-abdominal disease is encountered
at primary operation. In addition to an observed palliative effect of bulk resection, survival has been prolonged in patients with stage III disease if all gross tumor
is excised, or if there are no palpable masses postoperatively. (1,2,3,4)

The apparent inverse relationship between tumor volume and survival of ovarian cancer patients is consistent
with the natural history of the disease. Epithelial carcinomas of the ovary disseminate by implantation of clon-
igenic cells on peritoneal surfaces. Lymphatic spread to
para-aortic lymph nodes is common, but extra-abdominal
dissemination by this route is slow. Hematogenous spread
is usually a late manifestation and in nearly half of
those who succumb to the disease the tumor has not extend-

ed beyond the abdominal cavity or retroperitoneal lymph
nodes. Although the under surface of the right hemidia-
phragm may be involved early in the course of the disease,
the density of tumor implantation is greatest in proximity to the primary tumor. Consequently, pelvic peritoneum,
sigmoid colon, omentum, cecum and terminal ileum are most
frequently and extensively involved. Occasionally conti -
guous growth within the omentum predominates; bulky tumor
occupying the anterior abdomen extends over the transverse
colon to the greater curvature of the stomach and along
the gastrocolic and gastrosplenic ligaments to involve the
splenic pedicle.

As a group the epithelial carcinomas are relatively
non-invasive and destruction of vital organs is infrequent
With increasing tumor growth, however, there is progressive mechanical interference with gastrointestinal function
Disordered small bowel motility secondary to tumor implantation and interference with neural transmission through
myenteric plexus results in a segmental ileus which may
simulate partial small bowel obstruction. Metabolic effects of an enlarging tumor bulk are no less inimical. As
a parasite the tumor has an avidity for glucose and amino
acids which transcends that of host tissues. In the ox-
ygen-poor microenvironment of the tumor, energy is derived
by anerobic glycolysis (Embden-Meyerhof pathway), which is
not only an inefficient energy source but also leads to an
accumulation of lactic acid. The energy-dependent conver-
sion of excess lactic acid to glucose in the liver (Cori
cycle) further depletes energy stores. The predominant
catabolic effect of the tumor on the host is protein deficiency. With diminished oral intake and increasing demand by proliferating tumor for glucose and amino acids,
proteolysis of skeletal muscle protein maintains the pool
of free amino acids necessary for gluconeogenesis and visceral protein synthesis by the liver. This translocation
of skeletal to visceral protein is further exaggerated by
the additional requirement for visceral protein imposed by
ascites formation. The net result of these mechanical and

metabolic tumor effects is a borderline state of nutritional compensation which may be clinically inapparent for a considerable period of time. Cognizance of these adverse nutritional effects is critical, since the sudden imposition of a new demand for protein, e.g. a surgical wound may tip the balance and result in a rapidly decompensating phase in which the depleted skeletal muscle stores are unable to keep pace with the large amino acid requirement for wound healing. Visceral protein synthesis is sharply curtailed resulting in rapid reaccumulation of ascites, gross anasarca and a depleted blood volume. Without surgical intervention death follows a protracted period of progressive inanition. In general the proximity of death appears to be related to the volume of proliferating tumor within the abdominal cavity.

In 1964 we undertook a retrospective analysis of 103 patients with stages II and III ovarian cancer in order to answer the following questions: 1) What is the relationship between size of residual tumor masses and survival? 2) Is residual mass size an independent determinant of survival, or is it simply representative of the extent and agressiveness of the tumor? 3) Will the surgical excision of masses above a certain size limit favorably affect survival? If so, what is that size limit?

We used a multiple linear regression equation with survival as the dependent variable to control simultaneously for multiple therapeutic and biologic variables.(5) As an independent determinant of survival the diameter of the largest residual mass was statistically significant at the two percent level. Regardless of other prognostic factors survival time was uniformly poor if the diameter of the largest residual tumor mass exceeded 1.0 ± 0.5 cm, but increased in proportion to decrements in mass size below that range. Approximately half of those patients whose largest mass size was below 1.5 cm in diameter had undergone resection of larger metastatic lesions. This group fared as well as those whose largest metastatic les-

ions were below the 1.5 cm limit at the outset. We concluded that surgical "debulking" would be valueless unless
all tumor masses larger than 1.5 cm in diameter were excised and that a further reduction in largest mass size
below this limit would further enhance survival. For the
purpose of discussion we have termed these operations "optimal," but, since others have used a diameter of 2 cm as
the critical limit, it seems appropriate to expand our definition of "optimal" to this extent. The assumption that
an optimal operation prolongs survival by relieving or delaying the adverse nutritional effects imposed by a massive tumor burden seems reasonable.

Current evidence suggests that a more important result
of an optimal operation is the reduction in tumor mass
size to a point where chemotherapy or irradiation will exert a maximal effect. The value of cytoreductive operations for a chemotherapy sensitive tumor as well as the
necessity for near complete tumor excision was clearly demonstrated by Magrath et al in 1974.(6) After removal of
at least 90 percent of abdominal tumor in Burkitt's lymphoma, patients treated with cyclophospamide achieved remission and long term survival comparable to those of patients with jaw involvement only. Excision of greater
than 50 percent but less than 90 percent of tumor bulk
failed to improve remission and survival rates beyond
those observed without surgical resection. In a prospective trial of postoperative therapy reported from the
Princess Margaret Hospital, Toronto, the survival curve
of patients receiving whole abdominal radiation was significantly better than that of patients receiving pelvic
irradiation plus chlorambucil, only when the comparison
was made among patients with a small tumor residuum (those
who had undergone total abdominal hysterectomy and bilateral salpingo-oophorectomy.) Furthermore the survival
of those patients without gross residual disease surpassed
that of patients with a small tumor residuum.(7)

The association between a complete response to chemotherapy and a prolongation of survival has been well es-

tablished (8,9,10,11,12). Furthermore two recent studies
suggest that more than 50 percent of patients with stage
III disease in whom chemotherapy has induced complete remissions confirmed by multiple intraperitoneal biopsies
will survive four to five years from diagnosis (12,13).
These figures contrast sharply with the five to seven percent five year survival rates usually reported (9). Table
1 illustrates the dependence of a complete remission on
residual mass size, but equal dependence on the use of
combination chemotherapy rather than single agent therapy
is also apparent. In the report from the M.D. Anderson
Hospital the overall response rate to hexamethylmelamine
was independent of mass size, but the three patients with
biopsy confirmed complete responses (CR) had masses less
than 2 cm in diameter at the outset. (11) In contrast,
melphalan (as the control arm in the National Cancer Institute HEXACAF study) induced a greater proportion of
overall responses in patients with masses under 2 cm than
in those with larger masses; the CR rate was the same.(13)
The effect of mass size on the incidence of confirmed complete responses was readily apparent when effective drug
combinations were employed. In the NCI study hexamethyl-
melamine-cyclophosphamide-methotrexate-fluoruracil(HEXACAF)
induced complete responses in all eight patients with
masses under 2 cm whereas only five of 32 patients with
larger masses were complete responders. At the Sidney
Farber Cancer Institute and the Boston Hospital for
Women 11 of 12 patients with masses less than 2 cm in diameter had complete responses as compared with only one of
29 patients with larger masses. (12)

By 1974 we were encouraged by our preliminary results
with combined adriamycin-cyclophosphamide therapy and were
satisfied that our multivariate analysis had defined a
practical surgical objective. As a result, we undertook
a project to assess the feasibility of performing optimal
surgical operations on an unselected series of patients.
Equally important was a careful evaluation by laparoscopy
of the effect of post-operative combination chemotherapy

on residual tumor.

Our operative approach which has been described in detail (14) is based upon the relative noninvasiveness of ovarian epithelial carcinoma, the routes of tumor spread within the abdomen and basic anatomic concepts. Since lines of cleavage between tumor-bearing peritoneum and normal tissue usually exist, isolated masses may be safely removed from the surface of the liver, diaphragm, bowel and parietal peritoneum. Often an apparently hopeless situation may be dealt with simply, as in the case of contiguous omental involvement to the greater curvature of the stomach. Although the transverse colon may appear to be massively involved, excision of the omentum from the greater curvature with exposure of the lesser sac and transverse mesocolon followed by caudal dissection of tumor laden omentum within a lamellar plane usually reveals a transverse colon with surprisingly little adherent tumor. Excision of all gross tumor in the pelvis is facilitated by a lateral retroperitoneal dissection along the iliac vessels from the pelvic brim to the lower limit of tumor growth. By incising the bladder and rectal serosa the entire tumor bearing parietal and visceral peritoneum of the pelvis can be removed in continuity with the internal genitalia. Because of the proximity of the sigmoid colon and terminal ileum to the primary tumor, resection of these bowel segments is occasionally necessary. Patients have been considered inoperable in the presence of tumors greater than 1.5 cm in diameter which involve suprarenal para-aortic lymph nodes, lesser omentum, porta hepatis, or splenic pedicle, unless the splenic vessels can be safely isolated and ligated.

From December 1974 to December 1977, 28 operative procedures were performed on 26 consecutive patients with stage III or stage IV (three patients) ovarian epithelial adenocarcinoma. The results of this project have been reported in detail elsewhere. (14) Fifteen patients including two with stage IV disease underwent primary operation and secondary chemotherapy. (Group I) An optimal operation was carried out in twelve or 80 percent. Following operation eleven of the fifteen patients received adriamycin 45 mg/M^2 and cyclophosphamide 500 mg/M^2 intravenously every three weeks until the total cumulative dose of adriamycin reached 450 mg/M^2. Three of the remaining four patients were treated with melphalan alone because of advanced age and the final patient died of adrenal failure two months postoperatively after a single course of combination chemotherapy at another institution. Nine patients had extirpative operations after receiving apparently successful combination chemotherapy as primary treatment (Group II). Two of the three Group I patients who were operative failures were included in this category. Optimal operations were carried in seven patients (77 percent) including the two previously inoperable patients. Only four of the nine patients received combination chemotherapy postoperatively, because the remaining five had reached the total cumulative dose of adriamycin allowed. Group III consisted of four patients with recurrent disease after successful primary therapy. Optimal operations were possible in three of these (75 percent) and only one patient was eligible for adriamycin-cyclophosphamide thereafter.

There were no operative deaths in this series and only two major complications. We attribute the paucity of major complications to our all but routine use of total parenteral nutrition in the immediate postoperative period.

At the time of last analysis, ten patients in Group I were alive (six without disease) and the median survival time had not been reached at 18 months. In contrast only four of the nine patients in Group II were alive, two without disease, and the median survival time from secondary operation was nine months. In Group III two of four patients were alive, one without disease and the median survival time was twelve months. These results indicate that patients treated with primary resection and secondary chemotherapy (Group I) have fared the best. Since other prognostic variables (age, stage and grade) tended to weigh against Group I and the operability was the same for all groups, the superior results in Group I were attributable to the higher proportion of patients treated with combination chemotherapy. In considering only those patients who had optimal operations (all groups), 12 of the 14 patients who received postoperative combination chemotherapy were alive in excess of 19 months and eight patients had no evidence of disease. In contrast only two patients of eight who received single agent chemotherapy were alive, both with disease, and the median survival time was 14 months.

The effect of adriamycin-cyclophosphamide chemotherapy after optimal operation was determined by laparoscopies at three-month intervals in 12 patients who had gross tumor. The laparoscopy performed at the conclusion of chemotherapy (six-month treatment period) was the determinant of response. The results are compatible with those obtained in the NCI study with HEXACAF (Table 1).

Table 1.

Response to chemotherapy by diameter of largest mass

Agents	No. Patients	Objective Response	CR*
HXM(11)			
<2 cm	17	35%	18%
>2 cm	37	30%	0%
L-PAM(13)			
<2 cm	11	73%	18%
>2 cm	26	46%	15%
HEXACAF(13)			
<2 cm	8	100%	100%
>2 cm	32	69%	16%
ADRIA-CTX(12)			
<2 cm	12	100%	90%
>2 cm	29	38%	3%

* = biopsy confirmed

ABBREV: HXM = hexamethylmelamine
         L-PAM = melphalan
         HEXACAF = HXM + cyclophosphamide + methotrexate
                 + fluorouracil
         ADRIA-CTX = adriamycin + cyclophosphamide

In conclusion, cytoreductive surgical procedures will result in a modest but significant improvement in the survival time of patients with stage III ovarian cancer providing all tumor masses larger than 1½-2 cm in diameter are excised. Relief from direct tumor insult, however, is less important than reduction in mass size to a point where chemotherapy will exert a maximal effect. The attainment of a complete remission confirmed by intraperitoneal biopsy has been associated with median survival times (actuarial) in excess of four to five years. Complete remissions have been achieved in most patients who have undergone optimal cytoreductive operations and effective combination chemotherapy (Table 1).

REFERENCES

1. Declos L and Quinlan EJ: Malignant tumors of the ovary managed with postoperative megavoltage irradiation. Radiology 93:659, 1969.
2. Parker RT, Parker CH and Wilbanks GD: Cancer of the ovary. Am J Obstet Gynecol 108:878, 1970.
3. Aure JC, Hoeg K and Kolstad P: Clinical and histologic studies of ovarian carcinoma. Obstet Gynecol 37:1, 1971.
4. Griffiths CT, Grogan RH and Hall TC: Advanced ovarian cancer: Primary treatment with operation, radiotherapy and chemotherapy. Cancer 29:1, 1972.
5. Griffiths CT: Surgical resection of tumor bulk in the primary treatment of ovarian carcinoma. Symposium on Ovarian Cancer. Natl Cancer Inst Monogr   42:101, 1975.
6. Magrath IT: Surgical reduction of tumour bulk in management of abdominal Burkitt's lymphoma.   Br Med J 2:308, 1974.
7. Dembo AJ, Bush RS, Beale FA et al: Ovarian carcinoma: Improved survival following abdominopelvic irradiation in patients with a completed pelvic operation. Am J Obstet Gynecol 134:793, 1979.
8. Smith JP, Rutledge F and Wharton JT: Chemotherapy of ovarian cancer: New Approaches to treatment. Cancer 30:1565, 1972.
9. Tobias JS and Griffiths CT: Management of ovarian carcinoma: Current concepts and future prospects. N Engl J Med 294:818 and 877, 1976.
10. Young RC, Canellos GP, Chabner BA et al: Chemotherapy of advanced ovarian carcinoma: A prospective randomized comparison of phenylalamine mustard and high dose cyclophosphamide. Gynecol Oncol, 2:489, 1974.

11. Wharton JT, Rutledge F, Smith JP et al: Hexamethyl-melamine: An evaluation of its role in the treatment of ovarian cancer. Am J Obstet Gynecol 133;833, 1979.
12. Parker LM, Griffiths CT, Yankee RA et al: Combination chemotherapy with adriamycin-cyclophosphamide for advanced ovarian carcinoma. Cancer (in press).
13. Young RC, Chabner BA, Hubbard SP et al: Prospective trial of melphalan versus combination chemotherapy (HEXACAF) in ovarian adenocarcinoma. N Engl J Med 299:1261, 1978.
14. Griffiths CT and Fuller AF: Intensive surgical and chemotherapeutic management of advanced ovarian cancer. Surg Clin North Am 58:131, 1978.
15. Griffiths CT, Parker LM and Fuller AF: Role of Cyto-reductive surgical treatment in the management of advanced ovarian cancer. Cancer Treat Rep 63:235, 1979.

2 POST-OPERATIVE RADIOTHERAPY IN OVARIAN CANCER STAGES I AND II

A. J. Dembo, R. S. Bush, J. F. G. Sturgeon

INTRODUCTION

A rational approach to the therapy of ovarian cancer has been confounded by the many prognostic variables characteristic of the disease, and the use of inappropriate parameters to measure the outcome of treatment. Comment is necessary on both of these issues to permit an understanding of data pertaining to the title of this paper.

The limited value of staging classifications

> "At any era in the history of science, the further advance of science has been retarded by certain fundamental concepts that were enlightening when introduced, but that later, after persisting too long, became barriers to future progress."
>
> Feinstein (6).

In the last decade it has become quite clear that the extent of disease encountered at operation, i.e., the anatomic stage, is a wholly inadequate method of describing patient groups for purposes of prognostication or choice of therapy. (1,2)

The factors which have been shown to have greater prognostic significance are the amount of tumor residual after operation (3), the histologic grade (2,4), and the surgical technique used in staging (1,5). Recognition of the importance of these factors makes it essential to interpret data by multivariate techniques of analysis, examining outcome in subgroups defined according to patient and tumor characteristics. It also detracts greatly from the value of any staging classification. We believe that the use of any staging classification as the prime method of grouping patients for choice of treatment, prognostication, analysis of data, etc., is likely to obscure a clear appreciation of the events under consideration and is obstructing progress in understanding this disease.

A.T. van Oosterom et al. (eds.), Therapeutic Progress in Ovarian Cancer, Testicular Cancer and the Sarcomas, pp. 13-26. All rights reserved.
Copyright 1980 by Martinus Nijhoff Publishers, The Hague/Boston/London.

The FIGO staging classification, and the UICC and AJCC (TNM) staging classifications derived from it, suffer from several artificial distinctions between the staging categories. As a result staging conventions will differ from center to center. For example when does the degree of adherence of the tumor to the pelvic sidewall represent extension beyond the ovary (Stage IA versus IIB)? Applying the criterion of the need for sharp rather than blunt dissection to remove the tumor, relies on the technique of the surgeon rather than the extent of the tumor to define the stage! Should there be a distinction between Stage II and Stage III if the peritoneal cavity is continuous between the pelvis and abdomen? Evidence discussed below would indicate not (1,3).

Depending on the amount of residual disease, its grade, and the type of post-operative treatment, the prospects for long term survival within Stage II or III may range from less than 5% to greater than 80% (2). If tumor characteristics can be clearly defined, and they can, to permit the recognition of subgroups of Stage III patients with a better prognosis than clearly recognizable subgroups of Stage II patients, then why cling to the use of Stage to choose therapy or define prognosis?

Smith has demonstrated that 5 year survival rates for Stage II and Stage III patients are virtually identical, provided they are stratified by the size of the largest residual tumor mass (3). Thus for patients with no gross residuum or with gross residuum 1 cm or less, 5 year survival rates were 43.9% and 45.2% respectively for Stages IIB and III. When the residuum is 2 cm or greater, these figures fall to 18.9% and 6.9% respectively. Taken together with the evidence that the entire peritoneal cavity is at risk for implantation metastasis once disease has spread beyond the ovary (1-5), a strong argument can be made for approaching post-operative therapy in Stages II and III not on the basis of Stage, but on the extent of residual tumor present. Moreover, for patients with localized disease presentations, the histologic grade exerts a powerful prognostic influence (2).

The matter is further confounded by the technique of staging. The more meticulously the abdomen is explored, the more frequently will one encounter tumor spread beyond the pelvis (5). The effect of this is to classify as Stage III a considerable proportion of patients that would be considered to be Stage I or II on pelvic operation. The consequences are shown in Fig 1, where a theoretical disease is discussed. This disease has two stages: Stage A (confined to pelvis) and Stage B (spread to abdomen). Using 'older' staging techniques half of the patients belong in Stage A (75% cured) and half in Stage B (15% cured). Overall, 45% of patients are cured.

Theoretical Disease

Stage A = Pelvis   Stage B = Abdomen

	A=75	B=15	A+B = 45
Old staging:			
(% cures)	90 : 60	15	mean = 45
New staging:	A=90	B=30	A+B = 45

Figure 1.

With newer staging techniques that explore the upper abdomen, it is discovered that there are in fact 2 (equal) subpopulations of Stage A: a group with a cure rate of 90% in whom there is no detectable evidence of upper abdominal spread, and another group with a cure rate of 60% in whom minimal evidence of gross abdominal spread can be found. When this latter group is classified in Stage B of the theoretical disease, the cure rate for Stage A becomes 90% and of Stage B 30%. The cure rate for Stage A and B combined unfortunately is still only 45%. This "improvement" in the cure rate in each stage has resulted from the reclassification of patients and not the treatment given. In ovarian cancer, treatment results in a given Stage using the newer techniques of classification are sometimes incorrectly contrasted with those obtained using the older staging technique. This is prone to occur when protocols are designed to examine a particular stage of the disease rather than the whole population. The safeguard against this pitfall is to study all stages and to report the result obtained in each individual stage as well as the result obtained for all stages combined.

Perhaps a graver error than ascribing improved results to therapy rather than reclassification, is to prescribe treatment for the patients classified using new staging techniques by applying concepts founded on experience with patients classified by less meticulous explorations. We have previously presented evidence that treating patients with minimally detectable upper abdominal disease in the same way as those who have large unresected upper abdominal masses may deny a proportion of the minimal disease patients the chance of being cured (1).

Endpoints for evaluating therapy

The answers clinicians really require from phase III clinical trials relate to the questions: does this treatment method CURE a higher proportion of patients, or does it better PALLIATE patients than the standard therapy (4)? Unfortunately the measurable parameters currently available do not assay cure or palliation directly. In general cure can be inferred from long term survival and disease-free or relapse-free survival rates. Prolongation of survival for patients who are not cured can be measured from median survival times. The duration of survival is one aspect of palliation that can be measured. Ideally of course we would like to measure quality-adjusted duration of survival. However, the quality of survival cannot be measured. This is a serious deficiency in our ability to measure the palliative worth of a therapy: investigators usually choose to ignore the impact on quality of life that treatment has even when studying clearly palliative situations.

The confusion that has arisen from use of measurable tumor regressions (i.e., response rates) as an endpoint of phase III trials is considerable. Tumor response is a parameter which measures the activity of a treatment method. As such its applicability should be restricted to phase II trials. Positive tumor responses do not reliably predict for patient cure. At best they predict prolongation of survival, a palliative endpoint, which is much better measured from the shape of the survival curve, and sometimes the median survival time, in a phase III situation (4). When investigators draw "phase III" conclusions (i.e., preferability of one treatment method over another) from data on response rates, a phase II endpoint, they are potentially doing a disservice to patients and to community physicians who rely on their con-

clusions. We regret that some investigators and Journal editors
consider this acceptable practice: it is not.

The most satisfactory way of comparing therapeutic outcomes in phase
III studies is by means of survival curves, or relapse-free survival
curves as an interim measure (4). The shape of the curve also gives
more information than a survival rate at a given time (e.g., 2, 5, or
10 years); or than a time at which a given proportion of patients are
alive (e.g., median or 3rd quartile survival times). As shown in Fig 2
the effect of treatment can result in a difference in the survival
curves by virtue either of increasing the <u>proportion</u> of long term survivors (Fig 2a), or of prolonging <u>duration</u> of survival without increasing the proportion of long term survivors (Fig 2b).

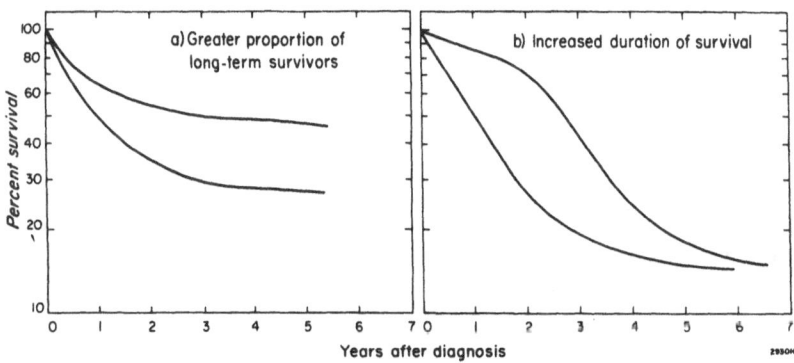

Figure 2.

If the curves differ significantly in the manner shown in Fig 2b, then
the therapy which produced the longer duration of survival may be regarded as the superior therapy in a palliative context, provided that
the toxicity of the therapy did not abrogate the benefit of prolonged
survival. Unless a treatment which produced a significantly greater
response rate also produces a significantly improved survival curve of
the type shown in Fig 2b, the observed effect on the tumor masses cannot be considered to have resulted in any gain at the clinical level (4),

Again; tumor response is not an appropriate endpoint for phase III studies.

In the setting of ovarian cancer, treatments which produce superior survival curves of the type shown in Fig 2a are usually curing a higher proportion of patients. The implications of a result of the type shown in Fig 2a usually make the choice between the two therapies a crucial one, as failure to appreciate this difference may result in the cure of fewer patients.

Finally, in ovarian cancer, when results of treatment are being compared by whatever endpoints, the comparison is only valid if the patient groups are closely matched by extent of residual disease, tumor grade, stage, staging technique, patient age and time at risk since diagnosis.

POST-OPERATIVE IRRADIATION FOR STAGES I AND II

The applicability of the foregoing discussion to the post-operative management of patients with Stages I and II ovarian cancer is twofold. First, stage designation alone should not form the basis for choice of post-operative therapy (2). The prognostic factors mentioned above, particularly the extent of residual disease and tumor grade must be considered as well. Second, the objective of therapy for these patients is cure. Since this objective can be successfully realized in the majority of cases, the endpoints used in any evaluation of a treatment method must be parameters that assay cure (4).

In Fig 3 the uncorrected actuarial relapse free survival curves are shown for all patients with Stage I and II presentations treated on the Princess Margaret Hospital (PMH) study between 1971 and 1977, all treatment methods. For the 78 Stage I cases studied, the 5-year relapse free survival rate (RFS_5) was 77.5%. Tumor grade appeared to be the dominant prognostic factor, with all relapses to date occurring in the patients with poorly or moderately differentiated tumors (2,4).

The RFS_5 for the 164 Stage II patients studied was 50% (Fig 3). However, Stage II is considerably more heterogeneous than Stage I. The

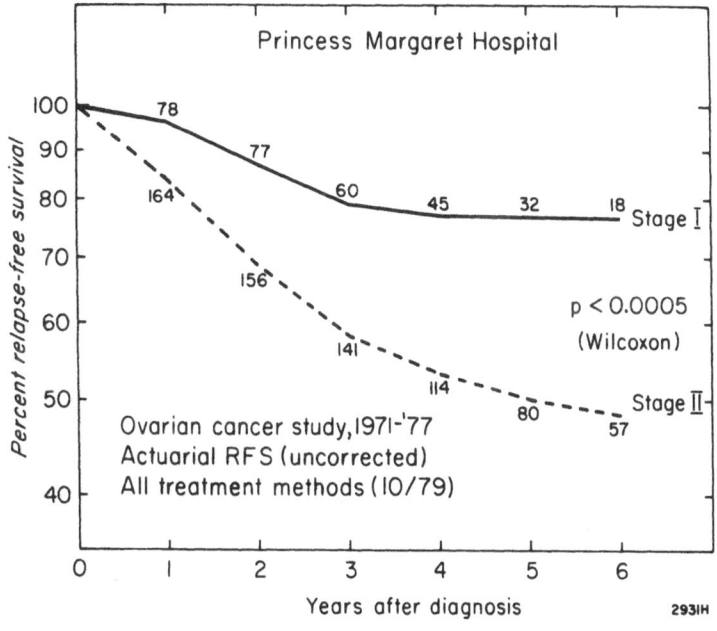

Figure 3.

dominant prognostic factor appears to be the amount of residual disease. Our first stratification, shown in Fig 4, depends on whether the pelvic tumor permitted completion of bilateral salpingo-oophorectomy and hysterectomy (BSOH)(1). The RFS_5 for 24 incomplete BSOH patients with residual tumor, usually much larger than 2 cm, was 8%, and the median survival time was 1 year. In contrast, the RFS_5 for 140 patients with BSOH incomplete but no gross tumor residuum, or with BSOH completed with and without gross residual tumor, was 57% (p < 0.0005). Data below suggests that, just as the prognosis of these two clearly defin-able subgroups of Stage II patients is vastly different, the choice of the therapy they receive should be different, too.

Amongst the therapeutic modalities with which considerable experience has been gained in the management of ovarian carcinoma, three major possibilities exist in the approach to the post-operative management of Stages I and II. These are: No Treatment, Radiotherapy and Chemo-therapy. The roles of combined modality treatment and immunotherapy remain to be defined.

20

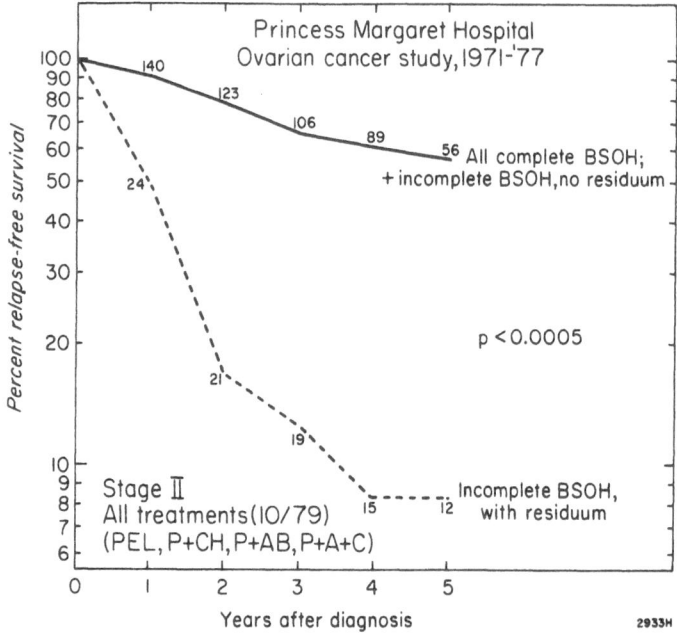

Figure 4.

Post-operative observation

A proportion of patients are cured by their operation. If the characteristics of these patients could be clearly defined, no post-operative
therapy would be required for them. It is likely this group is derived
from patients who presented with localized disease, who had all gross
disease excised and usually whose carcinoma was well differentiated(4).

Between 1971 and 1977, 55 patients with Stage IA were prospectively
studied at the PMH (2,4). Randomization was between pelvic irradiation
or observation. The frequency and sites of tumor relapse did not differ
significantly between the two groups, indicating that the pelvic irradiation did not afford any improvement over the result attainable with
observation alone (2). Analysis was in October 1979, with a median
period at risk exceeding 5 years. No relapses have occurred in the
patients with well differentiated (WD) carcinoma. These patients com-

prise 5% of all cases referred to the PMH; their RFS_5 was 100% (2). Histologic grading was based on the worst differentiated elements of the tumor, and 'borderline malignant' cases were not included. On the basis of these results we believe observation alone is appropriate post-operative therapy in Stage IA WD cases. The RFS_5 was 67% for the Stage IA patients with PD tumors. They require post-operative therapy and we prefer pelvic plus abdominopelvic irradiation, since tumor relapse is as likely to occur in the upper abdomen as in the pelvis.

Although the study design was different for Stage IB, none of the 6 cases with WD tumors has relapsed, and we are currently studying the question of whether any post-operative therapy is required for these patients. The RFS_5 for the Stage IB cases with PD tumors was 63%. Six of 17 Stage IB cases with PD tumors have relapsed (4/5 in the treatment groups which did not include abdominopelvic irradiation, and 2/12 in the groups which did). We believe adjuvant therapy is required for Stage IB patients with PD tumors and have found P+AB to be highly effective (see below)(2).

The Gynecology Oncology Group (GOG) compared observation with either pelvic irradiation or melphalan in a randomized study of Stage I cases (8). Nearly 50% of patients entered were excluded from the analysis (borderline histology, protocol violations) and rigid staging criteria were not applied in this multi-center study. No significant difference exists in survival between the treatment groups but there is a significantly higher proportion of relapses in the patients receiving pelvic radiation than those receiving melphalan (8/22 vs 2/30, p=0.02, Fisher 2 tail). However, one cannot use this data to conclude that melphalan is more effective therapy than pelvic irradiation in Stage I because relapses were not significantly higher in the control group than in the melphalan group (5/24 vs 2/30, p=0.3). Moreover, the numbers of evaluable patients in the melphalan group exceeds that in the radiation group by 37%. This suggests that the large number of patients excluded invalidate the usual statistical assumptions which depend on the process of randomization to ensure that the populations being compared are prognostically similar.

Post-operative irradiation

In a stratified, randomized study at the PMH of 132 patients with
Stages IB, II and III, in whom BSOH had been completed, we showed that
pelvic plus abdominopelvic irradiation (P+AB) was more effective than
pelvic irradiation alone (PEL) or followed with chlorambucil (P+CH)(1).
Patients were staged on referral to our Institute based on findings
contained in the operative report. Meticulous upper abdominal exploration was rarely carried out, but if it had been, one would expect 20-
40% of the cases classed in Stages I and II might have been assigned
to Stage III (1,5). This implies that conclusions drawn from the study
of these cases with Stages I and II applies to cases who are Stage III
by virtue of minimal upper abdominal involvement, detectable only by
meticulous staging. Thirty-six per cent of patients had known residual
disease usually inferred to be less than 2 cm diameter.

With a median period at risk of 62 months, actuarial 5 year relapse
free survival rates for PEL, P+CH and P+AB are 38%, 44% and 77% respectively. Relapse was assessed clinically and confirmed by radiologic
or sonographic means. Patients were rarely subjected to 'second-look'
surgical procedures or peritoneoscopy. The improved survival obtained
with P+AB ($p < 0.01$) was shown on failure analysis to be due to control
of occult upper abdominal disease in approximately 25% more patients
than that achieved with P+CH, or PEL ($p < 0.001$) (1). The effectiveness
of P+AB was most striking in 32 patients with no gross tumor residuum
(RFS_5 = 90% compared with 52% for 30 P+CH patients, p=0.003). For no-
residuum patients with poorly and moderately differentiated tumors,
P+AB significantly reduced the risk of relapse (3/23 P+AB, vs 12/18
P+CH; p=0.001). The efficacy of P+AB was thus not apparently influenced by tumor grade (2). The benefit resulting from P+AB in the above
subgroup of patients is reflected in an improved overall survival of
approximately 10% for post-operative patients of all stages treated
within our institution.

In Fig 5 the relapse free survival is shown for Stage II patients with
BSOH completed. These patients were treated with post-operative irradiation to the pelvis and whole abdomen between 1971 and 1975, and in

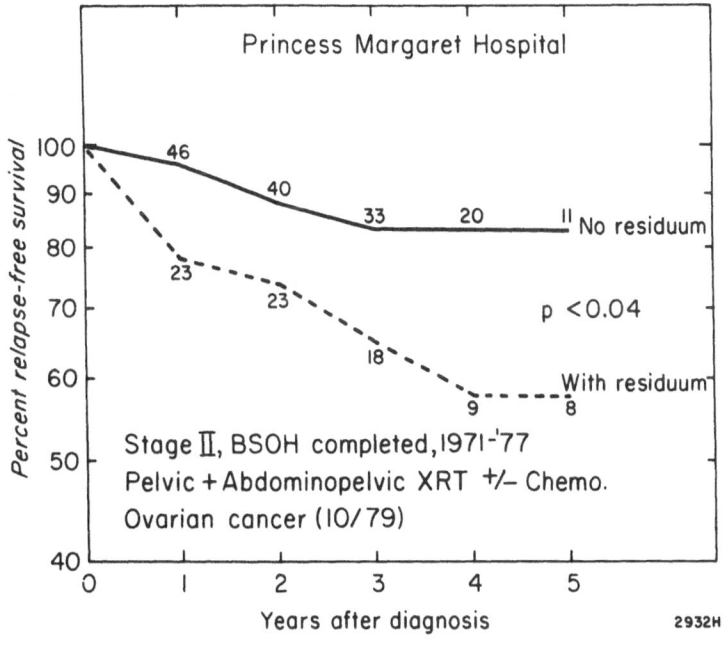

Figure 5.

1976-77, the radiotherapy was followed with 2 years of daily oral chemotherapy (chlorambucil or cyclophosphamide, (P+A+C). We have been unable to demonstrate any benefit resulting from use of the chemotherapy, which was poorly tolerated hematologically.) For patients with no known gross residuum, RFS_5 was 83%. When gross residuum was present, RFS_5 was 57% (p<0.04). Corresponding 5 year survival rates were 87% and 68.5%. Thus the BSOH completed group is not homogeneous and can be subgrouped by presence or absence of gross tumor residuum (Fig 5) and also by tumor grade (2,4).

The technique of abdominopelvic irradiation differs from that reported by others (7). Careful attention to anatomical detail and the use of a moderate radiation dose are critical factors in accounting for the results we obtained with P+AB. Serious toxicity was rare (1,7). After 2250 rads in 10 fractions to the pelvis, a downward moving strip was used to deliver 2250 rads in 10 fractions to the whole abdomen and pelvis. Radiographic verification was obtained to ensure the portals encompassed the diaphragm. No liver shielding was used, but the kidneys were shielded from the posterior beam (7).

In contrasting the positive PMH results for P+AB with the null outcome M.D. Anderson (MDAH) study which compared strip irradiation with melphalan for minimal disease cases, certain points emerge (4,9). First, there is evidence that the whole abdomen was not treated by the MDAH technique in all cases as in 23% of patients a field of only 30 cm or less was used (9,11). This implies that inclusion of the diaphragm in the irradiated field has a critical effect on the outcome of abdomino-pelvic irradiation. Second, at the MDAH a higher radiation dose resulted in more frequent serious and fatal complications. Third, there were more Stage I and fewer Stage II and III cases in the melphalan arm (11). Fourth, although all patients had residuum <2 cm, there was no stratification by whether gross disease was present or absent, a significant prognostic factor (2).

Another reason why the outcomes of the PMH and MDAH studies differ, might occur if P+CH produced inferior results than chemotherapy alone. However, analysis of data suggests that outcome in the P+CH is at least equal to results obtained by others using chemotherapy alone. Thus 10 of 21 BSOH-completed Stage II and III P+CH cases with known residual disease are relapse free. This is equivalent to a "complete response" rate of almost 50% sustained for a median period of 5 years. Furthermore, for the 26 BSOH-completed Stage II and III P+CH patients with no gross residuum, the RFS_5 rate is 54% (9). A Mayo Clinic study reported a 3 year RFS rate of 40% for Stage II and III patients with no residuum treated by cyclophosphamide alone or with adriamycin (9,10). At the MDAH the 5 year survival rates for similar cases was approximately 45% for a variety of treatment methods (3). Our RFS_5 for the 24 P+AB cases with similar features approaches 90% (2,9).

On the basis of the PMH results obtained with P+AB we conclude it is the post-operative treatment of choice in the following situations: Stage IA PD; Stage IB; Stage II and III no residuum, or small pelvic residuum (BSOH completed); and probably Stage III cases with small occasional foci of upper abdominal residual disease.

Post-operative chemotherapy

From the foregoing it can be concluded that our present recommendation
for post-operative chemotherapy in Stages I and II is restricted to
those cases with large amounts of residual disease (BSOH incomplete).
With PEL, P+CH or P+AB our RFS_5 for such cases at the PMH is 8% with the
median at one year (Fig 4). The role of radiation in such cases is limited. Certainly we would not recommend P+AB. The mainstay of therapy
is chemotherapy, though adjunctive pelvic irradiation may have a role
in some cases. For the vast majority of these patients therapy is palliative. Despite claims to the contrary, combination chemotherapy has
not been shown to offer patients with extensive residual tumor a greater
chance of cure than single agent therapy (4). This has two important
implications. First, the added toxicity of the combinations must be
borne in mind when a choice of therapy is made. Second, the greatest
potential for long term survival in such cases occurs if it is technically feasible to debulk their residual tumor to less than 1.5 or 2 cm
by surgical means before commencing post-operative treatment (12).

The results obtained with Cis-Platinum containing chemotherapy combinations are encouraging. Most reports are of short-term follow-up and
have used response rates as the reported endpoint. Until we know how
these responses influence the long term survival rates, the place of
these combinations as curative therapy remains investigational, and
their superiority over single agent chemotherapy remains unproven. For
patients with small amounts of residual tumor, i.e., those with BSOH
completed, P+AB must be taken as the standard against which these therapies are to be compared, using treatment morbidity and the long-term
survival rates as the endpoints for study.

REFERENCES

1. Dembo, A.J., Bush, R.S., Beale, F.A., Bean, H.A., Pringle, J.F.,
    Sturgeon, J., and Reid, J.G. Ovarian carcinoma: improved survival
    following abdominopelvic irradiation in patients with a completed
    pelvic operation. Am.J.Obstet.Gynecol., 134: 793, 1979.

2. Dembo, A.J., Sturgeon, J.F,G., Bean, H.A., Beale, F.A., Pringle, J.F. Brown, T.C., Gospodarowicz, M., and Bush, R.S. The effectiveness of adjuvant abdominopelvic irradiation in ovarian cancer. Adjuvant Therapy of Cancer II, Eds Jones and Salmon, Grune & Stratton, 1979.

3. Smith, J.P. Treatment of ovarian cancer. Advances in Chemotherapy, Japan Sci.Soc.Press, Tokyo/Univ.Park Press,Baltimore, 493, 1978.

4. Bush, R.S. and Dembo, A.J. Current status of treatment for patients with ovarian cancer. Proc.International Symposium of Ovarian Cancer, Birmingham UK, Pergamon Press, 1979 (in press).

5. Rosenoff, S.H., DeVita, V.T., Hubbard, S., and Young, R.C. Peritoneoscopy in the staging and follow-up of ovarian cancer. Semin.Oncol. 2: 223, 1975.

6. Feinstein, A. Clinical Biostatistics - XII: On exorcizing the ghost of Gauss and the curse of Kelvin. Clin.Pharmacol.Ther. 12: 1003, 1971.

7. Dembo, A.J., VanDyk, J., Japp, B., Bean, H.A., Beale, F.Å., Pringle, J.F., and Bush, R.S. Whole abdominal irradiation by a moving-strip technique for patients with ovarian cancer. Intl.J.Rad.Oncol.Biol. Phys. 1979 (in press, November).

8. Hreshchyshyn, M.M., Norris, H.J., Park, R., Lagasse, L.D., Blessing, J. Post-operative treatment of women with resectable malignant and possibly malignant epithelial ovarian tumors with radiotherapy, melphalan or no further treatment. Abstract 9W57, Proc.XII Int'l. Cancer Congress, 174, 1978.

9. Bush, R.S. Problems related to the evaluation of reported results in cancer of the ovary. Int.J.Radiat.Oncol.Biol.Phys. 1979 (in press, November).

10.Edmonson, J.H., Fleming, T.R., Decker, D.G., Malkasian, G.D., Jorgensen, E.O., Jefferies, J.A., Webb, M.J, and Kvols, L.K. Different chemotherapeutic sensitivities and host factors affecting prognosis in advanced ovarian carcinoma versus minimal residual disease. Cancer Treat.Rep., 63: 241,1979.

11.Smith, J.P., Rutledge, F.N., Delclos, L. Postoperative treatment of early cancer of the ovary: A random trial between postoperative irradiation and chemotherapy. Natl.Cancer Inst.Monogr. 42: 149,1975.

12.Griffiths, C.T., Parker, L.M., and Fuller, A.F. Role of cytoreductive surgical treatment in the management of advanced ovarian cancer. Cancer Treat. Rep., 63: 235, 1979.

3 RADIOTHERAPY IN THE TREATMENT OF STAGES III AND IV

D. Chassagne

The place of radiotherapy in the treatment of stage
III and IV ovarian cancer is a controversial subject
for many reasons (3-15-26).

1. Stage III and IV are well defined by FIGO or UICC
classification, but the importance of disease can be
very much different. The immediate outcome certainly
depends on the amount of residual disease left after
surgery ; final prognosis also depends on the size of
the residual tumor, providing that an appropriate
treatment has been given. There is certainly a need
to subdivise stage III in at least three categories:

- No apparent residual (and last FIGO
classification individualizes a minimal
stage III).
- Residual disease less than 2 cm.
- Bulky tumor remaining (or $>$ 2 cm)

Some other propositions have been made,
for instance $\leqslant 0.5$ cm, > 0.5 cm $\leqslant 1$ cm, > 1 cm $\leqslant 1.5$ cm
$> 1,5$ cm $\leqslant 2$ cm and it is a truism to say that both the
effect of radiotherapy and chemotherapy vary according to
the number of cells present at the start of treatment.

For many years, radiotherapy was the only
weapon after surgery, in stages III and IV dealing
with 10 to 15% and 0% five year survival respectively.
These poor results are not surprising if one considers
that no special effort was made by surgeons to debulk
the tumor. Conversely, radiotherapy was able to cure
minimal stage III and prove to be successful in some
cases (2-4-7-8-18-22-29).

A.T. van Oosterom et al. (eds.), Therapeutic Progress in Ovarian Cancer,
Testicular Cancer and the Sarcomas, pp. 27-40. All rights reserved.
Copyright 1980 by Martinus Nijhoff Publishers, The Hague/Boston/London.

The M.D. ANDERSON team has clearly shown, many years ago, that radiotherapy was only able to cure disease less than 2 cm in diameter (8-9).

2. There are many other prognostic factors which have been described by many authors (5-10-14--30).

a) Histological type - WHO recommends three types of adenocarcinomas: serous, mucinous and endometrioid. But it is curious to note the wide variations in the relative importance of these three types from one institution to another. Obviously there is a need for unanimously accepted criteria of definition.

b) Differentiation or grading (11-21) - This factor is probably more important than histological variety and should be combined with it.

In our experience there is practically no cure in undifferentiated carcinoma.

c) Age is also a prognostic factor which should be more documented in all reports (5). It is well known that many aggressive therapies can be used in young women, while there are obvious limitations in the elderly.

3. Published data is also controversial.

a) Historical series are numerous, most of them deal with whole abdomen irradiation with or without monochemotherapy, usually melphalan or thiotepa or chlorambucil (see excellent review of Fuks - 15).

These kind of treatment is now considered old fashioned.

However historical series provide an excellent reference basis. Some of the series will deserve a retrospective study to present the data according to new prognostic factors (tumor size, differentiation for instance).

b) There are now reports of several randomized studies in Stage III which unfortunately only compare chemotherapeutic regimens. Few data have been published either on radiotherapy itself, or on the comparison of radiotherapy and chemotherapy.

Three studies (27, 11, 29) must be mentioned:

a) The M.D. ANDERSON trial entered 187 patients from 1969 till Nov. 1975. Chemotherapy with melphalan was compared to total abdominal irradiation by the moving strip technique. Unfortunately no attempt was made to stratify by stage, and finally few stage III were included in the trial (approximately 25% of the total). The study only included minimal residual masses < 2 cm, no ascites and no tumor implants in those areas where irradiation had to be limited.

There were no differences in either survival or free of disease survival (NED) between the two groups. This important study shows that a monochemotherapy is able to do as well (that is to say 30% at 5 years NED) as radiotherapy conducted in the classical moving strip technique: 2600 - 2800 rad to each strip in about 2½ weeks. However, it should be pointed out that the stage III cases included in the trial were rather favourable ones and in spite of this, 70 percent failed.

The conclusion of the investigators that as a postoperative adjuvant, chemotherapy alone is at least as effective as either irradiation alone or irradiation plus chemotherapy cannot be drawn from this study.

In the M.D. ANDERSON study the complication rate in both arms was carefully followed. The eight percent radiation enteritis in the radiotherapy arm of the study was considered worse than the one leukemia and one pre-leukemia in the melphalan arm. The follow-up period is too short to warrant such conclusions.

b) The Princess MARGARET Hospital trial was carefully designed with the best stratification ever made, taking into account all parameters, especially differentiation, type of performed surgery and age (5-10-11).

The same type of favourable stage III cases as in the M.D. ANDERSON study were included in the trial: the so-called asymptomatic stage III. The radiation technique was different: 2250 rad of total abdominal irradiation being delivered in ten fractions by a moving trip technique,

24 to 30 cm wide by 10 cm long. The upper border of the abdominal fields was chosen above the domes of the diaphragm and no liver shielding was employed.

The results are outstanding for the 50 cases (85% living at 4 years) treated by abdomino-pelvic radiation only. It should be stressed that all stage III cases in this arm were asymptomatic and that only 2 cases have had a 4 years follow-up.

This study demonstrates that careful irradiation may cure small tumor implants spread in the abdominal cavity. But reports from the same institution (85 asymptomatic stage III cases, with only 12 at 4 years, and 6 at 5 years), however, show a five-year survival of only 30 percent.

c) In the Norwegian Radium Hospital a four-arm randomized study was conducted among two groups of patients with stage III ovarian carcinoma. The first group consisted of 157 patients who had radical surgery, the second group consisted of 145 patients with inoperable disease. The aim of the trial was to compare the results of 5000 rads given on a large abdominal field, and the results of a dose of 3000 rads followed by thiotepa. These treatments were assigned to both groups of patients.

It should be emphazised that these results of 30% in resectable stage III cases, and under 10% in unresectable cases, are exactly the same as the results obtained in other institutions with any kind of treatment.

The results of the treatments were identical within the two groups: 3000 rads gave the same poor result (less than ten percent five year survival) as 5000 rads in the inoperable group. Five thousand rads resulted in a 30% five year survival in the group that underwent radical surgery, the same 30% was obtained by 3000 rads plus thiotepa. From our point of view, these results do not mean that thiotepa replaces 2000 rads of abdominal radiation. We believe that 5000 rads were not delivered to the whole abdomen, and that the domes of the diaphragm were not included in the radiation field. It is therefore likely that not all abdominal tumor was covered by this irradiation.

4. The techniques of irradiation used in various centres might greatly differ. The three studies considered above refer to pelvic-abdominal radiation, are quite different in terms of treated and shielded volumes, as well as delivered dose to the tumor. The M.D. ANDERSON Hospital and the Princess MARGARET Hospital techniques are both Strip Techniques. In Toronto the strip width is larger, the liver is never shielded and the total dose is lower. Therefore the potential effect on peritoneal implants could be very different.

Is there a difference in result of strip technique and open-field technique. Results of a comparative randomized trial published by MAIER and FAZEKAS (12) failed to show such a difference.

The reproducibility of a certain radiation technique in different institutions is a far more important problem than the arguments among radiotherapists about the advantages or disadvantages of strip technique over open-field technique.

The Gynecological Oncology Group (19) designed a four-arm randomized trial for stage III ovarian cancer, with 2 stratifications in residual tumor sizes $>$ 3 cm and $\leqslant$ 3 cm. The four arms were the following: post-operative abdominal radiation alone, melphalan alone, radiation plus melphalan, and melphalan plus radiation. Three hundred and forty patients have been entered, but unfortunately no definitive conclusions could be drawn because of too many protocol violations. It is particularly interesting to quote the entire paragraph which deals with radiation techniques (19):

"Possibly the greatest major drawback in this whole study was the fact that total abdominal radiation was not given for one-third of the patients as called for in the protocol. A review of portal films indicates that the upper margins fell below the diaphragms, and restricted lateral margins left gutters of the abdomen on each side untreated; the lower margins fell short of the most inferior portions of the pelvic cavity. In a few cases, there was apparent excessive blocking of liver and kidneys.

When the protocols were set up, it was assumed that the total abdomen and pelvis were well-defined potential tumor-bearing volumes familiar to surgeons and radiation therapists alike. Unfortunately, this assumption delayed quality checking of portal films. A lesson was learned that the clinical research protocol can teach us that all therapy may not be as ideal as it is supposed to be".

HOW CAN WE DEFINE THE PROPER PLACE OF RADIOTHERAPY IN STAGE III OVARIAN CARCINOMA?

1. One should never forget the "Basic Truths" of radiotherapy:

   . Ionizing radiation can only destroy cancer cells inside the target volume.
   . Prescribed dose should be adapted to the number of cells or tumor volume present inside the target volume.

In order to fulfill these basic principles in stage III ovarian cancer we should improve by all means our knowledge of the distribution of the disease inside the peritoneal cavity. The first requirement is to improve the surgical staging. Practically, that means a better education of all gynecologists and general surgeons who first operate ovarian cancer. The second requirement is to routinely use the C.T. scan, the peritoneoscopy, the lymphangiography etc., in order to detect any amount of hidden disease which has not been detected by the surgeon at the time of the operative procedure. Many excellent papers recently stressed the frequency of the involvement of para-aortic nodes and/or diaphragmatic domes (13-14-24-25).

2. We should stratify our studies according to all known prognostic parameters. For the radiotherapist, it is particularly important to know the size of the tumor implants. (5-13-17-30).

3. We should improve our radiation techniques in three ways.

   a. The classical techniques of pelvic-abdominal radiation should be described with all relevant details.

b. More care should be given to individualize the treatment according to the location and size of the tumor implant. This individualization is somewhat conflicting with the above statement of the classical technique. This problem could easily be solved by careful planning and description of optional boost (5-15-).

c. New techniques have to be studied in phases I or II. For instance, the treatment of diaphragm proposed by Glatstein et al. (16) should be evaluated. This technique allows to deliver 4500 rad over 5-6 weeks to the para-aortic nodes and medial hemidiaphragms. As it is stressed by the authors: "more patients and longer follow-up will be necessary to assess both the long term safety of the technique and the possibility of underdosing critical areas of the posterior or lateral peritoneal surfaces".

As prospective studies, one can foresee the use of multiple daily schedules (already in use in our institution) low dose-rate continuous irradiation, radiosensitizers and hyperthermia.

AS A BASIS FOR DISCUSSION WE PROPOSE SOME PROTOCOLS WHICH COULD BE TRANSFORMED IN RANDOMIZED CLINICAL TRIALS.

Assuming that the patients are stratified by age, histological type, and furthermore differentiation we propose three tumor size categories.

1. No residual tumor

Bilateral salpingo-oophorectomy and hysterectomy and removal of all apparent disease in the pelvic cavity. In the peritoneal cavity two schematic situations can be distinguished:

a. No apparent disease at the time of the exploration, but pathological reports of microscopic implant, for instance in the omentum. This situation is not uncommon. In our experience of 62 systematic omentectomies we have found 12 cases of microscopic involvements, 12 cases of a normal omentum and 38 cases of widespread peritoneal implants (20).

This situation is now defined as minimal stage III.

b. Apparent disease was seen at the time of the exploration, but these implants were limited and could be apparently completely removed. This situation is well outlined in a recent paper by C.T. GRIFFITHS on the role of cytoreductive surgery in the management of advanced ovarian cancer (17).

In both situations, there was no apparent residual tumor, but recurrences will certainly appear if no further treatment is given. There is a trend to only advocate chemotherapy, but no one knows when the chemotherapy should be stopped and upon what criteria. Furthermore, few long term follow-up studies have been reported.

On the other hand, we know that radiation therapy is able to definitively destroy this subclinical disease with a relatively low dose, for instance 3.000 rad in 4 weeks. Data from DEMBO and BUSH (11) are strongly in favor of radiotherapy, with a 80% cure rate at four years.

In this conflicting situation, we think that there is a place for a randomized trial between chemotherapy alone and pelvic-abdominal radiotherapy alone at a low dose level.

2. Minimal residual disease

The definition of minimal residual disease has to be precised. In the literature we found less than 3,0 cm, less than 2 cm, less than 1,5 cm etc. M.D. ANDERSON data clearly show that the curative effect of radiotherapy is closely related to the size of the residual tumor (8-9).

The radiotherapeutist should irradiate a tumor implant that is as small as possible. Chemotherapy is the best technique to decrease tumor size and it seems logical to combine both modalities. Chemotherapy should be started as soon as possible after operation, and radiotherapy can be used as a means "to kill the last cell", and is probably a much better tool than chemotherapy alone. Nevertheless problems are numerous in this combination:

a) Tolerance of radiotherapy after 5 to 6 courses of combinations of 4 to 5 drugs. From our experience this tolerance has never been an insoluble problem, providing that individualized care is given to each patient. We have treated 56 patients with stage III ovarian cancer after chemotherapy given at "full dose" for at least 3 courses, without major problems.

b) Is a second-look operation necessary or not after 6 to 12 months of chemotherapy? (14-17).

The scientific purpose of this second-look is obvious, but every radiotherapist knows that second-laparotomy will impair the tolerance to radiation, already decreased by the first laparotomy.

c) Some authors still believe that radiotherapy is able to cure minimal residual disease without the help of chemotherapy. That is certainly true at the pelvic level where a 5000 rad dose can be delivered. That remains to be proven at the upper abdominal level, but the proposed techniques may solve this problem at the para-aortic and/ or diaphragmatic level (1-6-16).

From the above considerations, it seems logical to propose the following three arm randomized trial:

OVARIAN CANCER

LOGICAL PROTOCOLS IN STAGE III

2. Minimal Residual Disease [x]
Less than 2 cm

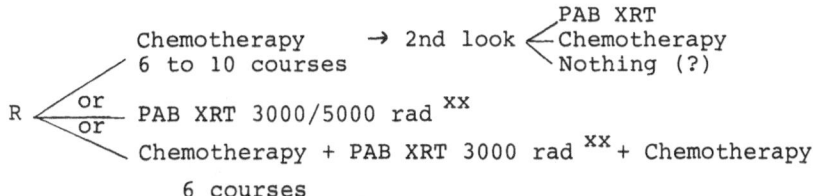

[x] One may stratify by 0.5 cm, $<$ 1 cm, $<$ 2 cm
[xx] Pelvic boost 5000 rad + individualized boost

3. Bulky residual disease

There is hardly a place for radiotherapy.

However, if a second-look operation is performed after at least 6 months of chemotherapy, the use of radiotherapy can be discussed in some favourable circumstances. For instance, if all traces of the disease were removed the role of radiotherapy at a low dose level could be considered.

On the contrary, if no results are obtained with the chemotherapy, external radiation could be proposed as a palliative measure.

The long-term value of this palliative radiotherapy is generally very poor, but occasionally it may benefit the patient.

4. Metastases outside the abdomen (Stage IV)

Here again, the treatment of choice is chemotherapy. Some stage IV, can be easily "reduced" to stage III, for instance pleural effusion may disappear after one to three courses of chemotherapy.

External radiation can be helpful to treat supra-clavi-cular metastases or the rare bony metastases. Usually a 3000 rad dose is sufficient to obtain an excellent palliative effect.

In summary, the use of radiotherapy in the treatment of Stage III ovarian carcinoma has to be specified by careful well-planned studies.
We believe, from our own experience and from the literature that radiotherapy can be used to advantage together with or complementary to chemotherapy.

REFERENCES

1. AISEM, S., BRUNETI MONTENEGRO C.R., MIOLA U.S.,
   MALAGUTI SCAFF L.A.
   Irradiaçao do abdomen no tratamento do carcinoma de
   ovario: Modificaçao e technica
   Rev. Bras. de Cancerologia 28, 17-21 (1978).

2. BARBER H.R.K., KWON T.H.
   Current status of the treatment of gynecologic cancer
   by site - ovary.
   Cancer 38, 610-619 (1976).

3. BRADY L.W.
   Future prospect of radiotherapy in gynecologic oncology.
   Cancer 38, 553-565 (1976).

4. BUCHLER, D.A.
   Stage III ovarian carcinomas: treatment and result
   Radiology 122, 469-472 (1977).

5. BUSH R.S., ALLT W.E.C., BEALE F.A., BEAN H.A., PRINGLE
   J.F., STURGEON J.
   Treatment of epithelial carcinoma of the ovary:
   Operation, irradiation and chemotherapy
   AM. J. Obstet. Gynecol. 127, 692-704 (1977).

6. CHASSAGNE D., WOLFF J.P.
   Radiotherapy in ovarian cancer for post-surgical minimal
   residual disease.
   In Recent Results in Cancer Research 68, 152-156 (1979).

7. DARGENT M., DARGENT D., LANSAC J.
   Traitement des tumeurs malignes primitives de l'ovaire.
   Etude rétrospective de 349 observations recueillies
   entre 1946 et 1966 au Centre Anti-Cancéreux de Lyon.
   J. Gynecol. Obstet. Biol. Reprod. (Paris) 2, 421-431
   (1972).

8. DELCLOS L., QUINLAN E.J.
   Malignant tumors of the ovary managed with post-opera-
   tive megavoltage irradiation.
   Radiology 93, 659-663 (1969).

9. DELCLOS L., SMITH J.P.
   Ovarian cancer with special regards to types of radio-
   therapy.
   Natl. Cancer Inst. Monogr. 42, 129-135 (1975).

10. DEMBO A.J., BUSH R.S., BEALE F.A., BEAN H.A. PRINGLE
    J.F., STURGEON J., REID J.G.
    Ovarian Carcinoma: improved survival following abdomino-
    pelvic irradiation in patients with a completed pelvic
    operation.
    Am. J. Obstet. Gynecol. 134, 793-800 (1979).

11. DEMBO A.J., BUSH R.S., BEALE F.A., BEAN H.A., PRINGLE
    S.F., STURGEON J.F.G.
    The Princess Margaret Hospital Study of Ovarian Cancer:
    Stages I, II and asymptomatic III presentations.
    Cancer Treatment Reports 63, 249-254 (1979)

12. FAZEKAS, V.T., MAIER V.G.
    Irradiation of ovarian carcinomas. A prospective com-
    parison of the open field and moving-strip techniques.
    Am. J. Roentgenol. 120, 118-123 (1974).

13. FISHER R.I., YOUNG R.C.
    Advances in the staging and treatment of ovarian cancer.
    Cancer 39, 967-972 (1977).

14. FRICK G., JOHNSSON J.E., LANDBERG T., SNORRADOTIR M.
    Relaparatomy in advanced ovarian carcinoma
    Acta Obstet. Gynecol. Scand. 57, 165-168 (1978).

15. FUKS Z.
    External radiotherapy of ovarian cancer: Standard
    approaches and new frontiers.
    Semin. Oncol. 2, 253-266 (1975).

16. GLATSTEIN E., FUKS Z., BAGSHAW M.A.
    Diaphragmatic treatment in ovarian carcinoma: A new
    radiotherapeutic technique.
    Int. J. Radiat. Oncol. Biol. Phys. 2, 357-362 (1977).

17. GRIFFITHS C.T., PARKER L.M., FULLER A.F.
    Role of cytoreductive surgical treatment in the
    management of advanced ovarian cancer.
    Cancer Treatment Reports 63, 235-240 (1979)

18. HINTZ B.L., FUKS Z., KEMPSON R.L., ELTRINGHAM J.,
    ZALOVDEK C., WILLIAMSON T.J., BAGSHAW M.A.
    Results of post-operative megavoltage radiotherapy of
    malignant surface epithelial tumors of the ovary.
    Radiology 114, 695-700 (1975).

19. LEWIS G.C., BLESSING J.
    Ovarian cancer: Use of multiple modality programs
    involving surgery, radiation therapy and chemotherapy.
    Cancer 40, 588-594 (1977).

20. MICHEL G., PRADE M., CHARPENTIER P.
    Intérêt de l'omentectomie systématique chez les malades
    porteuses de tumeurs malignes de l'ovaire.
    Gynecol. 27, 455-457 (1976)

21. OZOLS R.G., GARVIN A.J., COSTA J., SIMON R.M.,
    YOUNG R.C.
    Histological grade in advanced ovarian cancer.
    Cancer Treatment Reports 63, 255-264 (1979).

22. PEREZ C.A., WALZ B.J., JACOBSON P.L.
    Radiation therapy in the management of carcinoma of
    the ovary.
    Natl. Cancer Inst. Monogr. 42, 119-126 (1975).

23. PEREZ L.A., KORBA A., ZIVNUSKA F. et AL.
    Co^{60} moving strip technique in the management of
    carcinoma of the ovary = analysis of tumour control and
    morbidity
    Int. J. Rad. Oncol. Biol. Phys. 4 379 (1978)

24. PIVER M.S., LOPEZ R.G., XYNOS F., BARLOW J.J.
    The value of pre-therapy peritoneoscopy in localized
    ovarian cancer.
    Am. J. Obstet. Gynecol. 127, 288-290 (1977).

25. ROSENOFF S.H., De Vita V.T., HUBBARD S., YOUNG R.C.
    Peritoneoscopy in the staging and follow-up of ovarian
    cancer.
    Semin. Oncol. 2, 223-228 (1975)

26. RUBIN P.
Understanding the problem of understaging in ovarian cancer.
Semin. Oncol. 2, 235-242 (1975).

27. SMITH J.P., RUTLEDGE F.N., DELCLOS L.
Results of chemotherapy as an adjunct to surgery in patients with localized ovarian cancer.
Semin. Oncol. 2, 277-282 (1975).

28. UNDERWOOD P.B., MERRIT J.O., HITZ L.H. WALLENCE K.H., MARKS R.D.
Carcinoma of the ovary: the adjunctive use of irradiation.
Gynecol. Oncol. 3, 298-307 (1976).

29. WELANDER C., KSORSTAD K.E., KOLSTAD P.
Post-operative irradiation and chemotherapy in patients with advanced ovarian cancer.
Acta Obstet. Gynecol. Scand. 57, 161-164 (1978).

30. YOUNG R.C.
Ovarian carcinoma: an optimistic epilogue.
Cancer Treatment Reports 63, 333-337 (1979)

4 CISPLATIN THERAPY OF OVARIAN CANCER

J. F. Holland, H. W. Bruckner, C. J. Cohen, R. C. Wallach,
S. B. Gusberg, E. M. Greenspan and J. Goldberg

During the course of our early investigations with cis-diamminodichloroplatinum II, we discovered and first reported its activity against testicular cancer.[1,2] Following this discovery, perhaps in the simplistic attempt to establish gonadal symmetry, we undertook a study of platinum in ovarian cancer. We had previously recognized the high activity of adriamycin (doxorubicin) in a variety of disease states including gynecologic cancer.[3] The combination of adriamycin and platinum was thus explored in a broad Phase II trial during which it was shown to demonstrate major efficacy against metastatic testicular neoplasia,[4] and, incidentally, against prostatic cancer. In patients with advanced ovarian cancer we thus undertook a prospective trial of adriamycin and platinum in combination versus platinum alone versus a standard chemotherapeutic regimen in use in our institutions,[5,6] consisting of an alkylating agent and an antimetabolite, thioTEPA and methotrexate.[7,8].

Our studies have involved women with FIGO classification Stages 3 and 4 ovarian cancer. The data derive from the Mount Sinai Hospital and the Beth Israel Hospital, both of the Mount Sinai School of Medicine in New York and

represent a collaborative undertaking of the Departments of
Neoplastic Diseases, Gynecology and of Medicine. We have
treated two groups of patients: as a rescue, second line
therapy after failure of a prior chemotherapeutic regimen,[9]
and as first line therapy following definitive diagnosis,
with or without debulking, dependent upon feasibility.

Among 132 previously treated and relapsed or refractory
patients with ovarian cancer platinum alone produced partial
regression in 5 of 23 (22%), but with no complete remissions.[10] This confirms and extends observations of Wiltshaw
and her colleagues who treated alkylating agent refractory
patients with cisplatin alone and attained comparable
results.[11] In combination with adriamycin in 41 patients
the total remission rate rose to 39%, and 5 of these
remissions were complete. Addition of cyclophosphamide to
the regimen did not improve it; the total remission rate
was 40% of 45 patients. The median survival for each of
these groups was 7 months. Upon the addition of hexamethylmelamine as a fourth drug to the cyclophosphamide-
containing regimen of adriamycin and platinum, however,
the four drug combination has a 52% total remission rate,
an equivalent complete remission rate (12% vs 9%) and a
median survival of 13 months.

The response frequency in the 3 combination treatment
regimens for refractory ovarian cancer is clearly related
to performance status. Thus, 17 of 24 patients with a
performance status of 0 or 1, representing ambulatory
patients, responded to combination chemotherapy (71%); 24
of 49 responders who spent up to half their waking time in
bed responded (49%), but only 3 of 23 who were bedridden
more than 50% of their waking time responded (13%).
Response was age independent, and independent of prior
radiotherapy. Those who had previously been radiated had
14 responses of 33 (42%), in contrast to 32 responses among
64 who had received other combination chemotherapeutic
regimens alone (50%). Among these relapsed patients, women
with tumors less than 5 cm. in diameter had nearly twice

the response rate of those with tumors that were larger.

Adriamycin and platinum containing regimens, particularly when cyclophosphamide and hexamethylmelamine are additional components, constitute an effective therapeutic approach to relapsed ovarian cancer.[9,10] The results from our studies of previously untreated ovarian cancer recommend the use of these regimens for primary therapy, however.

Our first study of primary chemotherapy involved the treatment of patients with ovarian cancer Stages 3 and 4, biopsy proven and where possible, surgically debulked. (Fig. 1) Adriamycin and platinum was one arm of the study program, platinum alone a second arm, and thioTEPA usually with methotrexate, the alkylating agent-antimetabolite combination which had been standard for more than 300 patients at Mount Sinai Hospital served as control. As a preview, the adriamycin and platinum arm proved the best, and was entered into subsequent studies in comparison with thioTEPA and platinum, which proved excessively myelotoxic. The two-drug combination also served as a comparison standard against adriamycin and platinum plus cyclophosphamide and hexamethylmelamine. The dose levels used in each of these combinations throughout, was 50 mg/m^2 of platinum and 50 mg/m^2 of adriamycin every 3 weeks intravenously.[2] When cyclophosphamide and hexamethylmelamine were added, only the adriamycin dose was decreased. In Figure 2 the results at one year are shown for the three trials. Patients with evaluable tumor are less than the number randomized because not all patients had palpable tumor masses which could be assessed clinically after surgical debulking. The number alive at one year in the adriamycin and platinum containing arms is 78 and 86%, compared to 47% for the control alkylating agent treatment and 55% for platinum alone in the first study. By 12 months, escape from chemotherapeutic effects had occurred in the less effective regimens; only 24% for the thioTEPA and 33% for the platinum alone arm continued to remain

44

OVARIAN CANCER

TREATMENT SCHEDULES

ADRIAMYCIN-PLATINUM VS. PLATINUM VS. THIOTEPA-METHOTREXATE

ADRIAMYCIN-PLATINUM VS. THIOTEPA-PLATINUM

ADRIAMYCIN-PLATINUM VS. CYTOXAN-HEXAMETHYLMELAMINE-ADRIAMYCIN-PLATINUM

Fig. 1

ONE YEAR RESULTS
CONTROLLED TRIALS OF INITIAL CHEMOTHERAPY
OF ADVANCED OVARIAN CANCER

REGIMEN	Trial I			Trial II		Trial III*	
	TSPA MTX	DDP	DDP ADM	DDP ADM	DDP TSPA	DDP ADM	CHAP
NO. PATIENTS RANDOMIZED	17	18	18	15	24	9	18
NO. ALIVE @ 12 MONTHS	8	10	14	13	18	8	15
NO. PROGRESSION FREE @ 12 MONTHS	4	6	14	11	12	7	14
NO. WITH EVALUABLE TUMOR	14	12	13	12	20	7	11
NO. WITH OBJECTIVE RESPONSE	5	4	10	10	12	6	9

*Trial continues to accrue patients.
Cis-diamminedichloroplatinum (DDP), Adriamycin (ADM), Triethylenethiophosphoramide
(TSPA), Cyclophosphamide (CYC), Hexamethylmelamine (HMM), CYC+HMM+ADM+DDP (CHAP)

Fig. 2

at one year. In contrast 78% and 73% of patients treated
with adriamycin and platinum in combination were progression-free in the two trials.

The remission duration was longest for the adriamycin
and platinum regimen, and it is significantly greater than
that for the alkylating agent antimetabolite combination.
(Fig. 3) A multivariate analysis of these data concerning
primary chemotherapy demonstrated that residual disease
bulk and histologic type did not influence outcome, whereas
age and performance status, in addition to treatment assign-
ment, did. After adjustment for age and performance, the
risk of progression or death on the adriamycin combination
was 1/3 that of the thioTEPA methotrexate group.

PROGRESSION – FREE SURVIVAL

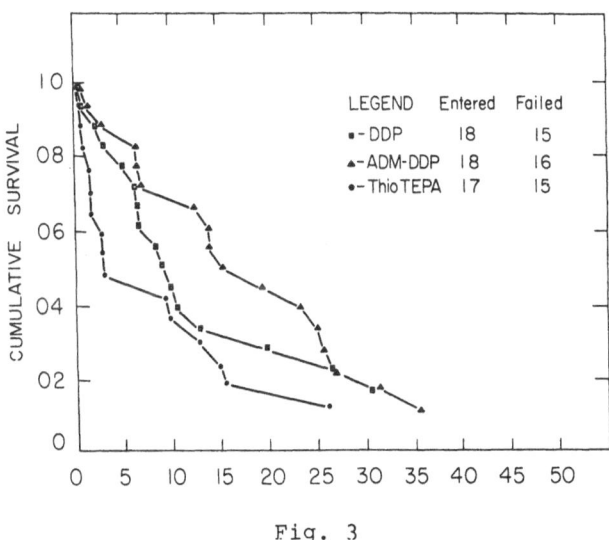

Fig. 3

The patient population under study was more typical of
a community medical center rather than of a selective
referral institution, with 44% in the adriamycin-platinum
arm 60 years or over, and 22% in performance status two or
worse. Only 28% had been debulked to lesions 2 cm. in
diameter or less. Survival showed superiority for patients
who had taken platinum alone or in combination as initial
treatment compared to those first exposed to alkylating
agents. (Fig. 4) The meager survival differences between
the three groups in Trial 1 may relate to crossover
responsiveness of patients to second line treatments who
had not received adriamycin and platinum as their primary
therapy.

Another less rigorous comparison of therapies has been
conducted in the Record Room at Mount Sinai.
Howard Bruckner was able to find an equal number of patients
by Record Room survey, with Stages 3 and 4 ovarian cancer
who had been contemporaneously treated by physicians who
were not members of the Department of Neoplastic Diseases
or Gynecologic Oncology, by conventional combination chemotherapy. Sometimes it seems that Mount Sinai is a
composite range of Alps, Pyrenees and Himalayas.

46

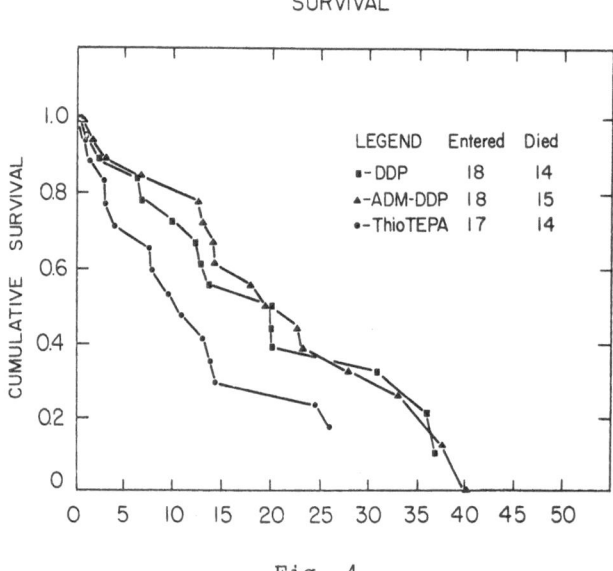

Fig. 4

Conventional chemotherapy at Mount Sinai might imply thio-
TEPA and methotrexate, or cyclophosphamide and fluorouracil.
By the time the 25th percentile of ovarian cancer patients
is dead, a major difference has already emerged, with the
conventional treatment intercepting at 2 months whereas the
adriamycin-platinum containing combinations are at 17
months. The median survival is 11 months on conventional
treatment but 24 months on the adriamycin-platinum
combination. To diminish the obvious possible bias that
exists in this comparison, an analysis was made on
condition that patients survived 3 months, which again
shows great superiority for the adriamycin-platinum
containing regimens.

In Trial 3 we have compared the 4 drugs-cyclophos-
phamide, hexamethylmelamine containing regimen to the 2
drug adriamycin and platinum regimen alone. Tumor size,
age and performance status are all shown to be variables
which influence outcome, but in which the cyclophosphamide,
hexamethylmelamine, adriamycin and platinum arm appears to
be favored. This is translated to survival, where the
homogeneity of our results of adriamycin and platinum

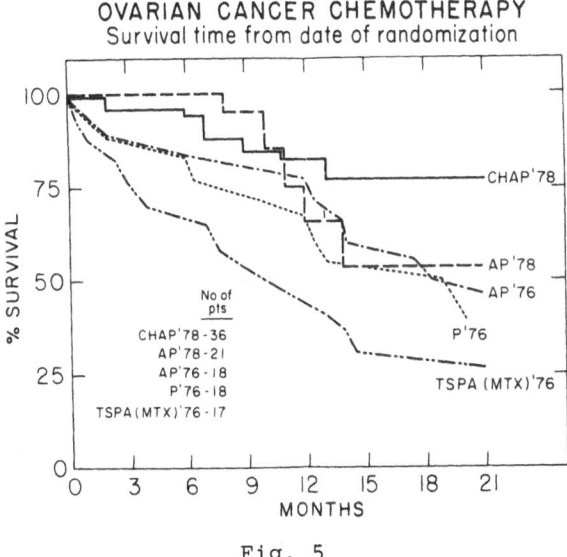

OVARIAN CANCER CHEMOTHERAPY
Survival time from date of randomization

Fig. 5

is shown as reproducible, and where there is a trend as yet insignificant favoring the 4 drug regimen. Fig. 5.

Complete responses, however, are the name of the game in clinical cancer investigation today, since from these are derived the potential for total eradication of disease by multimodality management. We have adopted the proposition that freedom from evidence of any clinical manifestation of disease at one year constitutes a continuing complete remission. Dr. Carmel Cohen and his colleagues, Drs. Gusberg and Wallach, have determined that laparoscopy is inadequate to establish freedom from disease. We have as an interim analysis, analyzed 41 laparotomies in patients who were clinically disease-free at one year. Dr. Cohen has established criteria for conduct of the laparotomy: a lengthy midline incision is made, not just an infraumbilical buttonhole. Washings are taken from beneath the diaphragms bilaterally, the subhepatic space, the lumbar gutters, and the pelvis. The inferior surfaces of the diaphragm are inspected and sampled. All the viscera are examined. Any suspicious area is biopsied.

Any area where tumor previously had been described is
biopsied. Any residual omentum or gynecologic organs not
excised at the first operative procedure are removed. The
para-aortic and iliac lymph node chains are biopsied bilaterally. A therapeutic end staging laparotomy obtains
30 to 50 independent histologic specimens. Only if all
these cytologic washings and biopsies are negative is the
patient considered in pathologically proved complete
remission, and at that point treatment is stopped. One
locus or more of demonstrable cancer cells constitutes
microscopic residual disease. Only 9 of the 41
patients had gross disease at exploration, 15 had
microscopic disease and 17 were disease-free after this
exhaustive search. (Figure 6) The bulk of these patients
came from the three adriamycin-platinum study populations,
only 3 from the 18 who received platinum alone, 3 from
the 24 who received thioTEPA and platinum, and 10 from the
4-drug combination, although the last study is early
because of the timing of the interim analysis, and the
denominator is small. None derives from the alkylating
agent series of thioTEPA and methotrexate.

These data compare with a literature estimate of
disease eradication by melphalan alone. (Figure 7) The
difference is striking. At the time of later analysis,
of 18 patients without evidence of disease at exploration, only a single individual had already relapsed. (Fig.
8) Furthermore, of those who had had microscopic residual
disease, thereafter maintained on an alkylating agent if
their adriamycin tolerance had been reached, progression
had been encountered in only a single patient. (Figure 9)

OVARIAN CANCER

Definitive Repeat Laparotomy

TREATMENT PROGRAM	NO. OF PATIENTS	RESIDUAL DISEASE		
		GROSS	MICROSCOPIC	NONE
Adriamycin-Platinum	25	4	10	11
Platinum	3	1	1	1
Thiotepa-Platinum	3	-	1	2
CHAP	10	4	3	3

Fig. 6

OVARIAN CANCER
Comparative Second Look Results

INSTITUTION	AGENT	NUMBER OF PATIENTS IN CLINICAL REMISSION		NUMBER OF "SECOND LOOK" PATIENTS NED	
M.D. Anderson	Melphalan	89/720 (?)	(12%)	17/89	(20%)
MSH	ADM-DDP	25/48	(52%)	11/25	(44%)

Fig. 7

50

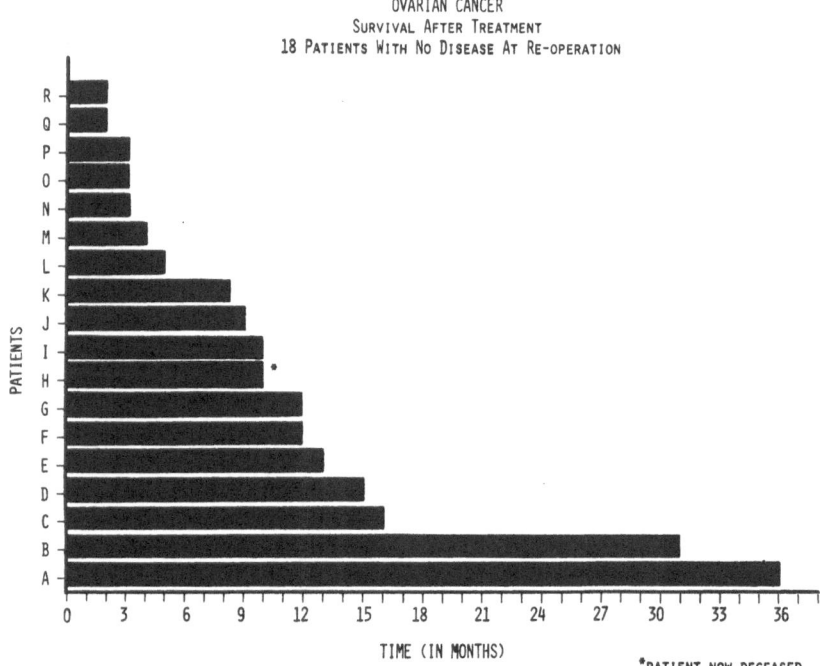

OVARIAN CANCER
SURVIVAL AFTER TREATMENT
18 PATIENTS WITH NO DISEASE AT RE-OPERATION

PATIENTS

TIME (IN MONTHS)

*PATIENT NOW DECEASED

Fig. 8

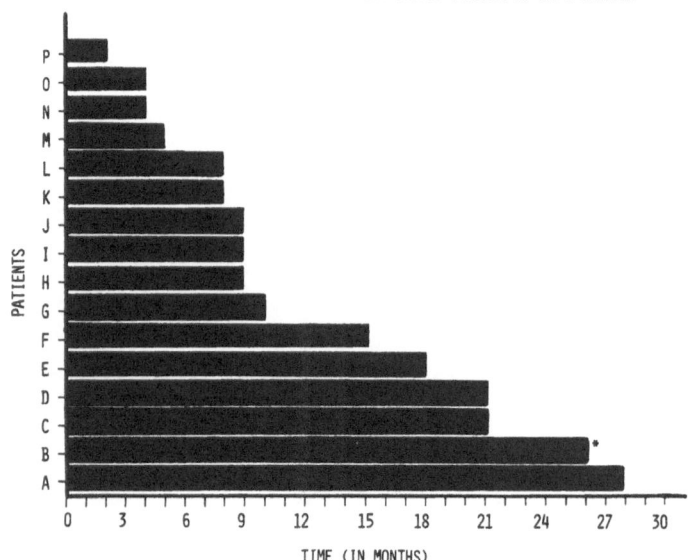

OVARIAN CANCER
SURVIVAL AFTER TREATMENT
16 PATIENTS WITH MICROSCOPIC DISEASE AT RE-OPERATION

PATIENTS

TIME (IN MONTHS)

*PATIENT NOW DECEASED

Fig. 9

We believe that the foundation of adriamycin and platinum, aggressive gynecologic oncologic surgery, and the evolution of additional chemotherapeutic components in the therapeutic regimen have provided the basis for an emerging curative treatment of disseminated ovarian cancer.

REFERENCES

1) Higby, D.J., Wallace, J.H., Jr., Albert, D.J. and Holland, J.F.: Diamminedichloroplatinum (DDP): A Phase I study showing responses in testicular and other tumors. Cancer Chemotherapy Reports 57:100, 1973.

2) Higby, D.J., Wallace, H.J., Albert, D. and Holland, J.F.: Diamminedichloroplatinum in the chemotherapy of testicular tumors. J. Urol. 112:100-104, 1974.

3) Barlow, J.J., Piver, M.S., Chuang, J.F., Cortes, E.P., Ohnuma, T. and Holland, J.F.: Adriamycin and bleomycin, alone and in combination, in gynecologic cancers. Cancer 32:735-743, 1973.

4) Vogl, S., Ohnuma, T., Perloff, M. and Holland, J.F.: Combination Chemotherapy with adriamycin and cis-diamminedichloroplatinum in patients with neoplastic diseases. Cancer 38:21-26, 1976.

5) Bruckner, H.W., Cohen, C.J., Gusberg, S.B., Wallach, R.C., Kabakow, B., Greenspan, E.M. and Holland, J.F.: Chemotherapy of ovarian cancer with adriamycin (ADM) and cis-platinum (DDP). Proc. ASCO 17:287, 1976.

6) Bruckner, H., Cohen, C., Goldberg, J., Kabakow, B., Wallach, R.C., Deppe, G., Greenspan, E., Gusberg,S.B.: Improved chemotherapy for ovarian cancer with cis-diamminedichloroplatinum and adriamycin (submitted).

7) Greenspan, E.M.: ThioTEPA and methotrexate chemotherapy of advanced ovarian carcinoma. J. Mt. Sinai 35:52-67, 1968.

8) Wallach, R.C., Kabakow, B., Blinick, G. and Antopol,W: ThioTEPA chemotherapy for ovarian carcinoma: Influence of remission and toxicity on survival. Obstet. & Gynec. 35:278-286, 1970.

9) Bruckner, H.W., Cohen, C.J., Wallach, R.C., Kabakow,
    B., Deppo, G., Greenspan, E.M. and Gusberg, S.B.:
    Treatment of advanced ovarian carcinoma with cis-
    dichlorodiammineplatinum (II). Poor-risk patients
    with intensive prior therapy. Cancer Treatment
    Reports 62:555-558, 1978.

10) Bruckner, H.W., Cohen, C.J., Deppe, G., Kabakow, B.,
    Wallach, R.C., Greenspan, E.M., Gusberg, S.B. and
    Holland, J.F.: Chemotherapy of gynecological tumors
    with platinum II. J. Clin. Hematol. & Oncol.
    7:619-632, 1977.

11) Wiltshaw, E. and Kroner, T.: Phase II study of
    cis-dichlorodiammineplatinum (II) (NSC-119875)
    in advanced adenocarcinoma of the ovary.
    Cancer Treatment Reports 60:55-60, 1976.

5 HEXAMETHYLMELAMINE AND CISPLATINUM COMBINATIONS IN THE TREATMENT OF OVARIAN CANCER

E. Wiltshaw

From 1975 to 1979 patients with FIGO stages III and IV adenocarcinoma, together with those patients of earlier stage that had relapsed following surgery with or without radiotherapy, were entered into a trial comparing Cisplatin plus chlorambucil, and Cisplatin, chlorambucil plus Adriamycin. Those patients (total 22) excluded from the trial on medical grounds (usually cardiac problems) or because of their refusal to risk alopecia were given HMM plus Cisplatin (see table 1).

Another group of patients (total 40) who had failed to respond or had relapsed on chemotherapy other than Cisplatin were given 100 mg/m^2 Cisplatin. After five courses, therapy was continued in all cases with single agent HMM.

Lastly, patients who had relapsed following Cisplatin therapy (total 14) were given a trial of the HexaCAF regimen (4) as a second or sometimes third-line attempt at useful chemotherapy.

(exclusions) P-HMM x6——laparotomy——P-HMM x6   HMM maintenance for 1 year

Stages III & IV, and Recurrences after Surgery and/or Radiotherapy   Randomise

Chemo Bx6——laparotomy——Chemo Bx6   chlorambucil maintenance for 1 year
Chemo Cx6——laparotomy——Chemo Cx6

Failures from previous chemotherapy:

No previous Pt——Pt high dose x5——laparotomy——HMM for 18m
Failed B&C <x6——Pt high dose x5——laparotomy——HMM for 18m
Failed B&C >x6 or Pt high dose (D)——HexaCAF x12 courses

Figure 1: Management plan for ovarian carcinoma

A.T. van Oosterom et al. (eds.), Therapeutic Progress in Ovarian Cancer, Testicular Cancer and the Sarcomas, pp. 53-60. All rights reserved.
Copyright 1980 by Martinus Nijhoff Publishers, The Hague/Boston/London.

MANAGEMENT OF STAGE III AND IV CASES AND TUMOURS RECURRENT
AFTER SURGERY AND/OR RADIOTHERAPY

Cisplatin 20 mg/m^2 together with HMM 300 mg/day was given
as first-line chemotherapy (Table 1). All regimens were
continued for one year followed by chlorambucil (0.2 mg/kg/
day for 14 days every 28 days) for a further year for regimens B and C, and HMM (300 mg/day for 14 days every 28 days)
maintenance for a further year for regimen P-HMM.

Table 1: Treatment Regimens

Code

B	Cisplatin	20 mg/m^2 IV day 1	} q. 21 days
	chlorambucil	0.15 mg/kg/day PO days 2-8	
C	Cisplatin	20 mg/m^2 IV day 1	
	chlorambucil	0.15 mg/kg/day PO days 2-8	} q. 28 days
	Adriamycin	50 mg/m^2 IV day 1	
P-HMM	Cisplatin	20 mg/m^2 IV day 1	} q. 21 days
	HMM	300 mg/day PO days 2-15	

The P-HMM regimen was given to patients excluded from
our main trial from 1976 to the close of the study in 1979.
In 1976 second-look operations (SLO) were introduced into
our management plan for all good partial responders or complete responders after 6 courses of combination chemotherapy.
At operation, remaining tumour was removed where possible,
multiple biopsies were taken and, if not excised previously,
the uterus, ovaries and omentum were removed even if they
appeared to be tumour-free.

RESULTS (Table 2)

Preliminary results show that complete and partial regressions on clinical examination, ultrasound, CT scan and X-ray
examinations occurred in 50% of 46 patients on Regimen B,
52% of 39 patients on Regimen C, and 50% of 22 patients on
P-HMM. Complete remissions were seen in 28% of 46 patients
on Regimen B, 28% of 39 patients on Regimen C and 27% of
22 patients on P-HMM, while median lengths of complete re-

mission were 16, 13 and 11 months respectively.

Second operations were performed on 7/22 (31.8%) patients given P-HMM (6 laparotomies and 1 laparoscopy). In 2, no tumour was found, while in 3 only one site of tumour remained and in the last 2 cases the amount of involvement had been greatly reduced by chemotherapy. In the case of Regimen B 12/46 (26%) were subjected to SLO and in the group having Regimen C 17/39 (43.9%) had an SLO. The difference between B and C in this respect is probably not significant since SLO was introduced in 1976 after many B patients had already been treated, whereas very few patients had started treatment with the C regimen. Details of the B and C regimens have been published elsewhere (3).

Table 2: Comparative figures for treatment regimens
          B, C and P-HMM

Characteristic	B	C	P-HMM
Total No treated	46	39	22
Response Rate	52%	54%	50%
Complete Remission	28%	28%	27%
Median length of CR	16 m	13 m	11 m
SLO performed	12 cases	17 cases	7 cases
Small bulk disease before chemotherapy	75%	41%	85%
Complete Remission after SLO	50%	41%	28%

Comparing these figures, regimens B, C and P-HMM appear to be of similar usefulness. However, the longest continued remissions were seen in patients who had no surgical or pathological evidence of tumour after SLO irrespective of chemotherapy used. The numbers are small but in the P-HMM group, while 85% of cases had relatively small amounts of tumour before chemotherapy was started, only 28% achieved complete "pathological" remission. Similar figures for B were 75% and 50%, and for C 41% had minimal disease before chemotherapy, but 41% were in "pathological" CR on completion of SLO. In other words, there is a suggestion that the

P-HMM regimen may be slightly less effective than the other
two combinations (Table 2).

MANAGEMENT OF PATIENTS WITH RECURRENT DISEASE AFTER PRE-VIOUS CHEMOTHERAPY

For patients who had received previous chemotherapy other
than Cisplatin and for patients who failed to respond to
Regimens B and C after less than 6 courses, Cisplatin 100 mg/
m^2 was given with appropriate hydration and IV mannitol
(Regimen D). Five courses were given followed by laparotomy
as in B and C. After 5 courses of Cisplatin, maintenance
treatment consisted of 300 mg/day HMM for 14 days every
month for 18 months or until relapse occurred (Table 3).

Table 3:   Treatment regimens after previous chemotherapy

Code

D	Cisplatin 100 mg/m^2 IV with IV hydration over 48 hours and mannitol infusion. q. 28 days for 5 courses, followed by HMM 300 mg PO daily for 14 days every month for a total of 2 years.
HexaCAF	HMM 100 mg/m^2 PO for 14 days cyclophosphamide 100 mg/m^2 PO for 14 days methotrexate 40 mg/m^2 days 1 and 8 IV 5-FU 600 mg/m^2 days 1 and 8 IV q. 28 days (Folinic acid 15 mg PO 6-hourly 24 hours after each dose of methotrexate) Continue for one year.

   Of the 9 patients previously exposed to B and C regimens
none maintained remission long enough to go on to HMM, but
31 patients had never been exposed to Cisplatin before and
of these, 19 have responded to treatment. Eight of the 19
either relapsed on Regimen D or have not yet been treated
long enough to start maintenance chemotherapy, leaving 11
for study. Of the 11 many have relapsed quickly on HMM and
it is difficult to say how useful the HMM has been in main-taining the longer remissions (table 4).

Table 4: Maintenance of remission by HMM after five courses
of schedule D

Partial Regressions: 1, 1, 1, 2, 5, 10 months
Complete Regressions: 1, 5+, 11+, 16+, 26+ months

Certainly in the patients attaining partial remission on the
Cisplatin none have exhibited further regression following
HMM.

CHEMOTHERAPY AFTER FAILURE ON CISPLATIN (REGIMENS B, C, or D)

Patients in this group constitute the most advanced cases
and the patients have already been exposed to chemotherapy.
In some, two or more drugs had already been used. We tried
to use the combination of HMM, cyclophosphamide, methotrexate
and 5-fluorouracil as described by Young and his colleagues
(4). This combination (Table 3) had been very effective in
their hands when used in relatively early stage disease and
immediately after the initial diagnostic operation.

Fourteen patients are evaluable for response having had
more than two courses. There were no measurable regressions
and myelosuppression, nausea and vomiting, as well as stomatitis, were all severe.

TOXICITY AND SIDE-EFFECTS OF HMM IN THE STUDY

Both HMM and Cisplatin have a high incidence of nausea and
vomiting following administration and we found it impossible
to increase the dose of HMM above 300 mg/day. However, at
this level the side-effects were just tolerable to most
patients, although therapy was easier on the B regimen. Only
one of the patients on low dose Cisplatin and HMM stopped
treatment because of side-effects. Neurotoxicity, however,
on the P-HMM regimen was seen more frequently than in patients
on the B or C schemes. Five patients had symptoms of peripheral neuropathy (22.7%) compared with none on the B and
C schemes. In one patient who suffered from Parkinson's
disease as well as ovarian carcinoma the symptoms and signs
of Parkinson's were worse on Cisplatin and HMM and improved

on two occasions when chlorambucil was substituted for HMM.

In patients having high dose Cisplatin it was our policy to stop at 5 doses because we had shown that neuropathy due to Cisplatin is cumulative (3). Nevertheless, after 5 courses of Regimen D only 3/26 cases (11%) had paraesthesiae and none had motor weakness. Two went on to HMM maintenance and in one the neuropathy progressed. In two other patients neuropathy developed for the first time while on HMM maintenance.

Thus, there is an impression that HMM, not unexpectedly, increases the likelihood of neuropathy when used in combination with Cisplatin. So far, the neurological signs have disappeared with time in all our cases.

DISCUSSION

Single agent activity of HMM in ovarian cancer was suggested by studies at the National Cancer Institute (4) and at the M D Anderson Hospital (1), while a more comprehensive study has recently been reported by Wharton et al (2). A summary of their results using HMM in doses of 6-8 mg/kg/day is shown in Table 5. Many of the patients had to have dose reductions due to side-effects or toxicity, but remissions were achieved in 31.5% of 54 patients.

Table 5: Single agent HMM in 54 cases of ovarian cancer stages III and IV (Wharton et al)

% of Cases	Characteristic
14.5	Complete Remissions
17.0	Partial Remissions
9.2	SLO at 12 months
48.1	Neurotoxicity
31.5	Platelets <100,000
5.5	Unacceptable Vomiting

Their patients had less tumour than ours when chemotherapy was applied because they attempted radical surgery at the first laparotomy. Thus, 32% of their cases had residual tumour masses of less than 2 cm at the start of chemotherapy, whereas all our cases had measurable residual disease by clinical, radiological or ultrasound techniques. Nevertheless, with the addition of Cisplatin 20 mg/m^2 to HMM we were able to produce 50% responses.

CONCLUSIONS

HMM is an active agent in the treatment of ovarian cancer but it is not certain yet what additional benefit it gives when given in combination with Cisplatin. Additional toxicity, especially neuropathy, is seen and can be avoided if alkylating agents such as chlorambucil are given instead. Since there is a suggestion that the combination of Cisplatin and chlorambucil with or without Adriamycin is more effective in reducing bulky tumour to the level where complete remissions can be produced at SLO, it is probably better not to combine this agent with another neurotoxic substance, namely Cisplatin.

HexaCAF, while apparently very useful at producing remissions in patients with small amounts of residual ovarian cancer, has proved ineffective as second or third-line chemotherapy.

The role of maintenance HMM following high dose Cisplatin is not clear but increased neurotoxicity should be expected.

ACKNOWLEDGEMENTS

We are grateful to the National Cancer Institute for the free supply of hexamethylmelamine (NSC-13875) for this study.

The work was supported in part by grants from Johnson Matthey and Bristol-Myers.

REFERENCES

1. SMITH, JP and RUTLEDGE, FN (1975) Random study of
    hexamethylmelamine, 5-fluorouracil and melphalan in
    the treatment of advanced carcinoma of the ovary.
    Nat Canc Inst Monographs 42:169

2. WHARTON, JT, RUTLEDGE, FN, SMITH, JP, HERSON, J, and
    HODGE, MP (1979) Hexamethylmelamine: an evaluation
    of its role in the treatment of ovarian cancer.
    Am J Obst Gynecol 133:833-841

3. WILTSHAW, E, SUBRAMANIAN, S, ALEXOPOULOS, C, and
    BARKER, GH (1979) Cancer of the ovary: a summary of
    experience with cis-platinum diamminedichloride (II)
    in the Royal Marsden Hospital. Cancer Treatment Reports,
    Vol 63, 1545-1548.

4. YOUNG, RC, CHABNER, BA, HUBBARD, SB, CANELOS, GP, and
    DeVITA, VT (1975) Preliminary results of trials of
    chemotherapy in advanced ovarian cancer. Nat Canc Inst
    Monographs 42:145-148

6 CURRENT TREATMENT AND NEW PROSPECTS

D. L. Longo and R. C. Young

INTRODUCTION

We are entering an exciting era in the treatment of epithelial ovarian neoplasms. Virtually unknown before the
industrial revolution, this form of cancer, which accounts
for 85% of all ovarian malignancies, had been increasing in
frequency until 1970 and has been stable the past ten years.
It claims a life every fifty minutes in the United States;
nearly 11,000 lives every year. Despite the use of surgery
radiation, and drug therapies with definable response rates,
the death rate has not decreased appreciably. We have no
important insights into its etiology but epidemiological
studies implicate hormonal (ovulatory) and environmental
influences. Much of the treatment data which has been
generated is difficult to interpret and studies are almost
impossible to compare because of variability in patient
selection techniques and response criteria. But that is
the bad news.

The good news is that a number of careful studies have
identified important aspects of the natural history of the
disease, defined necessary staging procedures, and deline-
ated prognostic factors, all of which lay the foundation
for a multi-disciplinary attack on this dreadful disease.
Progress is just beginning.

NATURAL HISTORY, PROGNOSTIC FACTORS AND STAGING

Ovarian cancer tends to remain intraperitoneal throughout
its course although distant lymphatic and hematogenous
metastases occasionally are seen. It kills its victims by
progressive inanition and gastrointestinal tract obstruction. The five year survival of patients treated with
surgery alone with Stage I disease (limited to ovaries) is
about 67%; for Stage II disease (limited to true pelvis)

A.T. van Oosterom et al. (eds.), Therapeutic Progress in Ovarian Cancer,
Testicular Cancer and the Sarcomas, pp. 61-76. All rights reserved.
Copyright 1980 by Martinus Nijhoff Publishers, The Hague/Boston/London.

about 25%; and for Stage III (intraperitoneal disease) and IV disease (spread to liver or extraperitoneal sites) about 5%. Thus, stage of disease is a key prognostic factor, making accurate staging a vital component of successful management.

The patterns of spread of ovarian cancer are primarily based upon the flow of tumor-cell-containing ascites and upon the lymphatic drainage of the ovary. Tumor involving lymphatic channels of the ovary drain through the para-aortic chain and up to the diaphragmatic nodes. They alter the flow of lymph and produce hydrostatic pressure changes which result in ascites formation. This ascitic fluid which bears tumor cells bathes the peritoneal cavity and hemidiaphragms often resulting in nodular growths on peritoneal surfaces. It has been shown that approximately 25% of patients felt to have localized pelvic disease had lymphangiographic evidence of extra-pelvic lymph node involvement by tumor (8). A similar percentage of patients with presumed localized disease undergoing peritoneoscopy were found to have subdiaphragmatic tumor nodules (18). Despite these findings, the majority of patients referred to Roswell Park Memorial Institute (83%) (17) and the National Cancer Institute (75%) have had subumbilical or other limited incisions through which adequate examination of the upper abdomen would be virtually impossible.

The histologic grade of the tumor, in addition to stage of disease, is an important prognostic factor. Studies using Broder's classification for degree of cellular atypia have recorded significant differences in survival between high and low grade tumors within each stage of disease. In one study, overall 5-year survival of Stage II patients was 38% but when stratified according to histologic grade, patients with low levels of atypia (Grade 1) had an 80% survival while patients with highly anaplastic tumors (Grades 3 and 4) had only a 10% 5-year survival (13).

In addition to stage and grade, the amount of residual disease after initial laparotomy is an important prognostic factor. Aggressive cytoreductive surgery which produces residual tumor deposits of less than 1.5 cm in diameter

results in improved survival (9). In fact, complete resection of Stage III disease results in longer survival than
patients with incompletely resected Stage II disease.

Thus, the definition of adequate staging surgery must
be modified to accommodate our better understanding of the
natural history and the important prognostic factors. Such
a procedure should include 1) resection of as much disease
as technically feasible to minimize residual disease and
assure adequate tissue specimens for histologic grading; 2)
examination and biopsy of para-aortic nodes; and 3) careful
inspection of the peritoneal surface including the posterior
gutters, both hemidiaphragms and the liver surface.

While accurate primary staging at surgery is important,
periodic restaging is critical both to assure that the 25%
of patients who present with Stage I and II disease are not
progressing, and to evaluate the effects of treatment in
the 75% of patients who present with advanced disease.
Data accumulated to date have stressed the differences
between clinical complete responses and pathologically-
documented disease-free status. Approximately one-third to
one-half of patients felt to be disease-free on clinical
grounds will have no documented tumor on repeat laparotomy.
Furthermore, it is only the pathologically confirmed complete responses which translate into prolonged survival.
The same features which cause the majority of patients to
seek medical attention only after the disease has become
advanced, make detection of residual disease by clinical
examination alone impossible. Detection of all but bulky
disease requires non-invasive and low risk invasive procedures in both staging and restaging evaluations. Intravenous pyelography and barium enema have established utility
in detecting ureteral and bowel encroachment and abdominal
computerized tomography is being studied as a non-invasive
replacement for more invasive tests. Ultrasonography may
aid in detecting small amounts of ascites, nodal enlarge-
ment and masses not felt on physical examination. Lymphangiography may provide early evidence of retroperitoneal
lymphatic spread, and nodes with persistent abnormal lymphangiographic contours can be safely sampled nonsurgically

by percutaneous aspiration of the node under fluoroscopic guidance (25). Peritoneoscopy allows inspection of all peritoneal surfaces, biopsy of suspicious lesions, and sampling of fluid for cytological inspection. We have employed this procedure safely both to stage patients inadequately staged surgically and to follow results of therapy. Thirty-seven percent (7 of 19) patients referred to the NCI as Stage I or II were upstaged by peritoneoscopy and 36% (24 of 66) patients in clinical complete remission after chemotherapy had findings of residual disease at peritoneoscopy necessitating continuation of therapy (16).

Because of the demonstrated importance of complete staging and thorough restaging proceeding all the way to repeat laparotomy if necessary, new standards for assessing therapeutic effects have been established. In addition, the histologic grade of the tumor should be used as a stratification factor in studies evaluating new treatments because of the demonstrated higher response rate of lower grade lesions. Finally, the amount of residual disease after primary surgery should be balanced between any treatment groups in clinical trials because of the better prognosis of patients with minimal residual disease. Applying the knowledge of the natural history and prognostic factors which have been learned in previous trials should result in the collection of more meaningful data on therapeutic efficacy in future trials.

THE ROLE OF CHEMOTHERAPY IN THE TREATMENT OF OVARIAN CANCER

The response rates of ovarian cancer to a variety of agents has been examined. Alkylating agents used singly produce responses in 35% to 65% of patients and are similar regardless of the specific alkylating agent used or its route of administration. L-phenylalanine mustard (L-PAM) has become the standard alkylating agent used because of its high response rate ($\sim$50%), the vast experience in its use, and its ease of administration (daily oral doses for five days every four to six weeks). Methotrexate (MTX) (25%), 5-fluorouracil (5-FU) (33%), adriamycin (36%), cis-platinum (cis-plat)(29%), and hexamethylmelamine (hex) (47%) all demonstrate significant antitumor effects as well. Let us now consider their use in each stage of disease.

A.   STAGES I AND II (EARLY STAGE)

The optimal therapy for early stage ovarian cancer is unsettled. The role of chemotherapy in the adjuvant setting or as an adjunct to surgery and/or radiation therapy is controversial.   Several randomized trials have been under-taken, but long-term follow-up is inadequate at this point to define the precise role of chemotherapy in early stage disease.   However, several ongoing trials are worthy of mention.

There is a suggestion that chemotherapy in Stage I disease is at least as good as intracavitary radioisotopes and external pelvic plus abdominal radiation therapy.   One single arm study employing adjuvant chlorambucil reported a 5-year survival of 94% in 14 Stage I patients (12).   Where single agent alkylators have been compared to radiation therapy, chemotherapy has been as good or better. In a study randomizing Stage I patients to L-PAM or pelvic plus abdominal radiotherapy, 3 to 6 years of followup has failed to show significant survival differences in the two treat-ments (20,14). Eighty-five percent of irradiated patients are disease-free as compared to 90% of patients receiving L-PAM.   In a Gynecologic Oncology Group study comparing pelvic irradiation to L-PAM or observation, no survival differences have been found among the groups, however, the group receiving pelvic irradiation has the highest relapse rate to date (36%) as compared to 17% relapse rate in the untreated group and 7% for patients receiving L-PAM (10). The Ovarian Cancer Study Group has two ongoing studies which should yield important information.   They are compar-ing L-PAM to observation in Stage I patients with well-differentiated or moderately differentiated grades of tumor, and are comparing L-PAM to ^{32}P in Stage I patients with ascites or tumor outside the ovarian capsule or with poorly differentiated grades of tumor.   No survival information is yet available from these trials.   But these studies should help define the utility of adjuvant therapy in Stage I di-sease.

The proper treatment of Stage II disease has been argued extensively. "Traditional" therapy consists of surgery followed by pelvic radiotherapy and has produced 5-year survival figures of 25-40%. At least part of the cause for this low figure for control of disease supposedly limited to the true pelvis is that many of the patients (up to 40%) can be upstaged by the rigorous procedures described above, especially patients with macroscopic residual disease. Thus, in some studies, Stage II and Stage III survivals are similar and are being considered together. Two recent studies have examined the effects of single agent chemotherapy and radiotherapy in patients with Stage II disease. Workers at the M.D. Anderson Hospital randomized patients with minimal residual disease after surgery to receive either L-PAM or pelvic plus abdominal radiotherapy. With 3-6 year followup, percentage of disease-free patients is 58% and 55%, respectively, and show no statistically significant differences (20,14). In a group of Stage II patients not rigorously staged, treatment consisted of either pelvic irradiation, pelvic irradiation followed by chlorambucil, or pelvic plus total abdominal radiotherapy with extended fields (above diaphragms) (3). There were no survival differences among the groups however, those patients undergoing total abdominal hysterectomy with bilateral salpingo-oophorectomy (TAH-BSO) at staging had a 70% 4-year survival as compared to 18% in patients undergoing incomplete surgical procedures. In the TAH-BSO group, the extended field total abdominal radiotherapy produced better survival than pelvic radiotherapy with or without chlorambucil.

With careful staging, the number of patients who remain with Stage II disease is quite small. Patient accrual to the Ovarian Cancer Study Group protocol comparing pelvic radiotherapy plus L-PAM to L-PAM alone suggests that determining the best treatment for these patients may be ten years away.

B.   STAGE III AND IV (ADVANCED DISEASE)

In advanced stage disease, the prolongation of survival by
single agent L-PAM (15-20% 5-year survival in Stages III
and IV disease) has established chemotherapy as the treatment of choice.   The history of chemotherapy has taught us
that when several independently active drugs are available,
using them in combination often results in prolonged survival.   Several studies have been reported employing combination chemotherapy in previously untreated patients with
advanced disease (Table 1).

One study reported a 60% (25 of 41 patients) response
rate from a regimen employing actinomycin D, 5-FU, cyclophosphamide, vincristine and prednisolone.   Median duration
of response was 8 months with only two patients disease-
free for more than one year (5).   A four-drug combination
regimen consisting of cyclophosphamide, hexamethylmelamine,
adriamycin, and cis-platinum gave a 67% (8 of 12 patients)
response rate but the short duration of followup does not
allow assessment of survival prolongation (23).   These and
other studies of combination regimens that have been carried
out do not take into account histologic grade or extent of
residual disease and none of these compares combination to
single drug regimens.   They do not address the key question
of whether combination regimens are superior to single
agents in the treatment of advanced disease.

Two studies comparing actinomycin D, 5-FU and cyclophosphamide (ACFUCY) to single agent L-PAM failed to translate slightly higher response rates to the combination
therapy into prolonged survival (19,2).   The adriamycin
plus cyclophosphamide regimen has beem compared to single
agent cyclophosphamide (7) and single agent L-PAM (22)
in separate studies.   In neither study was the combination
better than the single agent in bulky disease patients, but
in the former study adriamycin plus cyclophosphamide was
significantly more effective than single agent cyclophosphamide in patients with minimal residual disease (7).

The first prospective randomized trial to demonstrate
the superiority of a combination regimen over standard

TABLE 1

COMBINATION CHEMOTHERAPY FOR OVARIAN CANCER

Regimen	% Responses	% Complete Responses	Duration of Response/Survival	Ref.
actinomycin D 5-FU cyclophosphamide vincristine prednisolone	60% 25/41	5% 2/41	8 mos/-	5
cyclophosphamide hexamethylmelamine adriamycin cis-platinum	67% 8/12	25% 3/12	N/A	23
adriamycin cyclophosphamide vs.	36% 13/36	6% 2/36	6 mos/12 mos	7
cyclophosphamide	31% 11/35	0	6 mos/12 mos	
adriamycin cyclophosphamide vs.	73% 8/11	54% 6/11	-/10 mos	22
L-PAM	29% 4/14	7% 1/14	-/10 mos	
hexamethylmelamine cyclophosphamide methotrexate 5-FU vs.	75% 30/40	33% 13/40	>30 mos/29 mos CR	24
L-PAM	54% 20/37	16% 6/37	>25 mos/17 mos CR	
actinomycin D 5-FU cyclophosphamide vs.	53% 26/49	28.6% 14/49	-/>9 mos	2
L-PAM	35% 17/49	18.4% 9/49	-/>9 mos	

single agent alkylator therapy was done at the National
Cancer Institute (U.S.A.) and compared hexamethylmelamine,
cyclophosphamide, methotrexate and 5-FU (hexa-CAF) to L-PAM
(24). Hexa-CAF treated patients had a higher response rate
(75% vs. 54%), more complete remissions (33% vs. 16%) and a
prolonged median survival (29 vs. 17 mos). Patients with
minimal residual disease after initial surgery had a higher
overall response rate than patients with bulky disease (84%
vs. 53%) and histologic grade was confirmed to be an important factor in predicting response. The effectiveness of
the Hexa-CAF regimen has subsequently been confirmed by
other investigators (15). More recent preliminary reports
of combinations incorporating cis-platinum have appeared
which claim response rates between 50 and 90%. Hopefully,
such cis-platinum-containing regimens will improve on the
33% complete response rate confirmed by restaging seen with
HexaCAF, for it is these restaged complete responses which
have the greatest impact on survival.

C.   RESPONSE TO CHEMOTHERAPY OF INITIAL TREATMENT FAILURES

The optimistic preliminary response rates reported to cis-
platinum-containing regimens acquire even greater importance
when it is recognized that Hexa-CAF, which produces a 75%
response rate in previously untreated patients, caused
only partial responses in 23% (3 of 13) of patients after
relapse from single agent chemotherapy or radiotherapy
(15). In a large series of patients (360) at M. D. Anderson
Hospital who received a variety of treatments (including
the two combinations ACFUCY and cyclophosphamide plus
hexamethylmelamine) after failure of primary therapy, only
6% of patients responded to second or third line drugs
(21). Adriamycin, which has a 36% response rate in previously untreated ovarian cancer patients, caused partial
responses in 8% (3 of 38) patients in one trial, and this
low figure has been confirmed by two other groups. A
variety of combinations has been tried as salvage regimens
for primary treatment failures. Hexamethylmelamine plus
5-FU (36%), high dose methotrexate with or without vincristine (30%), adriamycin plus cis-platinum (33%), cyclophos-

phamide (or 5-FU) plus hexamethylmelamine plus adriamycin plus cis-platinum (48 to 67%) all have moderate response rates. However, complete responses are extremely rare, duration of followup is short, and the toxicity of the combination regimens is substantial in these previously heavily treated patients. Thus, until less toxic and more effective salvage regimens are found, complete response to initial therapy will be the major determinant of survival.

The net effect of all of these studies with salvage regimens is clear. Responses to combination chemotherapy are reduced in patients previously treated with either radiation or chemotherapy. Therefore, workers in this field must avoid grouping untreated and previously-treated patients together. The effectiveness of regimens as first line or salvage treatments must be ascertained separately.

The hope remains that precise staging, proper stratification of treatment variables, and pathologic documentation of remission will identify the most successful treatments and guide decisions for beginning and ending chemotherapy. Such careful use of effective agents may translate into prolonged disease-free survival.

IV. IMMUNOLOGICAL ENHANCEMENT OF CHEMOTHERAPY EFFECTS

Several studies have reported the use of a variety of nonspecific immunostimulants in conjunction with chemotherapy in the treatment of ovarian cancer. Most of these suffer from being single-arm studies of heterogeneous patient populations and no conclusive study exists which confirms that immunotherapy is useful.

Nevertheless, there are two studies which suggest a possible role for chemoimmunotherapy. The Gynecologic Oncology Group compared L-PAM plus intravenous Corynebacterium parvum to a historical group which received L-PAM alone. More patients receiving C. parvum responded (53% vs. 29% for L-PAM alone) and the progression-free interval was twice as long for patients receiving C. parvum (12 mos. vs. 6 mos for L-PAM alone), as was estimated median survival (24 mos vs. 12 mos for L-PAM alone) (4). The Southwest Oncology Group study randomized untreated patients

to adriamycin plus cyclophosphamide versus the same combination plus bacillus Calmette-Guerin (BCG) given by scarification to extremities. The patients receiving BCG had
higher response rates (53% vs. 36%), more complete responses
(seven patients or 12% vs. one patient or 2%), and median
survival nearly twice as long (24 months versus 13 months)
as the group receiving chemotherapy alone (1). These
studies provide hope that addition of immunoadjuvants to
effective combination chemotherapy regimens may improve
response rates and survival in advanced disease and raises
the issue of whether immune therapy might be useful in
early stage disease as well.

NEW APPROACHES TO THE THERAPY OF OVARIAN CANCER

Injection of radionuclides and chemotherapeutic agents
intraperitoneally has been attempted in the past with
variable results. Nevertheless, recent technical advances
in equipment for peritoneal dialysis, specifically the
introduction of the chronic indwelling intraperitoneal
catheter (Tenckhoff catheter) has allowed reconsideration
of this form of treatment. Intraperitoneal chemotherapy
for ovarian cancer has several attractive theoretical
advantages over systemic chemotherapy. Because ovarian
cancer generally remains confined to the peritoneal cavity,
intraperitoneal administration should enable higher concentrations of drugs to be maintained in direct contact with
the tumor for longer periods and with less systemic toxicity
than intravenous administration. Phase I trials with intraperitoneal methotrexate have shown that concentration gradi-
ents of 10-30 fold between peritoneum and plasma can be
achieved (11). Though some toxicity such as chemical peri-
tonitis and myelosuppression has been noted, intracavitary
administration of active drugs may be a unique approach to
the treatment of ovarian cancer. It may find its greatest
use in the adjuvant setting or in patients with minimal
residual disease.

The capacity to establish in vitro conditions for the
proliferation of ovarian tumor stem cells has allowed the
development of an in vitro predictor of clinical responses

to particular chemotherapeutic agents. This in vitro stem cell assay evaluates clonogenic potential after exposure to chemotherapy. In all 18 patients studied, results of in vitro testing accurately predicted clinical responsiveness. Only three patients demonstrated in vitro sensitivity to drugs, including one patient whose cells responded to vinblastine, a drug with very low activity in a population of ovarian cancer victims. All three patients were clinical responders to the drugs to which their stem cells had been sensitive in vitro. If more extensive application of this technique supports the contentions of this original report, it could significantly change the approach to ovarian cancer and other solid tumors. Treatment might be able to be individualized on the basis of in vitro testing much the same way that antibiotic susceptibility testing of bacterial isolates guides clinical decision-making in infectious diseases.

Despite the large number of agents which have been shown to be effective against ovarian cancer, new drug development and application of drugs active in other tumors which have not been adequately studied in ovarian cancer may bring important advances in its treatment. A list of potentially interesting older drugs is shown in Table 2. Drugs such as bleomycin, streptozotocin, and procarbazine whose dose-limiting toxicities are not bone marrow suppression are attractive candidates for new combinations. PALA, AMSA and pentamethylmelamine are all new drugs currently in phase I or II trials which have potential merit. Mitomycin C and its derivative Porfiromycin have been previously shown to be active in ovarian cancer but have been inadequately studied.

Basic science investigation has recently yielded an interesting finding which may ultimately lead to clinical utility. The cell from which most ovarian carcinomas arise is derived embryologically from Müllerian epithelium. In males, who have an extrordinarily low incidence of epithelial testicular tumors, Mullerian regression factor (MRF) causes involution of this cell type during sexual differentiation. It has now been demonstrated that MRF

TABLE 2

Drugs Not Yet Given Adequate Testing in Ovarian Cancer

Cytembena

Procarbazine

Porfiromycin

Streptozotocin

Chlorozotocin

Bleomycin

Hydroxyurea

Mithramycin

Mitomycin C

---

has cytotoxic activity against ovarian cancer cells _in vitro_ (6).

SUMMARY

A number of advances in the understanding of the biology and treatment of ovarian cancer over the past 5 years has changed the pessimistic view of this disease that was formerly commonplace. Systematic clinical investigation has yielded results which will have a beneficial impact on some victims of ovarian cancer. With continued efforts to define optimum treatment modalities, application of some of the new treatment ideas coming from the laboratory, development of methods of early diagnosis, and pursuit of knowledge on etiology and prevention, perhaps the dismal survival of patients with ovarian epithelial malignancies will be further improved.

REFERENCES

1. Alberts, DS, Moon TE, et al. Randomized study of chemoimmunotherapy for advanced ovarian carcinoma: a preliminary report of a Southwest Oncology Group study. Cancer Treat. Rep. 63: 325-332, 1979.

2. Barlow JJ, Piver MS. Single agent vs. combination chemotherapy in the treatment of ovarian cancer. Obstet and Gynecol 49: 609-611, 1977.

74

3. Bush RS, Allt, WEC, et al. Treatment of epithelial carcinoma of the ovary. Surgery irradiation, and chemotherapy. Amer. J. Obstet. Gynecol. 127: 692-704, 1977.

4. Creasman, WJ, Gall SA, et al. Chemoimmunotherapy in the management of primary Stage III ovarian cancer: A Gynecologic Oncology Group Study. Cancer Treat. Rep. 63: 319-324, 1979.

5. Dimitriades, M, Papadimitriou C et al. Chemotherapy of ovarian cancer. Int. Surg. 63/2: 81-84, 1978.

6. Donahue PK, Swann DA, et al. Mullerian duct regression in the embryo correlated with cytotoxic activity against human ovarian cancer. Science 205: 913-915, 1979.

7. Edmonson HJ, Fleming TR et al. Different chemotherapeutic sensitivities and host factors affecting prognosis in advanced ovarian carcinoma versus minimal residual disease. Cancer Treat. Rep. 63: 241-247, 1979.

8. Fuks, Z, Bagshaw MA The rationale for curative radiotherapy for ovarian cancer. Int. J. Rad. Oncol. Biol. Phys. 1: 21-32, 1975.

9. Griffiths CT, Fuller AF. Intensive surgical and chemotherapeutic management of advanced ovarian cancer. Surg. Clinics N.A. 58: 131-142, 1978.

10. Hreschchyshyn MH, Norris HG, et al. Postoperative treatment of resectable malignant and possibly malignant ovarian tumors with radiotherapy, melphalan or no further treatment. Abstract 9W57. Proc. of 12th Int. Cancer Cong., 157, 1978.

11. Jones RB, Myers CE, et al. High volume intraperitoneal chemotherapy ("belly bath") for ovarian cancer: pharmacologic basis and early results. Cancer Chemother. Pharmacol. 1: 161-166, 1978.

12. Julian CG, Woodruff SD. The role of chemotherapy in the treatment of primary ovarian malignancy. Obstet. Gynecol. Survey 11: 1307-1342, 1969.

13. Malkasian GD, Decker DG, Webb MJ: Histology of epithelial tumors of the ovary: clinical usefulness and prognostic significance of the histologic classification and grading. Semin. Oncol. 2: 191-201, 1975.

14. McGuire WP, Young RC. Ovarian cancer. In Randomized Trials in Cancer: A Critical Review by Sites. edited by M. J. Staquet, Raven Press, New York, 1978, p. 273-288.

15. Neijt JP, Van Lindert ACM, et al. Hexa-CAF combination chemotherapy and other multiple drug regimens in advanced ovarian carcinoma: present and future. Neth. J. Med. 22: 1, 1979.

16. Ozols RF, Fisher RI, Anderson T, Young RC. Manuscript in preparation.

17. Piver SM, Lele S, Barlow JJ. Preoperative and intraoperative evolution in ovarian malignancy. Obstet. and Gynecol. 48: 312-315, 1976.

18. Rosenoff SH, Young RC, et al. Peritoneoscopy: a valuable staging tool in ovarian cancer. Ann. Int. Med. 83: 37-41, 1975.

19. Smith JP, Rutledge F, Wharton JT. Chemotherapy of ovarian cancer: new approaches to treatment. Cancer 30: 1565-1571, 1972.

20. Smith JP, Rutledge F, Declos L. Postoperative treat-
     ment of early ovarian cancer: a random trial between
     postoperative irradiation and chemotherapy. Natl.
     Cancer Inst. Monog. 42: 149-153, 1975.
21. Stanhope RC, Smith JP, Rutledge F. Second trial drugs
     in ovarian cancer. Gynecol. Oncol. 5: 52-58, 1977.
22. Turbow MM, Fuks Z, Glatstein E. Chemotherapy of ovari-
     an carcinoma: randomization between between melphalan
     and adriamycin-cyclophosphamide. Proc. Amer. Assoc.
     Cancer Res. 19: 394, 1978.
23. Vogl SE, Berenzweig M, et al. The CHAD and HAD regi-
     mens in advanced ovarian cancer: combination chemothera-
     py including cyclophosphamide, hexamethylmelamine,
     adriamycin and cis-dichlorodiammine platinum (II).
     Cancer Treat.Rep. 63: 311-317, 1979
24. Young RC, Chabner BA, et al: Advanced ovarian adeno-
     carcinoma: a prospective clinical trial of melphalan
     (L-PAM) versus combination chemotherapy. New Eng. J.
     Med. 299: 1261-1266, 1978.
25. Zornosa J, Wallace S, et al. Transperitoneal percutan-
     eous retroperitoneal lymph node aspiration biopsy.
     Radiology 122: 111-115, 1977.

7 SECOND-LOOK LAPAROTOMY AND PROGNOSIS RELATED TO EXTENT OF RESIDUAL DISEASE

J. P. Smith and P. E. Schwartz

Abstract

One hundred forty-two patients with epithelial
tumors of the ovary managed at the M.D. Anderson
Hospital and Tumor Institute underwent an exploratory
operation (second-look operation) to assess the status
of their cancer. Thirty-one patients were found to
have no evidence of disease (NED) and chemotherapy was
discontinued. Eight patients with advanced ovarian
cancer are NED five or more years following negative
second-look surgery and are probable chemotherapy cures.
Seven patients found to have cancer at second-look
operations had their management changed as a results
of the surgery and are NED five or more years later.
The most important factors correlating with negative
second-look operations were the stage of cancer, amount
of residual tumor left at the initial surgery and the
number of courses of chemotherapy administered prior
to the second-look operation. Survival following positive second-look surgery varied directly with the
tumor volume found at the operation and the amount of
tumor left behind at the second-look surgery. Patients
treated with radiation therapy had a poorer survival
than those treated with chemotherapy following
positive second-look operations.

A.T. van Oosterom et al. (eds.), Therapeutic Progress in Ovarian Cancer,
Testicular Cancer and the Sarcomas, pp. 77-94. All rights reserved.
Copyright 1980 by Martinus Nijhoff Publishers, The Hague/Boston/London.

The management of patients with epithelial tumors
of the ovary is hampered by a lack of diagnostic tests
which are highly sensitive for detecting residual or
recurrent tumors following a course of radiation
therapy or an interval of chemotherapy. There are no
tumor markers[1], diagnostic radiographic techniques,
such as the various contrast studies or CAT scan or
other physical scanning techniques such as ultrasound[2]
that have proven reliable in demonstrating residual
tumor after treatment. Physicians who treat patients
with ovarian cancer must follow patients and direct
their treatment based on clinical findings such as
abdominal palpation, bimanual pelvic examination, chest
x-rays, laparoscopy and "second-look" operations.

Exploratory laparotomy to assess the status of a
patient's tumor in order to plan future treatment and
remove any tumor found if possible, a so-called "second-
look" operation is finding wide acceptance in the
management of patients with epithelial tumors of the
ovary. This operation has been used in patients
with epithelial cancer of the ovary at the M.D.
Anderson Hospital and Tumor Institute in Houston,
Texas, since 1960.

MATERIAL AND METHODS

One hundred and ninety-two patients had second-look
operations after an interval of chemotherapy during
a 14-year period between 1960 and 1974.
Forty-four of these patients received chemotherapy
prophylactically for Stage I and Stage II cancers and
will not be included in the subsequent material.
Six patients with Stage III cancer who had been included in
previous reports by the senior author[2] will not be included
in this report. These patients all developed abdominal or
pelvic masses after receiving post-operative radiation therapy and all received chemotherapy without having a laparotomy to prove that they had residual cancer.

The stages of the tumors are seen in Table 1.

TABLE 1

STAGE OF OVARIAN CANCER

STAGE	NO. OF PATIENTS
II	14
III	105
IV	23
TOTAL	142

Fourteen patients had Stage II, 105 had Stage III and 23 had Stage IV cancer. Two-thirds of the patients had serous carcinoma and the other third of the patients were divided among undifferentiated adenocarcinoma, mucinous carcinoma and endometroid carcinoma. Many of the patients with endometroid cancers or clear cell cancer of the ovary who were treated before 1970 were classified as serous tumors. Only 112 of the tumors were graded: however, among these tumors that were graded, 11 patients (10%) had Grade I; 33 patients (28%) had Grade II; and 68 patients (61%) had Grade III cancers.

Most of the patients in this report were treated before the policy of maximum tumor reduction was adopted. Only 13 of 128 patients with Stage III or Stage IV in this report had no residual tumor left after their original surgery. Thirty-one patients had residual tumor less than two centimeters but 83 patients had residual tumor greater than two centimeters in diameter. One patient's chart did not state the amount of residual cancer present when she began her chemotherapy. One hundred and twenty-three patients were treated with a single chemotherapy drug and 19 patients were treated with the three-drug combination of actinomycin, 5-fluorouracil and cyclophosphamide; 117 patients received melphalan; two received adriamycin; two received hexamethylmelamine; one received 5-fluorouracil and one received cyclophosphamide.

The first several patients who had a second-look operation had surgery when a significant change was observed in their tumors suggesting a previously

unresectable tumor could be excised. Following a review
of patients who had second-look surgery in 1969, all
patients have received 12 or more cycles of chemotherapy
before their second-look operations. This report
includes several patients who received adriamycin in a
clinical trial comparing several drugs in the post-
operative treatment of ovarian cancer. The patients
in this study who received adriamycin had second-look
surgery after they had received 540 mg/m^2 or after
approximately 27 weeks of treatment.

The surgical procedure described as a second-look
operation has changed significantly during the 14 years
included in this study. The present operation is performed with a vertical midline incision from the symphysis to approximately 5 - 7 centimeters above the
umbilicus. Immediately after opening the abdomen, saline
washings for cytologic evaluation and cell block for
histological studies are obtained from the pelvis and
both lateral paracolic spaces. Two biopsies then are
obtained from the peritoneum of the bladder, both
pelvic walls, the cul-de-sac, the paracolic spaces,
the right diaphragm and from the serosa of the recto-
sigmoid. If the uterus and ovaries are present, these
are removed and if the omentum is present, it is removed.
The entire small intestine and its mesentery and the
colon are examined and all irregularities and adhesions
are biopsied. Any irregularity seen in the peritoneum,
either visceral or parietal, is biopsied. The lymph
node areas in the pelvis and along the aorta are carefully palpated and all enlarged nodes are removed. If
no enlarged nodes are felt, the base of the mesentery
of the small bowel is opened and a group of nodes at,
or near, the renal vessels are removed for histological
study.
More than half of the lymph nodes in the paraaortic area
that are found to have metastatic cancer are normal by
palpation.

RESULTS

Stage II

Five of the 14 patients (36%) had negative second-look operations. Two of these patients had residual tumor less than two centimeters maximum diameter at their initial surgery and three had residual tumor greater than two centimeters. Two have survived 60 months or more without evidence of recurrent cancer and the other three are surviving more than 36 months following negative second-look surgery. All received 10 - 12 cycles of melphalan and all are presently living and well.

Stage III

Seventeen of 105 patients (16%) with Stage III tumor were free of cancer at the second-look operations. Two are without evidence of disease eight and nine years following negative second-look surgery. One patient has survived 37 months and nine are surviving 4 - 22 months following negative second-look surgery. Four patients had developed recurrent cancer 6, 7, 12 and 28 months following surgery and all are dead of their disease. One patient who received 18 courses of melphalan had a negative second-look operation and died of acute leukemia 16 months following surgery with no evidence of ovarian cancer seen at postmortem examination.

Fifteen of the patients who had negative second-look operations were treated with melphalan; one with 5-fluorouracil and one with cyclophosphamide. None of the four patients who developed recurrent cancer following negative second-look operations received 12 cycles of melphalan. They received 4, 5, 7 and 10 courses of melphalan, respectively, before their second-look operations.

Forty-two of the 80 patients who were found to have cancer at second-look surgery were clinically free of cancer by abdominal and pelvic examination immediately prior to surgery. Eleven of these patients are presently alive without evidence of cancer with six surviving more than five years. Four of these six patients had their treatment

changed because of the findings at second-look surgery;
one patient was continued on the same chemotherapy and one
patient had the only known focus of residual tumor removed.
The remaining five patients are living more than three years
following positive second-look surgery.

TABLE II

STAGE vs FINDINGS AT SECOND-LOOK SURGERY

STAGE	NO. PATIENTS NED	NO. PATIENST PERSISTENT CANCER	(% NED)
II	5	9	(35.7)
III	17	88	(16.2)
IV	9	14	(39.1)

Stage IV

Nine of 23 patients (39%) with Stage IV ovarian cancer
were found to be free of cancer at the time of their second-
look operations (Table II). Three patients are surviving
more than five years following the second-look operation and
three are surviving more than three years. Three patients
have developed recurrent cancer -- 7, 9 and 15 months --
following negative second-look operations.

All the patients with Stage IV cancer who were free of
disease at the time of their second-look operation had
received melphalan. Six received 10 - 35 courses of the
treatment. One of the patients who received 35 courses
prior to her second-look operations died 80 months after
surgery of acute granulocytic leukemia. The three patients
who developed recurrent cancer received 4, 12 and 15 courses
of melphalan.
Unfortunately, the patient who received 12 cycles of melphalan had only three biopsies at the time of her second-look
operation. She did not have paraaortic lymph nodes sampled
and developed a recurrence in this area.

TABLE III

FINDINGS AT SECOND-LOOK SURGERY

FINDINGS	NO. PATIENTS
NED	32
NED - + Cytology	0
Regression - Microscopic Tumor	19
Regression - Macroscopic Tumor	59
No Change	17
Progression	16
TOTAL	142

Thirty-one of the 142 patients were without evidence
of disease at second-look operation and had their chemotherapy stopped (Table III). No patient had cytological
evidence of malignancy in her abdominal washings with
negative random biopsies. Nineteen patients had no gross
evidence of disease at surgery but were found to have
microscopic disease in random biopsies. Several patients
had only a single biopsy site positive for microscopic
disease despite multiple random biopsies. Most of these
patients were continued on their previous chemotherapy.
Fifty-nine patients had significant response of their
tumors to chemotherapy but had visible cancer at surgery.
Seventeen patients demonstrated no change in the status
of their tumors from the original surgery. Sixteen patients
showed definite progression of their cancer as compared to
the findings at initial surgery. The percentage of patients
who were free of cancer at second-look surgery was directly
related to the number of courses of chemotherapy the patient
received.

TABLE IV

NUMBER OF COURSES MELPHALAN vs
NEGATIVE FINDINGS (NED) AT SECOND-LOOK SURGERY

NO. COURSES MELPHALAN	NO. PATIENTS NED	NO. PATIENTS PERSISTENT CANCER	(% NED)
2 - 9	7	41	(14.6)
10	8	21	(27.6)
11	0	2	(0)
12	8	11	(40.0)
13+	6	4	(60.0)

Seven of 48 patients (14.6%) completed 2 - 9 courses of melphalan and were found to be free of disease at second-look operation (Table IV). Eight of 29 patients (27.6%) received 10 cycles of melphalan and were free of disease and eight of 22 patients (36.4%) who received 11 or 12 courses of melphalan were without evidence of disease at second-look operations. Ten patients completed 13 or more cycles of melphalan and six (60%) were free of disease at second-look surgery.

The volume of residual tumor left at the initial surgery correlated directly with the incidence of negative second-look operations. Patients whose largest residual tumor mass was less than two centimeters had almost the same survival as patients who had no tumor remaining after initial surgery. Four of 13 patients (30.8%) who were without evidence of disease at the time of the original surgery had negative second-look operations and 12 of 38 patients (31.6%) with residual tumor less than two centimeters had negative second-look operations. Fifteen of 90 patients (16.7%)with residual tumor greater than two centimeters had negative second-look operations.

The patients with serous carcinoma who were free of tumor
at second-look operations totalled 18.8 percent, while 25
percent of patients with mucinous tumors, 37.5 percent of
patients with endometroid cancers and 28 percent of those
with classified adenocarcinoma had negative second-look
operations. Among the 112 patients whose histological grade
was known, two of 11 patients with Grade I lesions (18.2%),
six of 33 patients with Grade II lesions (18.2%) and 18 of
68 patients with Grade III lesions (26.5%) were free of
disease at the time of second-look surgery.

TABLE V

LOCATION OF RESIDUAL
TUMOR AT SECOND-LOOK

Site	No. of Patients
Ovary	53/56
Pelvic Peritoneum	58
Omentum	57
Bowel Serosa	63
Bowel Mesentery	20
Abdominal Gutters	23
Anterior Abdominal Peritoneum	21
Fallopian Tubes	16
Paraaortic Lymph Nodes	15
Liver Serosa	12
Uterus	11
Other	24

Sites where persistent disease were found at surgery
are seen in Table V. The serosa of the intestines, pelvic
peritoneum, ovaries and omentum are the most common sites.
Unfortunately, most of the patients in this series did not
have biopsies of the paraaortic lymph nodes or the diaphragm.
Fifty-three of the patients who had ovaries which were left

behind at the time of the initial surgery, had cancer in these ovaries. It is interesting that all patients who had either gross or microscopic cancer found in the diaphragm had positive biopsies from other intraperitoneal sites.

The survival following second-look surgery varied directly with the tumor volume found at that surgery (Fig 1) and the amount of tumor left behind at second-look operation (Fig 2). The five-year survival following second-look surgery for patients with no evidence of disease was 72 percent and in patients with only microscopic tumors, it was 38 percent. Patients found to have lesions which had regressed but were visible at the time of surgery, that is, patients with tumor masses larger than two centimeters, had a 15 percent five-year survival. Patients with no change in their tumor status compared to their initial surgery had a 17 percent five-year survival; and patients with progression of their tumors had an 18 percent five-year survival.

Resection of residual tumor at second-look surgery influences the survival rate (Fig 2). Five-year survival for patients who had all of their cancers removed at second-look surgery was 27 percent, and, if only a portion of the tumor was removed, leaving residual tumor masses smaller than two centimeters, the five-year survival was 29,5 per cent. The five-year survival for patients with residual cancer greater than two centimeters was 9.0 percent. Only one patient who had residual tumor greater than two centimeters diameter left at the time of second-look surgery is living more than 60 months following the operation.

Patients treated with chemotherapy after positive second-look operations had better two and five-year survivals than patients treated with radiation therapy (Fig 3). The survivals of two and five years with chemotherapy was 34.3 percent and 27.6 percent, respectively; whereas, the corresponding survival for patients treated with radiation therapy was 24.4 percent and 16.1 percent.

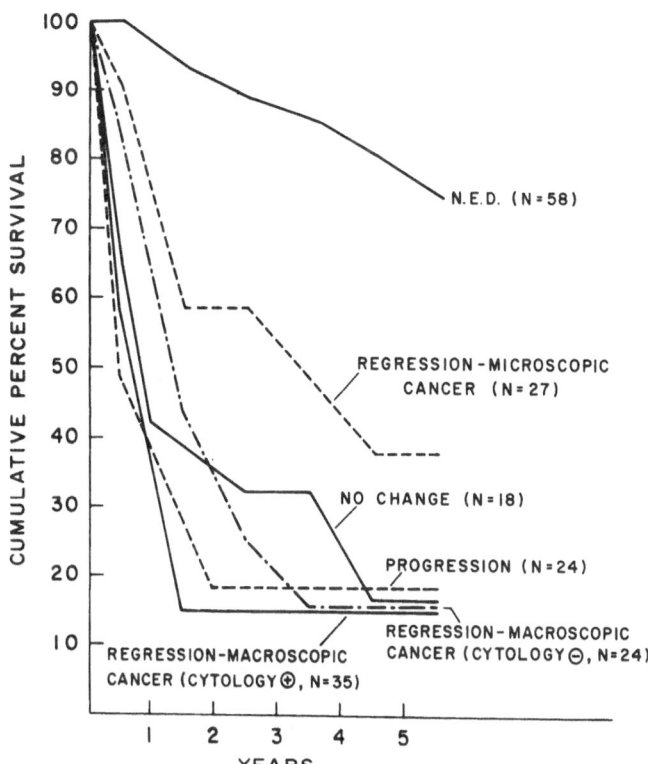

Fig. 1.

Survival from second-look surgery.

The chemotherapy response was determinded at second-look surgery.

N= number of patients;

cytology -= no malignant cells present in pelvic and para-colic space washings;

cytology += malignant cells present in washings.

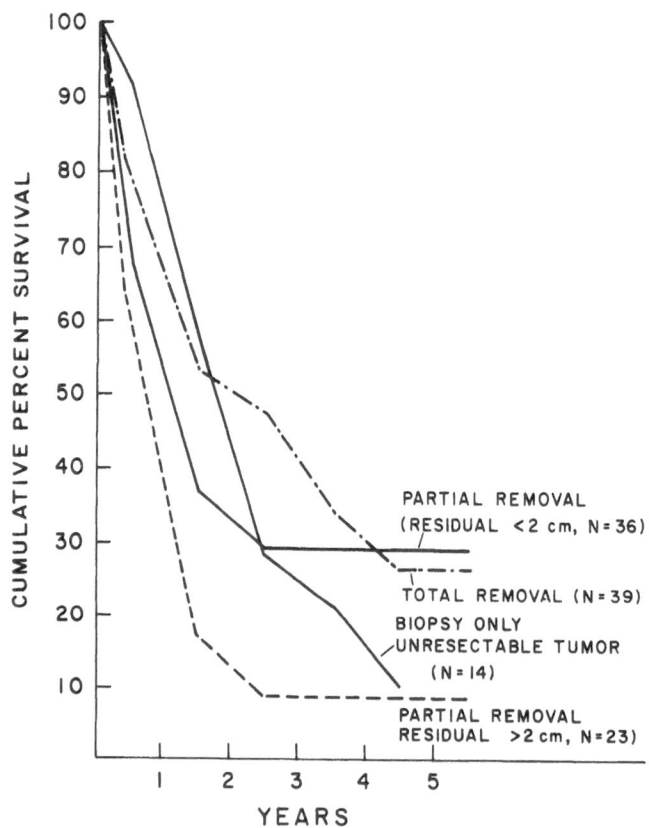

Fig. 2.
Survival from second-look surgery as determined by the
maximum diameter of the largest residual tumor mass upon
completion of the surgery.

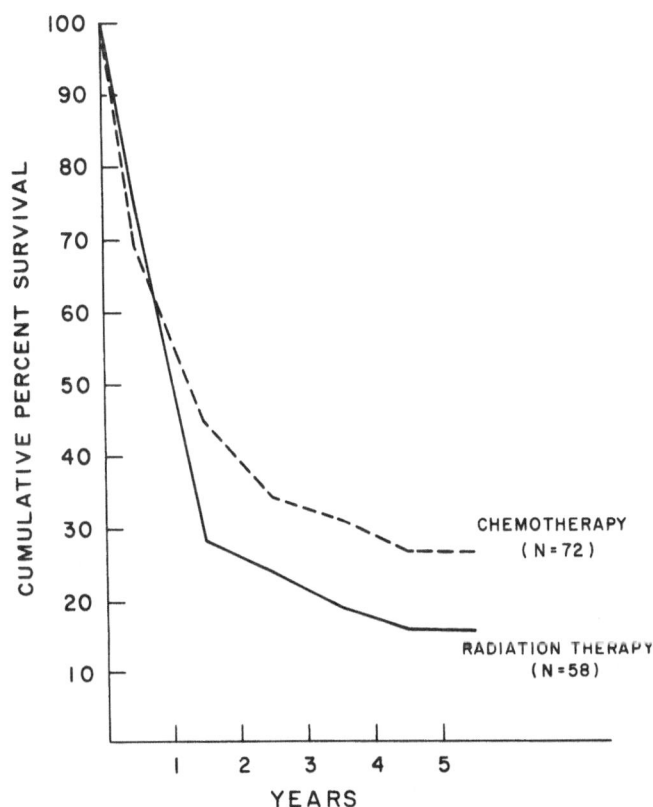

Fig. 3.
Survival from second-look surgery as influenced by subsequent therapy, radiation or chemotherapy

This is particularly significant because only patients with
residual tumors less than two centimeters at second-look
surgery were treated with irradiation. Patients with tumors
larger than two centimeters in diameter were treated with
chemotherapy.

The most common surgical complication in this group of
patients was wound infection. None of the patients in this
study died as a result of their surgery.

The most severe long-term complication in this group of
patients who had prolonged survivals was leukemia. Five
patients developed leukemia with three being diagnosed as
acute granulocyctic leukemia. All five patients had been long-
term survivors on chemotherapy with a range of 43 to 184
months. One patient developed subacute leukemia after
receiving nine courses of melphalan and then received
abdominal radiation by the moving strip technique with
additional radiation to the pelvis. The four patients with
acute leukemia received 18 to 44 courses of melphalan and
three had no evidence of ovarian cancer at the time of
their deaths. Three patients received chemotherapy for
their leukemia -- none survived more than three months from
the time of the diagnosis.

THIRD-LOOK PROCEDURES

Eight patients had a third-look operation after one or
more years of additional chemotherapy following a positive
second-look operation. Four patients were free of disease
at their third-look surgery; two of these patients, however,
have developed recurrent cancer 15 and 17 months following
their third-look surgery. The four patients who had persistent cancer at the time of the third-look surgery had their
treatment changed because of this finding.

COMMENTS

This series of patients demonstrates the shortcomings
of clinical examination in following patients with epithelial

cancer of the ovary.

Fifty-five of the 111 patients who were found to have residual tumor at second-look surgery were free of disease by abdominal or pelvic examinations prior to surgery. Conversely, five patients who were free of disease at second-look surgery had palpable masses prior to surgery which were thought to be cancer.

Eight of the patients in this report with advanced ovarian cancer are living and well without evidence of disease five or more years following a negative second-look operation and are probable chemotherapy cures. Ten patients with advanced ovarian cancer are living and well without evidence of disease more than three years following a negative second-look operation and are potential five-year cures. Thirty-one patients in this study would have been continued on chemotherapy without a second-look operation and would have been exposed unnecessarily to the possibilities of developing prolonged myelosuppression or, possibly, leukemia. Four of the 30 patients in this series who received more than 16 courses of melphalan developed acute granulocytic leukemia.

Laparoscopy has been proposed as an alternative to second-look surgery[4]. Nineteen patients in this series had no visible tumor at the time of second-look surgery but had microscopic cancer found on random biopsies of the peritoneal surfaces. Laparoscopy may be of value in patients who have extensive or unresectable cancers but it is doubtful that these surgeons would have correctly determined the status of these patients. In patients in whom it is possible to see metastatic cancer, confirmation by the means of the laparoscope is appropriate and treatment may be continued without a laparotomy. Should laparoscopy fail to demonstrate persistent cancer, a laparotomy and a meticulous search for tumor masses must be performed. Laparotomy is necessary for patients who have persistent cancer in the pelvis, mesentery or serosa of the small bowel, paracolic spaces, paraaortic lymph nodes and retroperitoneal areas.

These areas cannot be seen or biopsied with a laparoscope.

If localized cancer is seen at laparoscopy, a laparotomy may be indicated to remove this persistent cancer since patients who have all gross tumor removed at second-look surgery have an improved two and five-year survival (Fig 2).

The timing of second-look surgery in relation to the number of cycles of chemotherapy is extremely important. In this series, most patients who had surgery as soon as a nonresectable tumor mass became smaller were seldom benefitted by this surgery. The patients who had 12 or more cycles of chemotherapy had the best survivals. The time interval over which the chemotherapy was given did not influence prognosis. Seven patients have developed recurrent cancer following negative second-look surgery. Five of these patients received less than 12 cycles of chemotherapy.

Seven patients who had cancer at second-look surgery have survived five or more years free of disease and have clearly benefitted from the surgery. The presence of persistent disease was not appreciated clinically and the subsequent management of these patients was determined by the findings at second-look surgery.

Patients found to have tumor masses smaller than two centimeters in diameter at second-look surgery were initially treated with radiation therapy to the whole abdomen by the moving strip technique with additional radiation to the pelvis. Patients treated in this manner had a poorer survival (Fig 3) than patients with more extensive cancer who were treated with chemotherapy. Our current policy is to continue chemotherapy in all patients who are found to have cancer at second-look surgery.

REFERENCES

1. Samaan, N.A., Smith, J.P., Rutledge, F.N., and Schultz, P.N.: The significance of measurement of human placental lactogen, human chorionic gonadotropin and carcino embryonic antigen in patients with ovarian carcinoma. American Journal of Obstetrics and Gynecology, 126: 186-189, September, 1976.
2. Samuels, B.I.: Usefulness of ultrasound in patients with ovarian cancer. Seminars in Oncology, 2:229, 233, 1975.
3. Smith, J.P. Delgado, G., and Rutledge, F.N.: Second-look operation in ovarian carcinoma postchemotherapy. Cancer, 38: 1438-1441, 1976.
4. Smith, W.G., Day, T.G., Jr., and Smith J.P.: The use of laparoscopy to determine the results of chemotherapy for ovarian cancer. The Journal of Reproductive Medicine, 18: 257-260, 1977.

Authors addresses:

Julian P. Smith, Department of Gynecology and Obstetrics
Wayne State University School of Medicine
Hutzel Hospital, Detroit, Michigan 48201, USA

Peter E. Schwartz, Department of Obstetrics and Gynecology
Yale University School of Medicine
New Haven, Connecticut 06510, USA

8 LONG TERM SURVIVAL FOLLOWING CHEMOTHERAPY FOR ADVANCED EPITHELIAL OVARIAN CARCINOMA

J. T. Wharton, J. Herson, C. L. Edwards, J. Seski and M. P. Hodge

Abstract

Two hundred and seventy-eight patients with F.I.G.O. stage
III or IV epithelial ovarian carcinomas treated with surgery
followed by single or combination agent chemotherapy at
The M. D. Anderson Hospital and Tumor Institute at Houston,
Texas, during the interval July 1, 1972 and September 1,
1978, form the nucleus of this report. The effect of age
at diagnosis, F.I.G.O. stage, histologic grade, largest
tumor diameter remaining after surgery, and chemotherapy
treatment, on the frequency of 24 month or greater survival
($\geq$ 24 month) following chemotherapy initiation, were
analyzed by means of logistic regression analysis. The
chemotherapy treatments were placed into two treatment
groups on the basis of proportion of survivors observed on
each treatment. The final logistic regression equation
finds histologic grade, tumor diameter, and the interaction
of age and treatment group to be significant prognostic
factors for $\geq$ 24 month survival ($p < 0.10$). The logistic
regression equation predicts that a patient with histologic

This research was supported in part by Research Grants CA-6294 and
CA-11430 and Contract NO1-CM-33710 from the National Cancer Institute,
U. S. Department of Health, Education and Welfare.

Grade 1 carcinoma, 2 cm or less in diameter and age 45 or
less has 3.5 times the probability of surviving $\geq$ 24 months
than that of a patient with a histologic Grade 2 or 3
carcinoma, greater than 2 cm diameter and older than 45
years receiving the same treatments. The derived logistic
regression equation is shown to fit the observed data
quite well.

1. *Introduction*

The objective of this study is to determine how
initiating chemotherapy with a single agent or a
combination of agents in patients with various pretreatment characteristics affect the likelihood of
surviving with advanced ovarian cancer for 24 months
or longer ($\geq$ 24 months). The identification of the
pretreatment characteristics having a favorable or
unfavorable effect on survival may influence the design
of future clinical trials. The need for pretreatment
stratification for characteristics such as histologic
grade (1,5,9) and the amount of residual tumor prior
to initiating chemotherapy (2,3,4,7) have been recommended. Arguments concerning the need for stratification by other factors, sometimes without convincing
support data, abound.

A method for identifying which specific chemotherapy
program, single agent or combination of drugs, is best
suited for a patient with certain pretreatment characteristics is highly desirable. An understanding of
each of the characteristics' relative risk to the
patient would perhaps better define the need for
combination chemotherapy. Combination chemotherapy
has recently been shown highly active in patients with
advanced carcinoma, however, toxicity can be severe,
and reservation of this treatment modality for those
patients at higher risk might be desirable (6,7).

In this study, survival was the statistical end
point of interest. It should not be concluded that
all survivors had a response to the initial drug(s),

second line drug(s), or any other agents with which the
patient was treated. Patients received treatment
regimens in sequence—i.e., the regimen was continued
as long as activity was documentable and a switch to
another regimen was indicated for the following: growing
disease, stable disease after 2 or 3 courses of drug,
or dose limiting toxicity. Continuation of chemotherapy
was not necessary when multiple negative biopsies were
obtained at surgical second look laparotomy performed
after 12 courses of therapy. It should also be pointed
out that survival was credited to the first regimen the
patient received regardless of anti-tumor activity.

The 24 month interval was chosen for this report
since this allowed inclusion of the maximum number of
patients from the 3 studies analyzed. This interval
also appears to be reasonable for the identification
of favorable pretreatment characteristics or drugs with
superior activity since most series to date have near
or less than 50% 2 year overall survival rate for
patients with advanced carcinoma.

2. *Materials and Methods*

The 337 patients for this analysis were part of three
separate prospective randomized studies for patients
with advanced epithelial ovarian cancer conducted at
the M. D. Anderson Hospital and Tumor Institute,
Houston, Texas from July 1, 1972 to September 1,
1978 (Table 1 & 2). The objectives of these sequential
studies were to investigate the ability of certain
single agents or combination of active agents to induce
clinically detectable tumor regression.

Only patients with F.I.G.O. stage III or IV
epithelial ovarian carcinomas previously untreated with
chemotherapy or irradiation were included in this study.
The pattern grading system based on the degree to
which a carcinoma formed papillary structures or glands
versus solid areas was used. This system also considers

Table I

*Randomized Prospective Studies for Patients
with Advanced Ovarian Carcinoma*

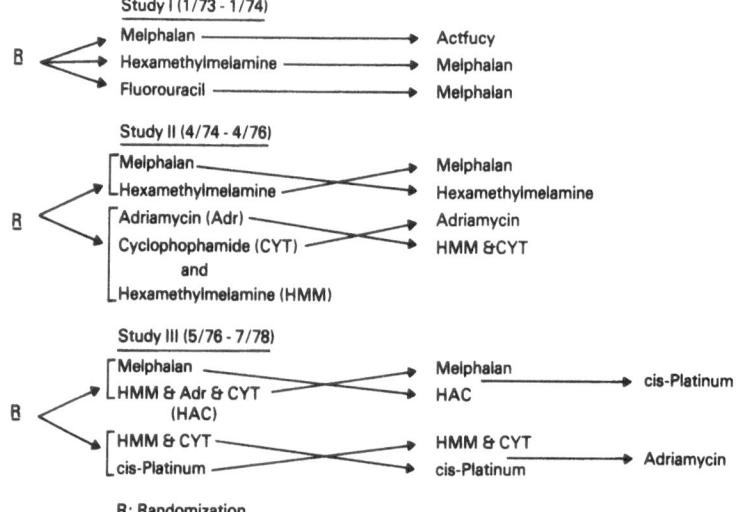

Study I (1/73 - 1/74)

R — Melphalan ——————→ Actfucy
— Hexamethylmelamine ——————→ Melphalan
— Fluorouracil ——————→ Melphalan

Study II (4/74 - 4/76)

R
┌ Melphalan ——————→ Melphalan
└ Hexamethylmelamine ——————→ Hexamethylmelamine
┌ Adriamycin (Adr) ——————→ Adriamycin
Cyclophophamide (CYT) ——————→ HMM &CYT
and
└ Hexamethylmelamine (HMM)

Study III (5/76 - 7/78)

R
┌ Melphalan ——————→ Melphalan ——————→ cis-Platinum
└ HMM & Adr & CYT ——————→ HAC
(HAC)
┌ HMM & CYT ——————→ HMM & CYT ——————→ Adriamycin
└ cis-Platinum ——————→ cis-Platinum

R: Randomization

Table 2

Chemotherapy Data

Agent(s)	Dose	Treatment Duration & Interval
Melphalan	1 mg/kg oral	divided over 5 days every 4 weeks
5-Fluorouracil	15 mg/kg I.V.	weekly
Hexamethylmelamine	8 mg/kg oral	daily and continuous
Adriamycin	60 mg/M^2 I.V.	day 1 and repeated every 3 weeks (1imit 550 mg/M^2)
DDP	30 mg/M^2 I.V.	daily x 3 repeated every 4 weeks
HMM and	4 mg/kg oral	daily 1 - 14
CYT	250 mg/M^2 oral	daily 1 - 5 (repeated every 4 weeks)
HMM and	4 mg/kg oral	daily 1 - 14
CYT and	200 mg/M^2 oral	daily 1 - 5
Adriamycin	40 mg/M^2 I.V.	day 1 (repeated every 4 weeks)

HMM: Hexamethylmelamine

CYT: Cyclophosphamide

DDP: cis-Dichlorodiammineplatinum

cell differentiation in that most solid areas consist of undifferentiated cells whereas better differentiated cells lined the well-formed papillary structures. Grade 1 carcinomas were well differentiated, Grade 2 moderately differentiated and Grade 3 carcinomas were poorly differentiated. Patients were selected at random for the various treatment arms and were given a full explanation of the nature of a randomized trial.

Table 3 displays the treatment arms for each study and the number of patients registered in each arm. Of the 337 patients registered on Studies I, II and III, 278 were eligible for this 24 month survival analysis.

In order to be eligible for statistical analysis these patients had to: 1) have the histologic grade of the carcinoma determined; 2) either have expired prior to 24 months or survived at least 24 months following the initiation of treatment and; 3) have started chemotherapy prior to September 1, 1977.

Table 3

Patient Distribution

Study	Treatment	Number Registered	Number Eligible for Study
Study I	Melphalan	50	49
	HMM	25	23
	5-FU	25	22
Study II	Melphalan	35	34
	HMM	34	31
	Adriamycin	34	33
	HMM & Cytoxan	34	28
Study III	Melphalan	25	18
	*H.A.C.	25	14
	HMM & Cytoxan	25	11
	DDP	25	15
Total		337	278

HMM: Hexamethylmelamine

DDP: cis-Platinum

*HAC: HMM & Adriamycin & Cytoxan

The following factors were considered as potential prognostic factors for survival: patient age at diagnosis, F.I.G.O. stage, histologic grade, tumor diameter at chemotherapy start and chemotherapy treatment. Each of these factors was studied separately for its effect on the frequency of $\geq$ 24 month survival. The statistical significance of this effect was tested by the chi square test.

Those factors that showed a significant effect on frequency of $\geq$ 24 month survival at the level $p = 0.10$ were called "candidate" prognostic factors and further analyzed using multiple logistic regression analysis (10,11). This type of analysis permits consideration of the importance of each factor in determining the likelihood of the patient surviving $\geq$ 24 months while adjusting for the simultaneous effects of the remaining factors. The method also permits study of the effect of the interaction between factors on $\geq$ 24 month survival. Those factors showing statistical significance at the level $p = 0.10$ in the logistic regression analysis were called prognostic factors. The goodness of fit of the multiple logistic model to the observed data was tested by a chi square test as described by Hosmer and Lemeshow (12).

3. *Results*

Figure 1 presents a survival curve for the 278 patients on this study. The curve was drawn using the Kaplan-Meier product limit method (13). Two hundred and twenty-eight of the 278 patients have expired to date. The product limit estimate of median survival time is 17 months.

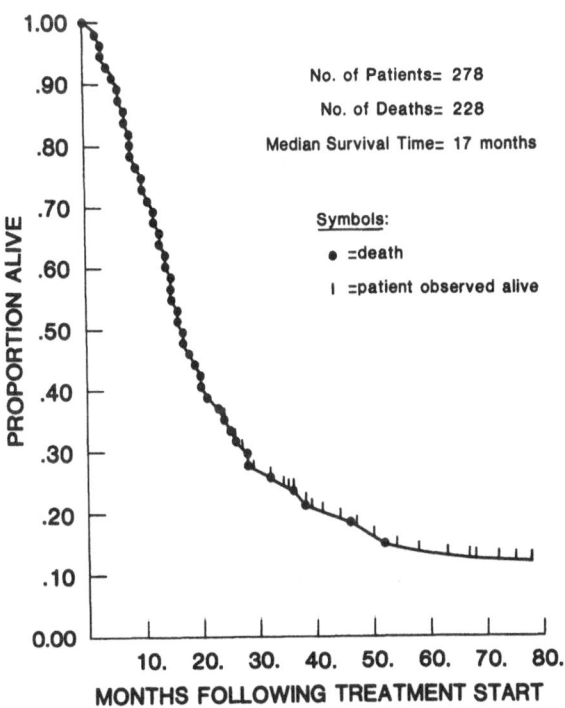

Figure 1. Survival time of advanced ovarian cancer patients,
Studies I-III, M. D. Anderson Hospital and Tumor Institute, 1973-78.

Table 4 presents the results of the analysis of potential prognostic factors. Age and tumor diameter were dichotomized for analysis purposes (age at 45 years and tumor diameter at 2 cm). The overall proportion of patients surviving $\geq$ 24 months was 0.371 (or equivalently 37.1%). There was no evidence of a significant difference in 24 month survival proportion between Grades 2 and 3 (p = 0.285) so these groups were combined for further analysis. Similarly, the 7 treatments were combined into two distinct groups: Group A, consisting of 5 fluorouracil (5 FU), Adriamycin, Hexamethylmelamine, (HMM), and HMM and Cytoxan and Group B, consisting of Melphalan, cis-Platinum (DDP) and Hexamethylmelamine, Adriamycin and Cytoxan (H.A.C.). Age, histologic grade, tumor diameter and treatment group all qualified as "candidate" prognostic factors (p < 0.10). There was no evidence of a significant effect of F.I.G.O. stage on $\geq$ 24 month survival proportion (p = 0.155).

The four candidate prognostic factors, age, grade, tumor diameter and treatment group, together with all six two-factor interactions were further analyzed by logistic regression. The results of this analysis are presented in Table 5. Grade, tumor diameter and the interaction of age and treatment group all emerged as significant prognostic factors (p < 0.10).

The significance of the interaction between age and treatment group is that the effect of these two factors on $\geq$ 24 month survival cannot be assessed separately but only in combination. This phenomenon can be illustrated with reference to Table 6. Here we see that the $\geq$ 24 month survival proportion for treatment group B patients is relatively good and about the same regardless of the patients age - 0.481 for $\leq$ 45 years and 0.437 for > 45 years, (p = 0.844). While for treatment group A the older patients (> 45 years) have a significantly lower survival proportion (0.248) than younger patients ($\leq$ 45 years) whose survival proportion is 0.486 (p = 0.014). Thus patients treated with the

Table 4

Analysis of Frequency of 24 Month Survival

Following Treatment Start by Selected Patient Characteristics

Characteristics	Number Patients	24 Month Survivors No. Patients	Proportion	p-Value
All Patients	278	103	0.371	
Age				
<45	62	30	0.484	0.051
>45	216	73	0.338	
FIGO Stage				
III	221	87	0.394	0.155
IV	57	16	0.281	
Grade				
1	22	17	0.773	2 vs 3=
2	108	32	0.296	0.285
3	148	54	0.365	1 vs (2+3)
(2+3)	(256)	(86)	(0.336)	=0.0001
Tumor Diameter				
<2cm	93	49	0.527	0.0002
>2cm	185	54	0.292	
Treatment				
Group A	(148)	(45)	(0.304)	Group A vs Group B =
5FU	22	5	0.227	0.018
Adriamycin	33	10	0.303	
HMM	54	17	0.315	
HMM & CYT	39	13	0.333	
Group B	(130)	(58)	(0.446)	
Melphalan	101	43	0.426	
cis-Platinum	15	7	0.467	
*H.A.C.	14	8	0.571	

*H.A.C.= Hexamethylmelamine, Adriamycin, Cytoxan

Table 5

Logisitic Regression Analysis

of Prognostic Factors

Factor	Regression Coefficient	p-Value	Favorable Prognosis Pt.	Unfavorable Prognosis Pt.	Ratio
			Predicted Probability of $\geq$ 24 month Survival		
Constant Term	-0.58				
Age (X_1)	-0.20				
Graded (X_2)	-0.45	0.001	.721	.329	2.2
Tumor Diameter (X_3)	-0.38	0.004	.489	.239	2.1
Treatment Group (X_4)	0.28				
Interaction: Age and Treatment Group ($X_1 . X_4$)	0.22	0.090	.479	.257	1.9
Composite			.866	.251	3.5

Details of the Logistic Regression Methods Utilized

a. logistic regression equation

Let a = probability the patient survives >24 months

ln = natural logarithm

The logistic regression equation linking a with prognostic factor

codes X_1, X_2, X_3 and X_4 is:

$$\ln \left(\frac{a}{1-a}\right) = -0.58 \quad -0.20X_1 \quad -0.45X_2 - 0.38X_3 + 0.28X_4 + 0.22X_1.X_4$$

b. prognostic factor codes

X_1 = age at diagnosis (yrs) = -1.868 if patient $\leq$45 yrs
= 0.536 if patient >45 yrs

X_2 = grade = -3.411 if grade 1 (favorable prognosis)
= 0.293 if grade 2 or 3 (unfavorable prognosis)

X_3 = tumor diameter = -1.409 if $\leq$2cm (favorable prognosis)
= .710 if >2cm (unfavorable prognosis)

X_4 = treatment group = -0.938 if group A (5-FU, Adria, HMM, HMM + Cytoxan)
= 1.066 if group B (Melphalan, DDP, HAC)

Interaction: age and treatment group

$X_1 . X_4$ = -1.991 if patient $\leq$45 yrs and treatment group B
-0.503 if patient >45 yrs and treatment group A (unfavorable prognosis)
-0.571 if patient >45 yrs and treatment group B
-1.752 if patient $\leq$45 yrs and treatment group A (favorable prognosis)

Table 6

Interactive Effect of Age and Treatment Group

on Probability of $\geq$24 Month Survival

Treatment Group	Age (yrs)	Observed	p-value	Proportion of 24 Month Survivors Predicted By Logistic Regression Equation
A	$\leq$ 45	0.486 (17/35)	0.014	0.479
	> 45	0.248 (28/113)		0.257
B	$\leq$ 45	0.481 (13/27)	0.844	0.417
	> 45	0.437 (45/103)		0.434

Treatment Group A: 5 FU, Adriamycin, HMM, HMM and Cytoxan

Treatment Group B: Melphalan, DDP, H.A.C.

H.A.C. = Hexamethylmelamine and Adriamycin and Cytoxan

DDP = cis-Dichlorodiammineplatinum

regimens in treatment group B have favorable survival regardless of age whereas younger patients treated with group A regimens have superior survival to older patients receiving the same treatments.

Returning to Table 5 the effect of the other factors may be assessed. The logistic regression equation is shown in section (a.) beneath Table 5. This model shows the contribution of each prognostic factor to the predicted probability that a patient with specified prognostic factors survives $\geq$ 24 months. The values of X_1, X_2, X_3 and X_4 represent codes for age, grade, tumor diameter and treatment group respectively. The prognostic factor codes utilized are shown in section (b.) Table 5. These codes were chosen so that each variable will be standardized—i.e., have a mean of 0 and a standard deviation of 1. The table shows that a favorable prognosis grade patient (i.e., Grade 1) has 2.2 times the likelihood of surviving $\geq$ 24 months than an unfavorable prognosis grade patient (i.e., Grade 2 or 3) (2.2 = .721/.329). Similarly the $\leq$ 2 cm tumor diameter patient has 2.1 times the probability of surviving 24 months than a > 2 cm tumor diameter patient.

A treatment group A ≤ 45 year old patient has 1.9 times the probability of surviving than a > 45 year old treatment group A patient. A distinct characteristic of the logistic analysis methods utilized is that they allow for the estimation of the effect of each factor on 24 month survival through the favorable-unfavorable ratios while correcting for the possible confounding effects of other factors. The model also estimates that the composite favorable prognosis patient (Grade 1, ≤ 2 cm diameter, ≤ 45 years old, treatment group A) has 3.5 times the probability of surviving ≥ 24 months than a composite unfavorable prognosis patient (Grade 2 or 3, > 2 cm diameter, > 45 years, treatment group A).

One measure of the usefulness of a logistic regression model is its "goodness of fit" or how well it fits the observed data. The data in Table 7 allow for the testing of the hypothesis of goodness of fit. The number of ≥ 24 month survivors predicted by the logistic regression equation and actually observed in each of 9 ordered categories of patients are presented.

Table 7

Goodness of Fit of Logistic Regression Equation

Group	Range of Predicted Probabilities of ≥ 24 month Survivals	Number Patients	Number of 24 month Survivors Predicted	Observed
1	0.189	31	5.86	5
2	0.189	31	5.86	5
3	0.189-0.323	31	7.47	11
4	0.323-0.339	31	10.49	10
5	0.339	31	10.51	10
6	0.340-0.385	31	10.77	9
7	0.385-0.532	31	13.85	10
8	0.532-0.553	31	16.51	20
9	0.553-0.881	30	21.86	23
Total		278	103.00	103

Test of significance of disparity between predicted and observed: chi square = 7.00 with 7 df, p >0.25

The chi square test shows that there is no evidence of
a statistically significant difference between predicted
and observed frequencies ($p > 0.25$).

4. *Discussion*

The probability of patient survival at 24 months is
significantly influenced by age, histologic grade,
tumor diameter and treatment. The logistic regression
results as shown in Table 5 give evidence that future
studies should be stratified for these factors.
Presumably patients could be assigned to stratum 1 if
the logistic regression equation in Table 5 predicts
their probability of $\geq$ 24 month survival to be $\leq$ 0.500
and to stratum 2 if > 0.500.

The proportion of Grade 1 carcinomas surviving
suggest that these patients form a subset that should
not be included in chemotherapy studies for advanced
carcinomas. It is most likely that studies including
only Grade 2 and 3 carcinomas or their equivalents
using other grading systems, would give more accurate
information concerning the effectiveness of combination
chemotherapy. Analysis of 24 month survival also allows
separation of regimens into what appear to be a weaker
group (treatment group A), and a stronger group (treatment group B). These initial prospective randomized
studies were correct in concept in that there does exist
a difference in single agent activity and melphalan
and cis-Platinum appear to be superior to the other
agents at this time. The survival proportion with
cis-Platinum is supported by a 52.4% complete response
plus partial response rate (14). This analysis with HMM
and Cytoxan in treatment group A may change as more
patients become eligible for inclusion. Further data
on the single agents will not be forthcoming because
present protocols use only drug combinations.

The detection of the significant interaction effect of age and treatment group (Table 6) may be the first step toward elucidating a treatment of choice for different subgroups of patients. The data from this study suggest that while there is no preference of treatment for patients $\leq$ 45 years those > 45 years have a survival advantage when receiving group B regimens rather than group A regimens.

This paper has focused on patient characteristics associated with $\geq$ 24 month survival in advanced ovarian cancer. The phenomenon of $\geq$ 48 month survival is also of interest and will be the subject of future investigations. Table 8 is a preliminary analysis of patient characteristics associated with $\geq$ 48 month survival. Analysis is restricted to patients who commenced chemotherapy treatment prior to September 1, 1975 (Study I and II). Among the 177 patients eligible for this analysis 29 survived $\geq$ 48 months (proportion 0.164). Age, grade and tumor diameter are all associated with $\geq$ 48 month survival in the same manner as they were associated with $\geq$ 24 month survival. In the present analysis Grade 2 and 3 tumors are not combined because their survival proportions are significantly different (p = 0.090). The phenomenon of Grade 3 tumors representing a separate subset was noted by Ozols, et.al. (1). In the case of age and grade, the ratio of survival proportions between favorable and unfavorable prognosis categories is greater, and that for tumor diameter is less in 48 month survival than in the 24 month case. Thus age and grade appear to exert a greater effect and tumor diameter a somewhat lesser effect on $\geq$ 48 month than $\geq$ 24 month survival. In both analyses, there was no evidence of a significant stage effect on survival. There is no evidence of a significant treatment effect on $\geq$ 48 month survival (p = 0.41). This latter statement is subject to change as much greater numbers of patients treated with combinations: HMM and Cytoxan, HMM,

Table 8

Analysis of Frequency of 48 Month Survival Following Treatment Start

By Patient Characteristics

Characteristic	Number	48 Month Survivors		p-Value
	Patients	No Patients	Proportion	
All Patients	177	29	.164	-
Age				
< 45	42	15	.357	.0003
> 45	135	14	.104	
F.I.G.O. Stage				
III	145	27	.186	.148
IV	32	2	.063	
Grade				
1	13	8	.615	
2	62	12	.194	.0001
3	102	9	.088	
Tumor Diameter				
< 2cm	48	12	.250	.097
> 2cm	129	17	.132	
Treatment				
5 FU	22	3	.136	
Adriamycin	24	4	.167	.488
HMM	45	4	.089	
HMM and Cytoxan	17	3	.176	
Melphalan	69	15	.217	

Adriamycin and Cytoxan (H.A.C.), and Melphalan and
cis-Platinum, become eligible for analysis. Since
Melphalan ranks as a strong single agent at 24 months and
is adequate in comparison at 48 months, it is a very
representative standard for measurement of drug combinations. The 48 month survival proportion for Grade 1
carcinomas (0.615) further emphasizes the need to delete
these patients from future clinical trials and limit
entry to Grade 2 and 3 patients with stratification

between the latter grades. Further analysis of the $\leq$ 45 year old group is necessary in view of the report by Edmonson, et.al., showing an influence related to the menopausal status (3).

It is of great interest to study the effect of tumor response as judged by surgical evaluations (complete response, partial response, no response) on survival time following surgical evaluation (15). Studies I - III required surgical evaluation after 12 courses of chemotherapy and many were delayed due to toxicity for considerably more than 12 months. As a result only 90 of the 278 patients in the 24 month analysis received a surgical evaluation and the time of the evaluation ranged from 7 to 25 months following treatment start. In the current advanced ovarian cancer clinical trial, Study IV, all patients receive surgical evaluation after 12 monthly chemotherapy courses. Reduced dose courses are administered in the presence of toxicity. The uniform timing of surgical evaluation will allow for future studies on the effect of surgically evaluated response on survival time. Adoption of the recommendations for chemotherapy dose reductions due to toxicity and format for reporting results as used by Young, et.al., will allow more precise comparison and interchange of data between study groups (7).

The goodness of fit test (Table 7) has shown the logistic equation to fit the observed data adequately. The best goodness of fit test will be to compare observed and predicted frequencies of $\geq$ 24 month survival among future patients using the equation from the present "learning sample".

REFERENCES

1. Ozols Robert F, Garvi Julian A, Costa Jose, Simon
   Richard M, Young Robert C; Histologic Grade in Advanced
   Ovarian Cancer. Cancer Treat Rep 63:255-263, 1979.
2. Day T G, Smith J P; Diagnosis and Staging of Ovarian
   Carcinoma. Semin Oncol 2:217-222, 1975.
3. Edmonson John H, Fleming Thomas R, Decker David G,
   et al; Different Chemotherapeutic Sensitivities and
   Host Factors Effecting Prognosis in Advanced Ovarian
   Carcinoma Versus Minimal Residual Disease. Cancer Treat
   Rep 63:241-247, 1979.
4. Griffith C Thomas, Parker Leroy M, Fuller Arlan F; Role
   of Cytoreductive Surgical Treatment in the Management
   of Advanced Ovarian Cancer. Cancer Treat Rep 63:235-
   240, 1979.
5. Dyson J L, Beilby J O W, Steele S J;Factors Influencing
   Survival in Carcinoma of the Ovary. Brit Jour of Cancer
   25:237-249, 1971.
6. Ehrlich C E, Einhorn L, Williams S D, Morgan J, Chemotherapy for Stage III-IV Epithelial Ovarian Cancer with
   cis-Dichlorodiammineplatinum (II), Adriamycin and
   Cyclophosphamide. A Prelimenary Report.
   Cancer Treatm. Rep. 63: 281-288,1979.
7. Young R C, Chabner B S, Hubbard S P, et al; Advanced
   Ovarian Adenocarcinoma: A Prospective Clinical Trial
   of Melphalan (L-PAM) vs Combination Chemotherapy
   (HEXA-CAF). N Eng J Med 299:1261-1266, 1978.
8. Griffiths C T, and Fuller A F; Intensive Surgical and
   Chemotherapeutic Management of Advanced Ovarian Cancer.
   Surg Clin North Am 58:131-141, 1978.
9. Decker D G, Massey E, Williams T J, et al; Grading of
   Gynecologic Malignancy: Epithelial Ovarian Cancer.
   Proceedings of the 7th National Cancer Conference 1973,
   pp 223-231.
10. Fleiss J; Statistical Methods for Rates and Proportions
    New York. John Wiley and Sons, 1973.

11. Lee E T, A Computer Program for Linear Logistic
    Regression Analysis. Computer Programs in Biomedicine.
    4:80-92, 1974.

12. Hosmer D, and Lemeshow S; A Goodness of Fit Test for
    the Multiple Logistic Regression Model. Biostatic
    Technical Report 79-1, School of Health Sciences,
    University of Massachusetts, Amherst, Massachusetts.

13. Kaplan E, and Meier P; Nonparametric Estimation from
    Incomplete Observations. J Am Stat Assoc 53:457-481,
    1958.

14. Gershenson David M, Wharton J Taylor, and Herson Jay,
    et al, (unpublished data).

15. Wharton J Taylor, Smith Julian P, Herson Jay, et al;
    Hexamethylmelamine. An Evaluation of Its Role in The
    Treatment of Ovarian Cancer. Am J. of Ob and Gynec
    No 7 133:838-841, April 1, 1979.

9 NEW DRUGS IN OVARIAN CANCER: *IN VITRO* PHASE II SCREENING WITH THE HUMAN TUMOR STEM CELL ASSAY

S. E. Salmon, B. Soehnlen and D. S. Alberts

INTRODUCTION

Development of new drugs for ovarian cancer or any other
specific type of cancer has thus far been a very arduous
and time-consuming procedure. The process, which initiates
from rational design, serendipitous discovery or a random
screening in a few signal mouse tumors has probably missed
a number of compounds which were inactive in L1210 or P388
leukemia, but would have had activity for other tumor types.
Even a broadened panel of 5-6 transplantable mouse tumors
of different histopathologies would be the conceptual equivalent of testing a new drug on 5-6 patients, each with a
different type of cancer. Viewed in that context, it is
perhaps remarkable that useful drugs have in fact been identified! In fact, many drugs have been identified through
other mechanisms in various countries. After a new drug
is found to be active in screening, it must pass preclinical
and clinical toxicology studies before it can be brought in
to large-scale clinical Phase II and Phase III studies in
various tumor types. We believe that the recent development of in vitro soft agar colony assays for human tumor
stem cells (1-10) now shows significant promise of shortening up and simplifying the entire drug testing procedure
including the preclinical drug screening for active compounds, clinical trials of new agents, and the final selection of treatment for individual patients. These comments
are particularly germain for ovarian cancer, because it is
so readily grown in the tumor stem cell assay starting with
either solid tumors or malignant effusions (3). Our initial

approach to drug testing in ovarian cancer with the stem
cell assay was to test drugs with known activity in patients
in relapse from standard drugs and correlate in vitro and
in vivo sensitivity (7,8). These correlation studies continue to be quite encouraging and will be updated in this
paper. However, our central focus will be the examination
of new Phase I-II agents to determine the frequency with
which significant inhibition of ovarian tumor colony formation is observed at pharmacologically achievable doses. In
that sense, we are conducting an "in vitro Phase II trial"
of new anticancer drugs. Additionally, we have applied the
assay to make some pharmacologic comparisons of 1 hour vs.
continuous contact to evaluate potential schedule dependen-
cy of some of these agents.

METHODS

Tumor biopsies and malignant effusions were obtained from
women with adenocarcinoma of the ovary. Techniques for pre-
paring single cell suspensions, drug incubations, and plating the cells in agar culture were as reported previously
from our laboratory (3,7,8), except that conditioned medium
was not utilized as sufficient ovarian tumor colony growth
was obtained without this addition. In our standard drug
assay system, cells are exposed to varying concentrations
of drugs in tissue culture tubes for 1 hour at $37^{\circ}C$ followed by washing and plating in the upper layer of the 2-layer
agar cultures. Standard agents included adriamycin, melphalan, vinblastine, cis-platinum, methotrexate, bleomycin
and 5-fluorouracil which were all tested at low doses up to
an upper limit of the pharmacologically achievable concentration. New agents studied included mitomycin, vindesine,
m-AMSA, dihydroxyanthracenedione, pentamethylmelamine and
phosphonacetyl l-aspartate (PALA). Dose finding studies
for new agents on which pharmacokinetic data were not available were carried out over a 3-log concentration range from
.1 to 10 µg/ml. In the present study, some samples were
also plated in the presence of standard concentrations of

stable drugs incorporated into the agar. In most cases, 5×10^5 cells were plated in each 35 mm Petri dish. Freshly plated cultures were examined by inverted light microscopy to ascertain that aggregates were not present. Plates were cultured at $37^\circ C$ in 5% CO_2 in air in a humidified incubator. Clusters were apparent within 3-4 days and ovarian tumor colonies usually were present in sufficient numbers and size to be counted 7-10 days after plating. Representative plates were prepared for morphologic analysis using our recently described dried slide technique with Papanicolaou staining (9). Data from all experiments were entered into disc storage on a Wang 2300 laboratory computer which was used for data analysis and graphic output. Criteria for in vitro sensitivity for standard drugs were based on calculation of the area under linear survival-concentration curves and ranking relative areas based on an initial training set of patients who were studied in vitro and in vivo. For new drugs wherein pharmacologic parameters were less certain, we use an operational definition of sensitivity of at least 70% reduction in survival of ovarian tumor colony forming cells at a relatively low dose of the drug. In all instances, wherein pharmacokinetic data were available, the dose to achieve at least 70% inhibition had to be less than the maximally achievable concentration time product in vivo. Patients for whom clinical correlations were made in relation to in vitro sensitivity had to achieve at least 50% tumor regression (a partial remission) to be considered clinically sensitive to the agent tested in vitro.

RESULTS

Clinical Correlates of In Vitro Sensitivity

Tumor cell assays and drug sensitivity measurements were initiated on biopsy samples from over 80 patients with ovarian cancer. Overall, about 75% of specimens provided sufficient colony growth to permit assessment of drug-induced lethality. While drug sensitivity assays have been carried out successfully on 65 samples, correlative clinical trials are reported only for patients who (a) had sensitivity to multiple agents measured in vitro, and (b) had enough retrospective or prospective data available for independent clinical evaluation of therapeutic response in vivo. Thus, a total of 44 evaluable patients with ovarian carcinoma have now been studied both in vitro and in vivo with correlations made with respect to clinical response in relation to drugs which showed evidence of in vitro sensitivity or resistance. In the course of this work, a total of 99 correlative clinical trials were carried out in these 44 patients.

table 1

Ovarian Carcinoma:
In Vitro Drug Sensitivity/Clinical Drug Sensitivity

December 1979

Pts	Clinical Trials	S/S	S/R*	R/S	R/R
44	99	16	9*	1	73

	Predictive Accuracy		Correlative Accuracy	
Sensitivity (S)	$\left(\dfrac{S/S}{S/S + S/R}\right)$	64%	$\left(\dfrac{S/S}{S/S + R/S}\right)$	94%
Resistance (R)	$\left(\dfrac{R/R}{R/R + R/S}\right)$	99%	$\left(\dfrac{R/R}{R/R + S/R}\right)$	89%

*Includes 3 patients with 25-50% tumor regression (improved) but classified as resistant in this summary which requires 50% regression to be classed as sensitive. If these patients were considered sensitive, the predictive accuracy for sensitivity would be increased to 76%.

As is summarized in Table 1, using the criterion of at least 50% tumor regression, the tumor stem cell assay predicts in vivo sensitivity with 64% accuracy. The successful prediction of clinical response to this extent is encouraging, as it approaches the predictive accuracy of in vitro culture for identifying useful antibiotics for treatment of some of the more difficult bacterial infections.

Were we to classify 3 patients who were predicted to be sensitive but who clinically achieved only 25-50% tumor regression as "sensitive", then the predictive accuracy would be 76%. Impressively, the assay also predicted <u>in vivo</u> resistance with 99% accuracy. Thus, the assay has extraordinary capability for identifying inactive agents which can be deleted from clinical use and thereby obviate unneeded toxicity. The relatively high accuracy rates for <u>in vitro</u>-<u>in vivo</u> correlations suggest that the assay should prove useful when applied in the circumstance of an "<u>in vitro</u> Phase II trial" of new agents. We plan to initiate studies of simple two-drug combinations <u>in vitro</u> in the near future, however, this will require limitation in the number of drug concentrations which we can study in the <u>in vitro</u> system for such combinations. Platinum-based combinations would be of particular interest for such correlations in ovarian cancer.

Relation of Drug Schedule to Lethality on Ovarian Tumor Stem Cells

Studies comparing one-hour exposure prior to plating to continuous contact in the agar to drugs thought to be stable <u>in vitro</u> have only been recently initiated in our program. Figure 1 summarizes our experience with vinblastine.

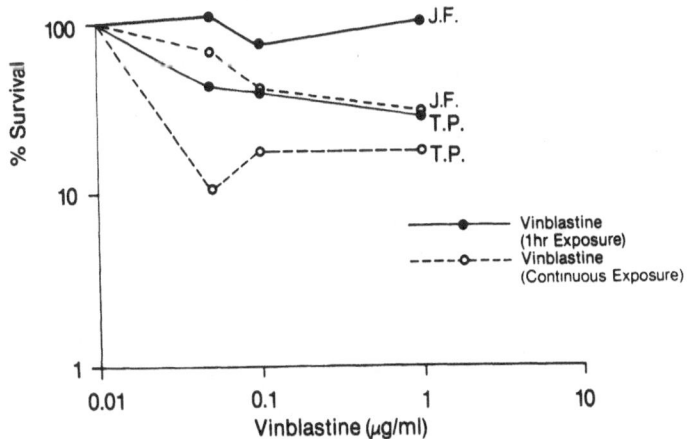

figure 1: Comparison of one-hour exposure (————) to continuous contact (-----) of two patients' ovarian tumor colony-forming cells to vinblastine. While there is slight augmentation in lethality at all dosage levels with continuous contact, this effect is relatively small, suggesting biochemical rather than kinetic resistance to this agent.

In the two patients studied in this system, there is somewhat greater _in vitro_ lethality observed with continuous
contact to vinblastine for the entire culture period
(approximately 10 days) in comparison to the one-hour exposure. However, in view of the fact that the effective
concentration time product of continuous contact would
appear to be at least 300 times as great as the one-hour
exposure, it would appear that prolonged contact is relatively ineffective in comparison to the potential toxicity
that might occur were such a schedule to be used _in vivo_.
Such observations would suggest that resistance to vinblastine may be more on a cellular uptake or biochemical basis
than on a cell kinetic basis. Inasmuch as lethality increased less than two-fold with the prolonged contact with
the drug, kinetic factors would appear to play a relatively
minor role in explaining _in vitro_ resistance to this agent
in that all clonogenic cells must pass through the cell
cycle multiple times in order to form tumor colonies _in
vitro_. Alternative explanations for this limited degree
of _in vitro_ lethality with prolonged exposure would include
(a) the possibility that even after short exposure times,
vinblastine might be stored intracellularly in host or tumor
cells and exert a prolonged effect despite the initial wash-
out or (b) the possibility that vinblastine might be un-
stable in this _in vitro_ system. Further studies will be
required to clarify these possibilities.

Mitomycin

A study of a relatively large number of anticancer drugs
which have not been extensively utilized in ovarian cancer
or are currently investigational agents on IND is now underway in our laboratories. Among standard agents that are
only rarely used for early or advanced ovarian cancer, we
have investigated mitomycin-C-induced lethality on tumor
samples from 11 patients. The results of these studies
summarized in Figure 2 indicate that only one of these 11
patients' cells had survival reduced to less than 30% of
the control at pharmacologically achievable doses of

mitomycin. However, four of the 11 patients had similar steep curves to the 0.1 µg/ml dosage level. Most of the patients who were studied were in relapse from prior alkylating agent therapy.

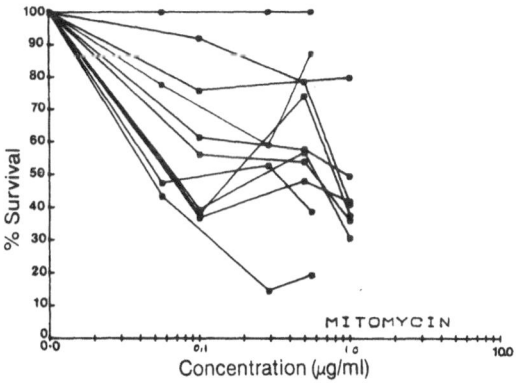

figure 2: Effect of a one-hour exposure of mitomycin on ovarian tumor colony formation. The 11 patients' cells studied manifest significant heterogeneity in response to this agent.

Pentamethylmelamine

Figure 3 summarizes our experience with <u>in vitro</u> assay of the new agent pentamethylmelamine (PMM).

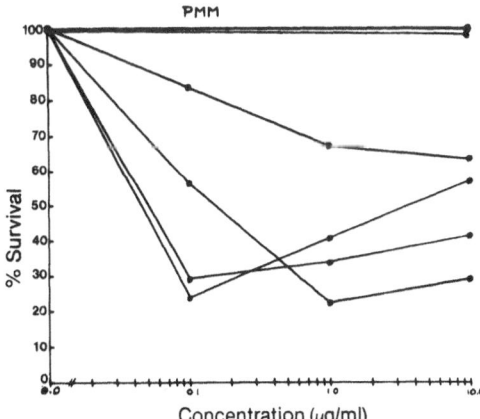

figure 3: Effect of a one-hour exposure of pentamethylmelamine on ovarian tumor stem cells. This new agent may prove to have utility in ovarian carcinoma.

This drug was formulated as an intravenous preparation to represent the active form of hexamethylmelamine (HMM) (which lacks sufficient solubility for intravenous use). PMM is under Phase I-II study in several centers, and is

120

of interest in ovarian cancer because HMM is known to be
active in this disorder (11,12). Of interest, three of the
five patients studied thus far in vitro have shown reduction to 30% survival of tumor colony-forming units in comparison to the control. While one of these assays showed
diminishing effect at increasing dose levels, this was not
observed in the other patients studied. These preliminary
data would suggest that pentamethylmelamine may prove to be
an active drug for use in ovarian cancer treatment. Selection of this agent in comparison to HMM will, in part, depend on comparative toxicology and clinical pharmacology
studies with both drugs.

Vindesine

The vinblastine analog, vindesine (desacetyl vinblastine)
(13) has been studied in vitro on 11 patients. Reduction
in survival to 30% of control values was observed at moderate dose levels in four of the 11 patients studied. Figure
4 depicts comparative lethality of vindesine and vinblastine
on ovarian tumor stem cells from 8 patients.

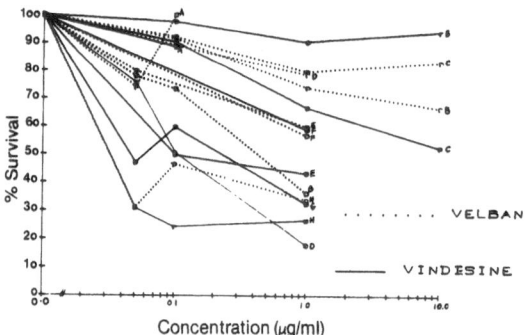

*figure 4: Comparative lethality of one-hour exposure of vindesine or
vinblastine on ovarian tumor colony formation. Both agents appear to
be of similar efficacy on the same 8 patients' (A-H) tumor stem cells
over the pharmacologically achievable dosage range.*

When studied simultaneously in vitro in this fashion, there
appeared to be no clear advantage to vindesine over vinblastine. We have observed occasional excellent objective
response in drug refractory ovarian patients treated with

vinblastine or vindesine. Our comparative _in vitro_ studies suggest the two drugs may have comparable clinical effects if the pharmacokinetics are similar.

MGBG

The investigational inhibitor of polyamine synthesis, methyl-glyoxal-bis(guanethylhydrazone)(methyl gag or MGBG) was also tested against ovarian tumor stem cells from 11 patients. This long-standing investigational agent has recently been revived and found active in renal and bladder cancer (14). In our _in vitro_ assays (Figure 5), MGBG had only intermediate lethality or less in most of the patients studied and only two of the 11 showed reduction to 30% of control at a relatively low dose _in vitro_.

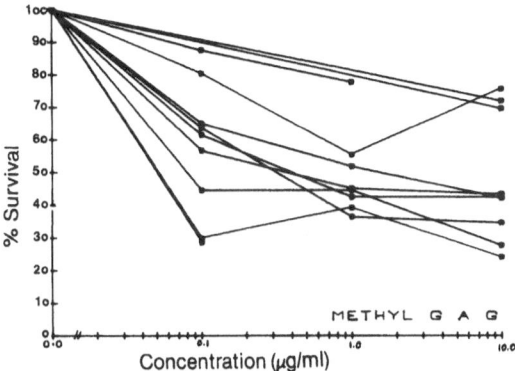

figure 5: Effect of a one-hour exposure of methylglyoxal bis guanethyl-hydrazone (methyl gag) on survival of ovarian tumor stem cells from 11 patients.

While some increasing lethality was observed with increasing dose, it seems unlikely that such high doses of methyl gag would be achievable _in vivo_ without excessive toxicity. Prior studies with high dose rates of administration of MGBG (in the 1960s) led to the premature abandonment of this drug. Our studies suggest that occasional patients with ovarian cancer may respond to MGBG (e.g., 10-20%).

AMSA

The new Phase II agent acridinylamino-methanesulfon-m-ansi-dide (AMSA) has been of considerable interest for investiga-

122

tion because of some antitumor effects which have been observed in epithelial tumors such as breast and ovarian cancer (15,16). While animal studies suggested that this agent is cross-resistant with adriamycin, some clinical observations in acute leukemia suggest that the drug may prove useful in patients who relapse from adriamycin. In our in vitro Phase II study of m-AMSA, some 17 patients were studied at in vitro doses ranging from .5 to 10 μg/ml for 1 hour. (Figure 6). We consider that 1 μg hour of

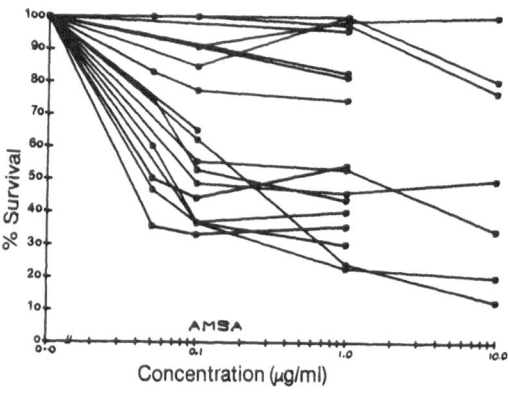

figure 6: Survival of ovarian tumor colony-forming units from 17 patients after one hour in vitro exposure to AMSA. Marked heterogeneity in sensitivity is apparent. Only 3 patients had reduction in survival to 30% of control, however, most cells studied were from patients in relapse from alkylating agents and anthracyclines.

exposure should be pharmacologically achievable in vivo. Substantial heterogeneity in response to this agent was observed and only two patients had reduction in cell survival to 30% of control with the 1 μg hour exposure to this agent. As with many of our other in vitro studies carried out to date, studies were on patients who had frequently received prior alkylating agents and anthracyclines. Additional studies on cells from patients who had not had previous drug exposure would be of extreme interest.

PALA

The new agent PALA (n-Phosphonacetyl-l-aspartate) is a transition state inhibitor of aspartate transcarbamylase which blocks de novo pyrimidine biosynthesis (17). The drug has undergone Phase I study (18) and recently entered Phase II clinical trials in the United States. We have completed in vitro studies in 8 ovarian cancer patients (Figure 7).

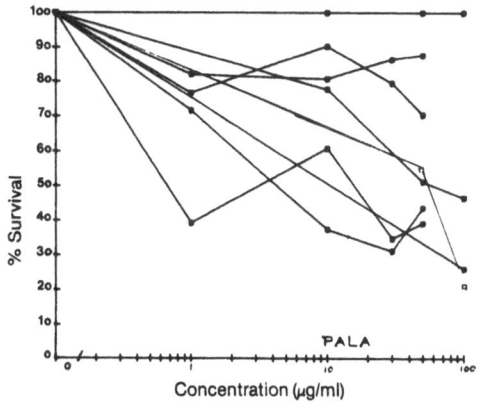

figure 7: Survival of ovarian tumor stem cells after one-hour exposure to 1-100 µg/ml of phosphonacetyl-l-aspartate (PALA). A few patients' cells showed significant lethality after exposure to very high doses of this agent.

A broad dose range was investigated (1-100 µg/ml) with one hour in vitro exposure prior to culture. The highest in vitro concentration (100 µg/ml) approximates the achievable plasma concentration attainable after a maximally tolerated clinical dose of 7.5 gm/M^2. At relatively high in vitro dosage exposures, 3 of 8 patients' tumor colony-forming cells had survival reduced to <30% of the control. Whether such high concentrations are achievable intratumorally remains to be established. In our predictive studies with standard cytotoxic drugs, we found that for in vivo activity, drugs had to exhibit substantial activity at 5-10% of the clinically achievable concentration time product or plasma concentration (8,10). If such criteria also apply to PALA, we would anticipate that this agent should be relatively inactive in ovarian cancer.

Dihydroxyanthracenedione

Certain anthraquinones have been studied as potential model

compounds analogous to anthracyclines such as adriamycin
and daunomycin. These new compounds have been designed
with the thought that cardiac toxicity might be averted and
therapeutic efficacy enhanced. Recently, a bis (hydroxy-
ethylamino-ethylamino) anthraquinone was found to possess
antitumor activity in several mouse tumors (19,20). The
new agent, dihydroxyanthracenedione has recently entered
Phase I clinical trial in San Antonio and Tucson. In conjunction with our Phase I trial, we have carried out preliminary observations of the in vitro lethality of dihydroxyanthracenedione in the tumor stem cell assay on cells from
seven patients with breast or gynecologic cancers. Results
of these in vitro survival curves are summarized in Figure
8.

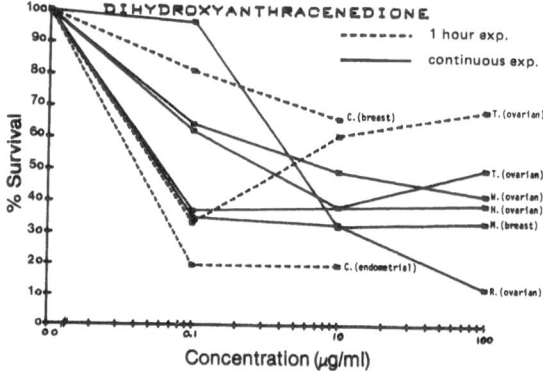

figure 8: Preliminary studies of one-hour exposure and continuous contact with dihydroxyanthracenedione on survival of ovarian tumor stem
cells

Survival of tumor colony-forming units was reduced to less
than 30% of the control with cells from one patient with
endometrial cancer (1 hour exposure) and one with ovarian
carcinoma (continuous contact). Pharmacokinetic data as
well as the results of Phase I studies will be required to
determine the achievable concentration time products in
vivo. However, in this pilot in vitro study, a log dose
response covering doses of dihydroxyanthracenedione from
1 to 100 μg hours of exposure should more than bracket the
pharmacokinetically achievable dosage exposure in vivo.

DISCUSSION

In this investigation of in vitro Phase II screening with
the human tumor stem cell assay, we have focused on some
of the new agents which are currently undergoing clinical
trials in ovarian cancer and other neoplasms. The feasibility of carrying out such in vitro studies rapidly on
multiple agents is confirmed by our studies inasmuch as we
have been able to conduct simultaneous studies on these
agents over the past nine months. It is obviously indeter-
minate at the present time whether our in vitro results
will correlate with the efficacy of these agents when
given to heavily pretreated patients with ovarian cancer.
Of greater interest in the future will be the application
of this assay system to ovarian tumor stem cells from
patients who have received no prior treatment. When such
data becomes available in assays carried out simultaneously with tests of standard agents known to be active (e.g.,
melphalan, adriamycin, and cis-platinum), it might be
possible to make a more realistic ranking of these drugs
and to predict potential in vivo utility of new versus
standard agents in such patients.

Our investigations of continuous contact of several
drugs versus one-hour exposure have not yet shown clearer
advantage for longer time exposures. This phenomenon will
clearly warrant further investigation in the course of
defining optimal drug exposures as well as validating such
observations through correlative clinical trials. The
data which we have obtained thus far correlating the results of one-hour exposure to results of clinical trials
continue to be quite promising, and it is likely that
studies from many other centers will also examine this
question independently in ovarian cancer over the next few
years.

While many of the new Phase I-II agents which we tested
showed heterogeneity of response on tumor colony-forming
cells from different patients with ovarian cancer, it must
be recognized that we have been carrying out "secondary"

screening of these agents. That is, the drugs were developed on the basis of animal models employing leukemias and other neoplasms and not because they had any particular utility in ovarian cancer. Recently, the National Cancer Institute (NCI) has decided to make a major test of the human tumor stem cell assay to determine whether it can be used for primary drug screening of new compounds sent to the NCI for screening evaluation. We believe that in primary screening, "positives" as defined with this assay should be identified when biopsy samples from the majority of a series (e.g., 5-6) of untreated patients with a given tumor type manifest substantial lethality with the new agent tested. At that point, the new drug could be introduced into toxicology testing followed by clinical trial for the appropriate tumor type. We anticipate that ovarian cancer will be a signal neoplasm in the new drug screening effort (because it can be grown so readily). It seems reasonable to expect that the assay will detect new structures with more consistent efficacy in ovarian cancer than those compounds which are currently available. The "proof of the pudding", of course, will be in the testing.

ACKNOWLEDGEMENTS

The authors thank Laurie Young for technical assistance, Dale Curtis and Dave Listowski for computer graphics assistance, H-S G. Chen, Ph.D. for correlative data assessment, and Thomas Moon, Ph.D. for statistical analysis of the data. Clinical assistance was kindly provided by the faculty, clinical fellows, pharmacy and nursing staff of The University of Arizona Cancer Center. This research was supported by Grants CA21839, CA17094 and CA23074 from the National Institutes of Health, Bethesda, MD.

Supported by Grants CA21839, CA17094 and CA23074.
From the National Institutes of Health, Bethesda, Maryland. 20205.

REFERENCES

1. Hamburger, AW and Salmon, SE. Primary bioassay of human tumor stem cells. Science 197:461-463, 1977.

2. Hamburger, AW and Salmon, SE. Primary bioassay of human myeloma stem cells. J. Clin. Invest. 60:846-854, 1977.

3. Hamburger, AW, Salmon, SE, Kim, MB, Trent, JM, Soehnlen, BJ, Alberts, DS and Schmidt, HJ. Direct cloning of human ovarian carcinoma cells in agar. Cancer Res. 38:3438-3443, 1978.

4. Jones, SE, Hamburger, AW, Kim, MB and Salmon, SE. The development of a bioassay for putative human lymphoma stem cells. Blood 53:294-303, 1979.

5. Meyskens, FL and Salmon, SE. Inhibition of human melanoma colony formation by retinoids. Cancer Res. 40:4055-4057, 1979.

6. Buick, RN, Stanisic, TH, Fry, SE, Salmon, SE, Trent, JM and Krasovich, P. Development of an agar/methylcellulose clonogenic assay for progenitor cells in transitional cell carcinoma of the human bladder. Cancer Res. 40, December, 1979.

7. Salmon, SE, Hamburger, AW, Soehnlen, BJ, Durie, BGM, Alberts, DS and Moon, TE. Quantitation of differential sensitivity of human tumor stem cells to anticancer drugs. New Engl. J. Med. 298:1321-1327, 1978.

8. Salmon, SE, Alberts, DS, Durie, BGM, Meyskens, FL, Soehnlen, BJ, Chen, H-SG and Moon, TE. Clinical correlations of drug sensitivity in the human tumor stem cell assay. In Proc. 1979 EORTC Plenary Session on Cancer Chemo- and Immunopharm., Paris, Recent Results in Cancer Research, in press, 1980.

9. Salmon, SE and Buick, RN. Preparation of permanent slides of intact soft-agar colony cultures of hematopoietic and tumor stem cells. Cancer Res. 39:1133-1136, 1979.

10. Salmon, SE (ed.) Cloning of Human Tumor Stem Cells. Alan Liss and Company, New York, in press, 1980.

11. Ames, MM. Pharmacologic studies of pentamethylmelamine and hexamethylmelamine. Proc. Amer. Assoc. Cancer Res. and Amer. Soc. Clin. Oncol. 20:636, 1979.

12. Morimoto, M, Schein, PS and Engle, R. Comparative pharmacology of pentamethylmelamine and hexamethylmelamine in mice. Proc. Amer. Assoc. Cancer Res. and Amer. Soc. Clin. Oncol. 20:980, 1979.

13. Currie, VE, Wong, PP, Krakoff, IH and Young, CW. Phase I trial of vindesine in patients with advanced cancer. Cancer Treatment Reports 62:1333-1336, 1978.

14. Knight, WA III, Livingston, RB, Fabian, C, Costanzi, J. methylglyoxal bis-guanethylhydrazone (methyl gag, MGBG) in advanced human malignancy. Proc. Amer. Assoc. Cancer Res. and Amer. Soc. Clin. Oncol. 20: C-115, 1979.

15. Legha, S, Gutterman, JU, Hall, SW, Benjamin, RS, Burgess, MA, Valdivieso, M and Bodey, GP. Phase I clinical investigation of 4'-(9-acridinylamino) methansulfon-m-aniside (NSC 249992), a new acridine derivative. Cancer Res. 38:3712-3716, 1978.

16. Von Hoff, DD, Howser, P, Gormley, P, Bender, RA, Claubiger, P, Levine, AS and Young, RC. Phase I study methansulfonamide, N-(4-(9-acridinylamino)-3-methoxyphenyl)-(m-AMSA) using a single dose schedule. Cancer Treatment Reports 62:1421-1426, 1978.

17. Johnson, RK, Inouye, T, Goldin, A and Stark, GR. Antitumor activity of N-(phosphonacetyl)-L-aspartic acid, a transition-state inhibitor of aspartate transcarbamylase. Cancer Res. 36:2720-2752, 1976.

18. Erlichman, C, Strong, J, Wiernik, P, Edwards, L, Cohen, M, Levine, A, Hubbard, S, Chabner, B. Phase I trial of PALA (N-phosphonacetyl-L-Aspartate). Proc. Amer. Assoc. Cancer Res. and Amer. Soc. Clin. Oncol. 20:C-98, 1978.

19. Zee-Cheng, RKY, Cheng, CC. Antineoplastic agents. Structure activity relationship study of bis (substituted aminoalkylamine) anthraquinones. J. Med. Chem. 21:290-294, 1978.

20. Johnson, RK, Zee-Cheng, RKY, Lee, WW, Acton, EM, Henry, DW and Cheng, CC. Experimental antitumor activity of aminoanthraquinones. Cancer Treatment Reports 63:425-439, 1979.

10 NEW DRUGS IN THE TREATMENT OF OVARIAN CANCER

F. M. Muggia

The identification of several drugs active against ovarian cancer other than the previously well known alkylating agents has opened the way for effective combination chemotherapy (1). Table 1 indicates the drugs of established efficacy and their principal dose-limiting toxicities. Since the initial HexaCAF combination was developed, cisplatin was shown to be a most effective drug against alkylating-resistant disease (2). It has therefore become incorporated into many new combinations which are currently used as the major therapeutic approach for patients presenting with Stages III and IV ovarian cancer. First-line combinations currently being tested are shown in Table 2.

TABLE 1

AGENTS ACTIVE AGAINST OVARIAN CANCER

Drug Category	Principal Toxicities
Alkylating agents	
L-Phenylalanine mustard	Myelosuppression, variable
Chlorambucil	GI intolerance
Thiotepa	
Cyclophosphamide	Same plus cystitis, alopecia
5-Fluorouracil	Myelosuppression, mucositis, enteritis
Methotrexate	Myelosuppression, mucositis
Hexamethylmelamine	Neurotoxicity, GI intolerance
Adriamycin	Myelosuppression, cardiotoxicity, alopecia
Cisplatin	GI intolerance, nephrotoxicity, neurotoxicity

A.T. van Oosterom et al. (eds.), Therapeutic Progress in Ovarian Cancer, Testicular Cancer and the Sarcomas, pp. 129-138. All rights reserved.
Copyright 1980 by Martinus Nijhoff Publishers, The Hague/Boston/London.

TABLE 2

FIRST-LINE COMBINATION CHEMOTHERAPY
REGIMENS IN OVARIAN CANCER

Acronym	Drugs	Dosage and Route	Days of Administration	Recyle Time	Institutions or Groups
AC	Adriamycin	$40/mg/m^2$ iv	d 1	3 wks	Mayo (3)
	Cyclophosphamide	50 mg/m^2 iv	d 1		
AC	Adriamycin	40 mg/m^2 iv	d 1	3-4 wks	SWOG (4)
	Cyclophosphamide	200 mg/m^2 po	d 3-6		
AP	Adriamycin	50 mg/m^2 iv	d 1	3 wks	Mt Sinai (5)
	Cisplatin	50 mg/m^2 iv	d 1		
PAC V or I	Cisplatin	V 20 mg/m^2 iv	d 1-5	4 wks	Indiana (6)
		I 50 mg/m^2 iv	d 1		
	Adriamycin	50 mg/m2	d 1		
	Cyclophosphamide	750 mg/m^2	d 1		
CHAP	Cyclophosphamide	150 mg/m^2 po	d 1-14	4 wks	Mt Sinai (5)
	Hexamethylmelamine	150 mg/m^2 po	d 1-14		
	Adriamycin	50 mg/m^2 iv	d 1		
	Cisplatin	30 mg/m^2 iv	d 1		
CHAD	Cyclophosphamide	600 mg/m^2 iv	d 1	3 wks	ECOG (7)
	Hexamethylmelamine	150 mg/m^2 po	d 8-21		
	Adriamycin	25 mg/m^2 iv	d 1		
	Cisplatin	50 mg/m^2 iv	d 1		
CHexUP	Cyclophosphamide	150 mg/m^2 po	d 2-8 + 9-16	4 wks	NCI (on going)
	Hexamethylmelamine	150 mg/m^2 po	d 2-8 + 9-16		
	5-Fluorouracil	600 mg/m^2 iv	d 1+8		
	Cisplatin	30 mg/m^2 iv	d 1+8		
Hexa-CAF	5-Fluorouracil	600 mg/m^2 iv	d 1+8	4 wks	NCI (1)
	Methotrexate	40 mg/m^2 iv	d 1+8		
	Cyclophosphamide	150 mg/m^2 po	d 1-15		
	Hexamethylmelamine	150 mg/m^2 po	d 1-15		

The circumstances for the evaluation of new agents in
ovarian cancer are highly dependent on the initial chemotherapeutic approach. Treatment with single alkylating
agents such as L-phenylalanine mustard (L-PAM), although
very well tolerated, is being replaced with treatment
utilizing more effective - albeit more toxic - cisplatin
containing regimens. As opposed to the chemotherapy of
testicular cancer, no single one of these combination
regimens can presently be considered a "standard". In
fact, combinations based on cyclophosphamide and adriamycin,

while promising, have not shown clear superiority over an alkylating agent alone (3). Such an experience, coupled with the steep dose response often seen with adriamycin and its grave toxic manifestations at high doses, argue against the routine use of this agent in the initial chemotherapy for ovarian cancer. On the other hand, hexamethylmelamine's contribution to currently used induction regimens has not been adequately assessed and its neurotoxicity may complicate its concomitant administration with cisplatin. Thus its role in induction regimens must be carefully considered. Finally, in developing new drug regimens, the concept that families of alkylating agents do not manifest absolute cross-resistance (8) must also be borne in mind. For completeness, one should also indicate that drugs with little demonstrable single agent activity, such as actinomycin D, had been introduced into some of the initial marginally successful combinations (9).

The initial treatment strategy is extremely important in determining the subsequent selection of new agents for evaluation in ovarian cancer, particularly since the extent and type of previous exposure to one or more drugs is likely to greatly influence the probability of a new response. Consequently both the search and the incorporation of new agents in such regimens is dependent on the strategy that one chooses for the treatment of advanced ovarian cancer. Other important factors to consider in the evaluation of new agents are the study of histologic grade, the residual tumor burden after surgery, the performance status, and methods of assessment prior to and after chemotherapy (10).

In general, one must consider four broad categories of investigative chemotherapy: 1) reassessment of drugs previously classified as "active", 2) alterations in dose-schedule and route of established drugs, 3) analogs of established drugs, both alkylating and non-alkylating types, and 4) new investigational drugs. Evaluation of any one of these approaches must be carefully planned in conjunction with the initial chemotherapeutic strategy. One must also consider other alternative therapies. Radiotherapy following failure to chemotherapy has been rarely used, but such treatment is likely to prove quite toxic and of borderline effectiveness. Local instillation of P^{32} colloidal suspensions, although popular in the past are no longer being explored in the advanced recurrent states because such treatment is unlikely to affect but the most superficial of serosal tumors. Other forms of local intra-peritoneal therapy are being explored as indicated subsequently. The possibility of utilizing a chemosensitivity test for treatment planning such as advocated by Salmon and co-workers (11) is particularly appealing in this disease because of the ready availability of tumor cells in many patients with relapsing disease. It must be recognized, however, that patients with recurrent ovarian cancer are often poor candidates for study. This stems from the fact that intestinal obstruction and nutritional derangements are common and assessment of disease status may be difficult. Peritoneoscopy is a valuable tool in aiding such assessment which is not always generally feasible or available.

I. Reassessment of drugs previously classified as active

With new initial chemotherapy regimens, it is necessary to reassess drugs previously known as active and to consider them in relation to new treatments being studied. This stems from these principal reasons: 1) methods of assessment of response have improved and 2) treatment strategies have changed considerably so that preceding evaluations do not apply to current circumstances. Chlorambucil and Thiotepa are two agents which now require reevaluation in drug-resistant disease. Experience with busulfan is not available, but its analog treosulfan has had extensive favorable trial outside the United States. Although Mitomycin C has not received evaluation in the United States as a single agent, it is part of a combination study with adriamycin and cyclophosphamide at Wayne State University. Ledacrine is a drug which has been studied in Poland, and further confirmation of its activity elsewhere is needed.

II. Alterations in dose-schedule and route of established drugs

This approach has particular appeal in the treatment of ovarian cancer. The serosal localization of the tumor and the frequent confinement of the disease to the peritoneal cavity lends itself to intraperitoneal drug administration (12). The National Cancer Institute (NCI) has initiated studies with intraperitoneal methotrexate and subsequently with 5FU and currently also with adriamycin. Administration of the latter agent via this route is particularly advantageous since high local concentrations may be achieved presumably without risking cardiotoxicity (12). Adriamycin by 24 hour continuous intravenous infusion also holds some interest. Preliminary experience indicates activity in breast cancer, and dose-limiting myelosuppression with likely attenuation of other toxic manifestations (13). Similarly, prolonged infusions with vinca alkaloids may have greater activity against solid tumors, and reevaluation in ovarian cancer by this schedule is warranted. High dose methotrexate with folinic acid rescue has received some attention because of preliminary reports of activity (14). However the regimen may be hazardous in the presence of ascites, and therefore the Sidney Farber Cancer Institute confined their trial to patients who had achieved complete remission. Their experience was disappointing, however, both in terms of maintenance of remissions and treatment of early failures (15). Intravenous melphalan may be of interest in view of the occasional erratic absorption orally. Also there is some interest in high dose alkylating agent therapy following priming doses of cyclophosphamide.

III. Analogs of established drugs

1) Alkylating agents - The extent of cross-resistance may be quite variable and conceivably sensitivity to drugs such as thioTEPA or cyclophosphamide may be retained after failure to melphalan (8). However, this has not been explored systematically, and in general, response rates have been poor to most agents after failure of any one of these. The Soviet drug, Dioxadet (a derivative of tri-ethylmelamine), has been reported quite active under these circumstances, and the hexitols and the aziridynil quinones (AZQ, Mitomycin C, carboquone) may also be worthy of testing (16). Ifosfamide is another agent undergoing trial as is the methanesulfonate derivative Yoshi-864. The latter showed some activity in the broad Phase II study of the Central Oncology Group. The nitrosoureas have shown some activity (17) but the marrow suppression render these drugs unattractive alone or in combination. BCNU with cyclophosphamide and adriamycin has been tested by the Southeastern Group (SEG) and a report in pending.

2) Hexamethylmelamine derivatives. Pentamethylmelamine is currently in trial because of its greater solubility and intravenous administration, thus hopefully bypassing some of the gastrointestinal intolerance of the parent compound. However, the central nervous system toxicity observed during the Phase I trial may limit its use.

3) Other analogs. New anthracyclines and platinum compounds are other logical possibilities for new drug testing in ovarian cancer. Platinum analogs of the 1,2 diamino-cyclohexane variety may notable be less nephrotoxic and also show some lack of cross-resistance to cisplatin in experimental systems (18).

IV. New drugs

A number of recently introduced investigational drugs and other drugs not previously evaluated are receiving

TABLE 3

NEW DRUG EVALUATION IN OVARIAN CANCER

Drug	Category	Institution or Group (Ref)
Maytansine	Mitotic inhibitor	Wayne State University
VM-26	Semisynthetic podophyllum derivative	Wayne State University Finsen Institute (19,20)
Bleomycin	Antibiotic	EORTC 55775
VP-16-213	Semisynthetic podophyllum derivative	ECOG 2877, GOG 26D, Mayo (21) EORTC (22)
Cytembena	Synthetic	Mayo, NCI, Wayne State University (23)
Medroxyprogesterone acetate	Hormone	ECOG 2877
Pyrazofurin	Antibiotic, antimetabolite	Mayo
ICRF-159	Synthetic	Mayo
Methyl GBG	Synthetic	ECOG 2877
Phenesterin	Steroid + cytotoxic moiety	ECOG 2877
Prednimustine	Steroid + cytotoxic moiety	Sweden (24)

trial in disease-specific Phase II studies for ovarian cancer under sponsorship of the Division of Cancer Treatment, National Cancer Institute. Table 3 indicates those drugs which have been or are currently under study, and the institution or group performing the study. Full publication of some of these studies is still awaited. Activity shown in broad Phase II studies (20) requires confirmation before proceeding to trials in combination. Interest in progestational agents has also been forthcoming, and medroxyprogesterone acetate is being evaluated. Finally, prednimustine, which consists of alkylating cytotoxic moieties linked to a steroidal carrier, is also receiving evaluation (24).

V. Conclusions

New drug studies in ovarian cancer present inherent difficulties related to assessment of response and the advanced status of disease manifestations. Nevertheless the recent success of combination regimens have stimulated interest in the application of innovative approaches to advanced ovarian cancer on presentation or at recurrence. Considerations of importance in the evaluation of new drugs, the type of studies that have been recently carried out, and specific drugs studies which are in progress have been reviewed. Hopefully, well conducted studies in the area of clinical investigation will lay the foundations for additional future therapeutic progress.

REFERENCES

1. Young, R.C., Chabner, B.A., Hubbard, S.P., et al. Advanced ovarian adenocarcinoma: a prospective clinical trial of melphalan (L-PAM) vs. combination chemotherapy (Hexa-CAF). N. Eng. J. Med. 299:1261-1266, 1978.

2. Wiltshaw, E. A review of clinical experience with Cis-platinum diammine dichloride: 1972-1978. Biochimie. 60:925, 1978.

3. Edmondson, J.H. Fleming, T.R., Decker, J.G., et al. Different chemotherapeutic sensitivities and host factors affecting prognosis in advanced ovarian carcinoma versus minimal residual disease. Cancer Treat. Rep. 63:241-247, 1979.

4. Alberts, D.S., Moon, T.E., Stephens, R.A., Wilson, H., Oishi, N., Hilgers, R.D., O'Toole. R. and Thigpen, J.T. Randomized study of chemoimmunotherapy for advanced ovarian carcinoma: a preliminary report of a Southwest Oncology Group Study. Cancer Treat. Rep. 63:325-333, 1979.

5. Holland, J.F. Ovarian cancer chemotherapy. In: Current status and new developments with Cis-platin. Ed: S.T. Crooke and S.K.Carter, Academic Press, 1980.

6. Ehrlich, C.E., Einhorn, L., Williams, S.D., and Morgan, J. Chemotherapy for Stage III-IV epithelial ovarian cancer with cis-dichlorodiammineplatinum (II), Adriamycin, and cyclophosphamide: a preliminary report. Cancer Treat. Rep. 63:281-288, 1979.

7. Vogl, S.E., Berenzweig, M., Kaplan, B.H., Moukhtar, M., and Bulkin, W. The CHAD and HAD regimens in advanced ovarian cancer: combination chemotherapy including cyclophosphamide, hexamethylmelamine, adriamycin, and cis-dichlorodiammineplatinum (II). Cancer Treat. Rep. 63:311-317, 1979.

8. Schabel, F.M. Jr. In: Fundamentals in Cancer Chemotherapy: anticancer symposia held in connection with the 10th International Congress of Chemotherapy, Zurich Sept. 18-23, 1977, F.M. Schabel (ed.) S. Karger, Basel, 1978.

9. Barlow, J.J. and Piver, M.S. Single agent vs combination chemotherapy in the treatment of ovarian cancer. Obstet. Gynecol. 49:609-611, 1977.

10. Muggia, F.M., McGuire, W.P. and Rozencweig, M. Rationale, design and methodology of Phase II clinical trials. In: Methods in Cancer Research. Busch, H. and DeVita, V.T. (eds). Academic Press, New York Vol. XVII pp. 199-214, 1979.

11. Salmon, J.E., Hamburger, A.W., Soehlen, B., Dure, B.G., Alberts, D.S. and Moon, T.E. Quantiatation of differential sensitivity of human tumor stem cells to anticancer drugs. N. Eng. J. Med. 298:1321-1327, 1978.

12. Ozols, R.B., Locker, G.Y., Doroshow, J.H., et al. Chemotherapy of murine ovarian cancer: a rationale for IP therapy with adriamycin. Cancer Treat. Rep. 63:269-274, 1979.

13. Gercovich, F.G., Praga, C., Beretta, G., Morganfeld, M., Muchnik, J., Pesce, R., Ho, D.H.W., and Benjamin, R.S. 10 hour continuous infusion adriamycin. Proc. AACR and ASCO 20, (Abstract C337), 1979.

14. Barlow, J.H. and Piver, M.S. Methotrexate (NSC-740) with citrovorum factor (NSC-3590) rescue, alone and in combination with cyclophosphamide (NSC-7627) in ovarian cancer. Cancer Treat. Rep. 60:846-851, 1976.

15. Parker, L.M., Griffiths, C.T., Yankee, R.A., Knapp, R.C. and Canellos, G.P. High dose methotrexate with Leucovarin rescue in ovarian cancer: a Phase II study. Cancer Treat. Rep. 63:275-279, 1979.

16. Baker, L.H., Caoli, E.M., Izbicki, R.M., Opipari, M.I. and Vaitkevicus, V.K. A comparative study of mitomycin C and porfiromycin. Proc. AACR And ASCO 15: 182, 1974.

17. Wasserman, T.H., Comis, R.L., Goldsmith, M., Hendels-
    man, H., Penta, J.S., Slavik, M., Soper, W.T. and
    Carter, S.K. Tabular analysis of the clinical chemo-
    therapy of solid tumors. Cancer Chemo. Rep. (part 3)
    6:399-419, 1975.

18. Burchenal, J.H., Kalaher, K., O'Toole, T. and Chris-
    holm, J. Lack of cross-resistance between certain
    platinum coordination compounds in mouse leukemia.
    Cancer Res. 37:2455-2547, 1977.

19. Dombernowsky, P., Nissen, N.I. and Larsen, V. Clini-
    cal investigation of a new podophyllum derivative
    (NSC 122819) in patients with malignant lymphomas
    and solid tumors. Cancer Chemo. Rep. 56:71-82, 1972.

20. Radice, P.A., Bunn, P.A., Jr. and Ihde, D.C. Commen-
    tary - Therapeutic trials with VP-16-213 and VM-26:
    Active agents in small cell lung cancer, Non-Hodgkin's
    lymphomas and other malignancies. Cancer Treat. Rep.
    63:1231-1239, 1979.

21. Edmonson, J.H., Decker, D.G., Malkasian, G.D.,
    Webb, M.J. and Jorgensen, E.O. Phase II evaluation of
    VP-16-213 (NSC 141540) in patients with advanced
    ovarian cancer resistant to alkylating agents. Gyn.
    Onc. 6:7-9, 1978.

22. EORTC, Clinical Screening Group. Epipodophyllotoxin
    VP-16-213 in treatment of acute leukemias, haemato-
    sarcomas and solid tumors. Brit. Med. J. 3:199-202,
    1973.

23. Baker, L.H., Samson, M.K. and Izbicki, R.M. Phase I
    and II evaluation of cytembena (NSC 104801) in
    disseminated epithelial ovarian cancers and sarcomas.
    Cancer Treat. Rep. 60:1389, 1978.

24. Johnsson, J.E., Trope, C., Mattson, W., Grundrell,
    H., Aspegren, K. and Konyves, I. Phase II study of
    Leo 1031 (prednimustine) in advanced ovarian carcin-
    oma. Cancer Treat. Rep. 63:421-424, 1979.

11 CURRENT AND FUTURE MANAGEMENT OF OVARIAN CANCER
Panel Discussion, held on December 7th, 1979

Chairman: R. C. Young (Bethesda)
Panel members: D. Chassagne (Paris), A. J. Dembo (Toronto),
C. T. Griffiths (Boston), J. F. Holland (New York),
F. M. Muggia (New York), S. E. Salmon (Tuczon), J. Seski (Houston),
J. P. Smith (Detroit), E. Wiltshaw (London)

CHAIRMAN:

We have outlined a series of approximately five major
headings:

1) initial surgery and staging

2) cytoreductive surgery or surgical debulking

3) initial therapeutic approaches both from a point of view
   of minimal and bulky residual disease

4) the duration of treatment and the need for maintenance
   and

5) new drugs and new approaches.

1. Initial surgery and staging

It would be worthwhile and appropriate to begin with some
comments regarding the initial surgery and the need for
staging procedures. One of the questions that frequently
comes up is: when the primary surgeon did not initially
suspect ovarian cancer, how can adequate surgical staging be
completed and what should that surgical staging include? I
would like to ask Dr. Julian Smith first to speak to the question of: what should a surgeon do when he explores a woman
in whom the diagnosis of ovarian cancer was not know in
advance, if it became clear that he was dealing with this
disease.

DR. SMITH: Most of the patients with ovarian cancer - at least in my experience in the United States - are explored by gynecologists. Very frequently in smaller hospitals, where he's not able to find somebody to help him; he's a bit frustated by what he finds, he's a little embarrassed by what he finds. At that time he's not sure he wants to call anybody else in to help him- at least not until maybe he's closed the patient and started thinking about it and then again becomes embarrassed of what he did. Maybe we should spread the word around that you shouldn't be embarrassed by what you do and go ahead and close the abdomen and send the patients to the centers where people are capable of looking into this problem more thoroughly. The patient with early disease. Stage I or Stage II disease - the ones that you and I both know that- quite often have disease spread beyond where it's been described and - are really in Stage III. That patient with very early disease which has spread is going to be a very favorable patient for combined treatment. Maybe all those patients from the outlying hospitals should be treated as though they were Stage III.

CHAIRMAN: What do the panel members feel is the optimal staging approach and - following up the comments that Dr. Smith made - who should perform that staging approach under optimal circumstances?

DR. GRIFFITHS: The appropriate staging procedure should begin, prior to laparotomy,with a uterine curettage. In our experience, many of our referred patients have had laparotomies for adnexal masses which were subsequently either excised or the patient closed and treated with chemotherapy. At the time that we've gone back to do a secondary debulking operation, we have found that the patient had endometrial cancer, corpus cancer, which may disseminate exactly as does ovarian cancer to the point of resulting in a large ovarian mass and then the typical implantational serosal surfaces. So, the first thing must be uterine curettage to rule out the possibility of endometrial or corpus cancer.

On opening the abdomen, once the determination of an adnexal mass is made, we look first into the cul-de-sac of
Douglas. If there's any free fluid there, it is aspirated;
if not, 150 cc of saline is directed into the peritoneal
cavity - 50 cc into each gutter and 50 cc over the bowel
surface. This eventually collects in the pelvic cavity and in
the gutters, when it is aspirated for cytologic examination.
Careful examination of all organs follows including careful
palpation of the undersurface of the diaphragms. There's
been some debate as to whether visualization of the diaphragms is important: I think this depends somewhat on one's
tactile sensitivity. In my experience I've tried both and
found that with the use of a proctoscope I could gain
magnification, but I have not yet found anything visible
that didn't have some slight elevation above the diaphragmatic surface. We do not biopsy the diaphragm routinely.
The bowel must be carefully searched, particularly deep
within the folds of the mesentery - a very likely place for
early tumor implantation. We believe that the omentum should
be biopsied. The tumor is apparently localized to one or
both ovaries. Usually the distal third of the omentum is
excised after biopsy. Following this, we excise the primary
tumor: this usually consists of a hysterectomy, bilateral
salpingo-oophorectomy. Careful inspection and palpation of
the pelvis is of course carried out to exclude the possibility of tumor implantation on serosal or parietal peritoneal
surfaces. We have found that there may be a relatively high
percentage of patients who have positive aortic nodes on
histologic examination which are not palpable. This is
particularly true in the poorly differentiated tumors. My
final step in the procedure is to incise the peritoneum over
the aorta, beginning with the right common iliac vessel. I
don't necessarily do a complete per-aortic dissection. I
do mobilize the duodenum, get well up towards the left
ovarian vein and then sample the fibro-fatty tissue, which
will almost include a few lymph nodes in that area, usually
bringing the dissection down to the bifurcation. I feel that
with this procedure one can gain a far better staging concept and one which, I think, should demonstrate itself as

valid in subsequent follow-up and survival, and recurrence.

DR. CHASSAGNE: I suppose Dr. Griffiths did not routinely perform omentectomy, just biopsy.

DR. GRIFFITHS: Yes, we do not feel that routine removal, o-mentectomy (and these are almost always infra-colic omen-tectomies or partial omentectomies) changes the prognosis in well-staged Stage I patients. If one looks at a number of poorly staged "Stage I" patients, it may well appear to improve prognosis because, if microscopic disease is found in the omentum, that patient is then relegated to a Stage III category thereby improving the quality of the Stage I patients.

HOSSFELD (Essen, Fed. Rep. Germany): Should we include lym-phangiography in the routine work-up of patients with - what seems to be - clinical Stage I and II disease at the time of initial evaluation?

DR. SESKI: We do not routinely use it and just use Dr. Griffith's approach.

CHAIRMAN: I'd like to make a comment about it. Around 10% to 15% of patients who seem to have clinical Stage I and Stage II disease will have positive lymphangiography. It must be considered in the context of how rigorous the surgical staging procedures have been. If the surgical staging has not been rigorous, then lymphangiography plays a significant role, and one can simply confirm the presence of metastatic disease by doing a trans-abdominal percutaneous biopsy of the nodes. If rigorous surgical procedure has been undertaken lymphangiography assumes less importance.

VAN HALL (Leyden): I have been surprised by the relatively high percentage of Stage I cases and even Stage II cases. In our experience, Stage I ovarian cancer is very rare. It's usually found by accident at laparotomy. I wonder how this difference is possible and how, perhaps in America, diag-nosis is made earlier than in our country.

DR. DEMBO: Perhaps you mean Canada. I made the point that most of our patients in that series did not have the kind of meticulous staging that Dr. Griffiths described. And this is why there was a much higher proportion of Stage I and Stage II cases in our series than in other series.

2.Cytoreductive surgery or surgical debulking

CHAIRMAN: We would like to move on the subject of surgical debulking or cytoreductive surgery - a fairly controversial subject. What is the panel's point of view on attempts at non-curative surgical cytoreduction in virtually every patient with ovarian cancer?

DR. WILTHSHAW: Our position would be that initial debulking operations take a long time. You heard Dr. Griffiths talking about this debulking operations. A long time in the theater may require a lot of support, both before and after surgery. And this would be quite impossible in our limited surgical time, with a large number of patients. The kind of debulking operations that we do   after chemotherapy takes an average of two-and-a half hours.This is feasible for us, but 8 hours, 12 hours, even 5½ hours per patient in the theater would mean that theater time would be too much used up with just a few patients. So, for the present time, we believe that not every patient should have debulking.

There is another problem. Some patients with ovarian cancer are nearly seventy or more and perhaps they could not take such a procedure. This should be restricted to certain patients. We are currently debulking patients who we know are sensitive to chemotherapy. If they are resistant to further treatment with chemotherapy, we are left with inadequate treatment in spite of debulking. If you can get down to a very small amount of tumor, then radiotherapy might be curative.

CHAIRMAN: Dr. Salmon, what is your view of the role of non-curative surgical cytoreductive surgery?

DR. SALMON: From my perspective, it has value only if the tumor can in fact be reduced to less than 1% of a its original volume. If you remove 50% of the tumor in a patient's abdomen; it has no value whatsoever. It's usually cutting

across tumor. Or, if the patient has invasion of the stomach and that area cannot be resected while another area can - it's foolish to undertake such procedures. When it's used as an adjunct to chemotherapy, you need to get a one - or two-log reduction in the amount of tumor present. We see patients who are referred after "debulking" when they've had half the tumor removed.
Often this will subject the patient to some jeopardy. I obviously concur with the idea of resecting an area that looks like there's an impending bowel obstruction. However, I would otherwise be opposed to carrying out a partial operation.

DR. SESKI:I think that would be a little bit naive.Anyone who has entered a patient's abdomen with ovarian cancer under-stands that it may take several hours before one even has an idea whether a tumor can be resected. Quite often at that point, the omentum has been removed, large pelvic masses have resected only to find that there may be a non-resectable residual in other areas. I still think that a patient has benefitted by having a 15 or 20 cm pelvic mass resected, pressure removed from the recto-sigmoid, or a segment of small intestine impending obstruction removed. The patient benefits by an improvement in the gastro-intestinal and urinary tract functions.

I would like to give an example. A patient with a 20-centi-meter pelvic mass and a large omental cake amounting to 5 or 10 pounds of tumor, may have   after debulking a signi-ficant residual of 5 to 10 centimeters in the peritoneal area. But that patient is able to take chemotherapy better, and is able to maintain her nutrition.

CHAIRMAN: The time at which surgical cytoreduction should be undertaken is also controversial. Obviously, one could consider using it before therapy, during induction, after induction, or at recurrence.

DR. GRIFFITHS: There are limitations in performing optimal debulking operations on individual patients. Most of these are related to co-morbid disease, rather than age and also to the involvement of certain anatomic sites. I would draw a limit at dense involvement of the splenic pedicle and tail of the pancreas. Dr. Seski was quick to point out that no such involvement would halt the intrepid surgeons of the M.D. Anderson Hospital. They would proceed to resect tumors in this area. We can get into a good deal of chest-beating about which surgeon can remove the most. But I think each surgeon must have in mind a definite plan, when he begins, as well as an idea of what he is not only capable of performing, but of what the patient is able to withstand. My final point in this regard is that debulking is of relatively little value, except for an immediate relief from the tumor insult, unless the patient is capable of taking effective combination chemotherapy of those regimens previously described. So, in the elderly patient in whom the chemotherapy will not be tolerated, I feel that even an effective optimal operation would be of little benefit.

As far as timing is concerned my figures suggest that an optimal operation is the most effective if performed initially. The tumor volume is the smallest at the time of induction chemotherapy. One does run into those patients who, in some surgeons hands, would be considered inoperable. I had two of those in my first group. After three courses of chemotherapy, we operated on them and they were indeed resectable. If the operation can conveniently be done at the first laparotomy, it should be so done. On the other hand, depending on the surgeon involved, and the condition of the patient, if it cannot be done at that time, it's worth a secondary try. This however, not after the induction course but rather mid-way in it, so that there will be effective combination chemotherapy available in the post-operative period.

3a. Initial therapeutic approaches:- minimal residual disease

CHAIRMAN: Some comments about therapy. We should consider two general groups of patients: those who, regardless of stage, are left with minimal residual disease; and those who are obviously, left with bulky disease. I think they constitute different management problems.

I would like to ask Dr. Dembo, first of all, about the use

of radiation therapy in the management of minimal residual disease.

DR. DEMBO: Our policy in general is to consider radiation as the treatment of first choice in this group of patients - which may, or may not come as a surprise. Our standard technique is to give radiation to the pelvis and the whole abdomen, using the moving-strip technique.
Pelvic radiation alone does not have a role to play, except possibly in very elderly patients with other reasons not to give whole abdominal radiation or not to give combination chemotherapy. With a well-differentiated tumor, Stage I or II, possibly then pelvic radiation alone is better than nothing. In general, however, if radiation is to be used, the pelvis and the whole abdomen should be treated.

Whether paraaortic areas should be boosted is only relevant to the situations in which retroperitoneal lymph-node disease dominates the clinical picture. Most of the patients, who have uncontrolled retroperitoneal disease, also have uncontrolled intraperitoneal and often extra-abdominal disease. It would add to morbidity and it's not been our practise to give a booster to the paraaortics, though we have not studied this.

Whether the moving strip is preferable to open-field whole abdominal radiation is, unanswered. The study of Fazekas and Mayer, was on small numbers of patients with many different tumor characteristics in each group. The conclusion that the two treatment were equivalent is really a Type II error. The statistical part of the test would not allow one to distinguish a difference between the two treatments.

We are now doing a randomized comparison to see whether the two therapies are significantly equivalent. This takes many more patients.

DR. HOLLAND: I'm surprised by your comment: that it comes as no surprise. It surprises me. It's my understanding that residual tumor, by all definition, is Stage III carcinoma, because one must assume that it's throughout the abdominal cavity. I didn't hear data that would allow me to recommend radiotherapy as a treatment of choice at this stage. You need more investigation to recommend it to the surgeon.

DR. DEMBO: It may beyond the scope of the panel to answer that fully; it brings up a whole lot of questions.
Is a treatment that produces
a five-year survival rate of 50% as good as a treatment that produces a 2-year complete response rate of 90%? We're comparing apples and oranges. Are patients, who are assigned to Stage III because of a random biopsy of small bowel mesentery that was grossly normal in appearance, in the same prognostic category as patients who've got disease plastering the diaphragm to the liver? Obviously not. Are patients, who are in Stage III because there is a recognizable growth in the abdomen, to be treated or approached in the same way as patients who are in Stage III only because meticulous exploration has identified them. Most of the members on this panel would agree that we should get away from Roman numerals in deciding how to treat our patients and treat them on the basis of the disease characteristics.

I showed a lot of evidence for patients with Stage II - on pelvic surgery- who in some subsets had a very long-term disease-free survival. More than half of them, would be Stage III, if they were properly staged. By long-term I mean 5 years, not 2 years or 1 year. That's why I don't think we're talking about experimental therapy. At the moment, looking at the data, I don't think there is evidence that for particular subsets of Stage III patients chemotherapy is more curative.

DR. WILTSHAW: Dr. Dembo wants to get away from Roman numerals - and to some extent I agree with him - but if the surgeons do meticulous staging and assign the patient with numeral "II", why would he want to irradiate the whole of the abdomen, why not just the pelvis and the paraaortics?

DR. DEMBO: Ovarian disease should be regarded as a disease of the whole peritoneal cavity. There's no lid on the

pelvis, there's nothing that distinghuishes or defines the
pelvis from the rest of the abdominal cavity - that's just
an artificial creation of the FIGO staging system. It's
impossible to adequately sample the whole peritoneum.

DR. MUGGIA: On this question of radiation versus chemotherapy, I just wanted to comment further on the Gynecology-
Oncology Group (GOG) study that was mentioned. It was
mentioned that in that study which looked at radiotherapy
versus melphalan versus the combination,one had to negate
the results because the radiotherapy contained several errors.
This could also be interpreted as the fact that one cannot
extrapolate from the experience at the Princess Margaret
and the experience that is going on elsewhere with radiotherapy treatments. Radiotherapy treatments are not delivered in the same way. Therefore, as a treatment for Stage
III it cannot be recommended except in specific institutions that have a track record of results that warrant a
further exploration.

DR. DEMBO: I hope I succeeded in stressing that technique
was extremely important. Some examples in published papers
and textbooks of how to treat the abdomen show that the
whole abdomen is clearly not being treated. This is something I would not recommend at all.

DR. HOLLAND: To Dr. Dembo or Dr. Chassagne: are there
improvements that you can anticipate in radiotherapy? Or
have you reached a zenith in radiotherapy? Because we're
jus beginning in chemotherapy and I am disappointed that
you are not persuaded by some of the disease-free extensively staged patients that Dr. Young and I have reported.

DR. DEMBO: It may be that the patients who have residual disease in the pelvis could be benefitted by having a higher
dose of radiation delivered to the pelvis. In other words,
the pelvic boosts are taken in a higher dose, also the
paraaortics, as previously mentioned.

Most of your data was very interesting. We're studying
platinum-containing combinations as well and are also
excited by the preliminary information. But, although you

were showing response rates that were dramatic - and I
made the point that I think there should be a Phase II end
point - the survival curves that you showed were all
super imposed one over the other and approximated or
approached the origin, as we would expect with patients
with bulky disease. It's too early to take as strong a
stand as you're taking.

DR. CHASSAGNE: In my paper, I had referred to the technique
advocated by Dr. Fuks (the Stanford technique) - irradia-
ting the domes of the diaphragm. I did not have time to
name all the improvements including the use of lateral
fields which are built into the Stanford technique, and also the CT scan for localization of the medial aspect of the
kidneys. Most radiotherapists probably shield too much
kidney. Many people could live with less kidney function
than we thought.

Other new developments include: radio-sensitizers and hyperthermia and the use of low-dose-rate continuous radiation.
At Gustave Roussy, we are treating many patients to the
whole abdomen with hyper-fractionation or low dose continuous
radiation.

We are not at the zenith. There are many projects for the
future.

DR. HOLLAND: I'm delighted to hear there is radiotherapy
research and I surely support that, but not necessarily
the dictum that one should apply that as the standard
treatment.

DR. CHASSAGNE: Most of the time we should combine chemotherapy and radiation therapy. Personally, I believe that
the task of the chemotherapist is to decrease the size
of the tumor to something which is microscopic. But, to
cure the microscopic disease, I do believe in radiotherapy.

CHAIRMAN: Dr. Smith, do you have some comments on the
combination of radiotherapy and chemotherapy in the
management of this group of patients, or other groups
of patients with this disease?

DR. SMITH: I'm concerned if we start with patients who are responders to chemotherapy, and then switch our treatment to radiation therapy. We've selected a group with favorable response to chemotherapy and then change the treatment on them: not everybody is going to be sensitive to the radiation therapy.

So, we put them back in the scheme, where maybe half would be and half wouldn't be. From results in the second look trial I would conclude that you had to be sensitive to chemotherapy to get this far. Then when you prove your sensitivity to chemotherapy, you stop the treatment that you know is working to do something you're not sure is going to work. I'm concerned about that.

CHAIRMAN: One of the subjects that we haven't covered, which is applicable to minimum residual disease patients is the use of radioisotopes intraperitoneally. While not applicable in bulky disease, it may play a substantial role in the management of patients with minimal residual disease.

Are there comments from the panel? No one believes in radioisotopes? Yes, everyone believes in them but no one uses them.

DR. GRIFFITHS: When one speaks of minimal residual disease here, it's all the more important to specifically define that term. If we use the most popular isotope available for this purpose today, ^{32}P chromic phosphate which is a pure Beta emitter, the penetrance of the radiation is little more than 3 to 4 millimeters. So certainly we cannot apply the previously used definitions of minimal residual disease, the i.e., 2 centimeters, because we will not have a sufficient-depth dose. I would submit that this apparently ideal agent is best tried in patients high-risk Stage I and patients who have very very small implants in the Stage II and III category.

DR. WILTSHAW: Only to agree with that, and to say that the consideration of radioactive isotopes in conjunction with other therapy, under particular circumstances, is very much on our minds. But we haven't done it.

CHAIRMAN: I would like to know if anybody in the audience has a large experience of using isotopes and has then looked laparoscopically. Dr. Griffiths says you can see very well after isotopes.

CHAIRMAN: Dr Davy is here who has considerable experience with radioisotopes. Would you like to educate the panel on the subject?

DR. DAVY: We have been using radioactive isotopes in the treatment of Stage I disease and Stage II disease where there is no residual disease. Therefore we have never laparoscopied the patients later. The only patients we've looked at have been those who have had complications of the therapy, such as subacute bowel obstructions.

CHAIRMAN: Are there questions from the audience regarding the management of patients with minimal residual disease? Dr. Salmon, not a member of the audience, but we'll let him talk anyhow.

DR. SALMON: It might interest you to know how we are applying the stem cell assay in patients with minimal residual disease. We test patients at the time of original surgery, when they undergo debulking.

In about 7 to 10 days after surgery when they might start on some form of systematic treatment we already have the results.We have seen some patients who have received no prior chemotherapy and yet manifest resistance to some of the standard drugs, including alkylating agents and adriamycin. We avoid those drugs to which there is proven resistance and use those for which there is some evidence of sensitivity. At least one patient, who expressed resistance to both adriamycin and alkylating agents showed sensitivity to cisplatinum, vinblastine and bleomycin and was treated with that program much in the fashion as used by Drs. Einhorn and Williams. At the time of second-look surgery and completion of treatment, the patient had no evidence of disease and has been off treatment.

3b. Initial therapeutic approaches- bulky disease

CHAIRMAN: The treatment of patients with bulky residual disease, advanced Stage III and IV, presents a major problem to all of us. It's appropriate to ask the panel members on the relative promise of the variety of modalities, singly or in combination.

Dr. Dembo, what is your view of the role of radiation therapy in bulky residual disease patients at presentation?

DR. DEMBO: It's rarely a curative form of treatment in this situation. There are times, it's appropriate to palliate the patient with a short course of radiation rather than chemotherapy. But, that's an individualized decision. However for most of the patients with Stage III and IV and large residual disease, radiation shouldn't be part of the initial management.

Prospects of cure, although small with chemotherapy, are probably better while the palliation and acute discomfort is potentially less.

CHAIRMAN: Comments regarding the role of chemotherapies, single agents versus combinations? I suspect there's no dearth of possible responders to that.

DR. MUGGIA: I've become convinced by the data that you and Dr. Holland presented, that new combinations are here to stay in the treatment of advanced ovarian cancer. You do obtain about 20 % long-term disease-free patients in those groups that have received platinum-containing regimens, or Hexa-CAF. At present my philosophy would be that we have to explore the most tolerable high-dose cisplatinum regimen, following what is considered to be optimal surgery.

CHAIRMAN: Another subject that we haven't mentioned yet is the role of immuno-therapy in the treatment of ovarian cancer. I wonder if there is any role for this modality.

DR. SALMON: One must point out a large-scale randomized clinical trial carried out by the Southwest Oncology Group (SWOG) on ovarian cancer, conducted by Dr. Alberts and the gynecology committee. It compared a combination of adriamycin plus cyclophosphamide for Stage III and IV

ovarian cancer patients as initial treatment versus the
same combination plus BCG (Pasteur) by scarification on
days 8 and 15. That trial has been reported in the NCI
Ovarian Cancer Symposium (Cancer Treatment Reports,
February 1979) and most recently updated in the Adjuvant
Therapy Book from the meeting in Tucson,March, 1979.
It has shown a consistent advantage in terms of overall
remission rate, remission duration and survival for
patients receiving BCG and chemotherapy. The difference
in median survival is close to a year. The groups are well
matched with regard to initial surgery, debulking and a number
of prognostic factors. Histo pathologic review, which is
not entirely complete, shows good balance as far as the
various tumor types. It needs to be accepted as a valid
observation.

There is also a pilottrial from a GOG institution adding
C-parvum to melphalan, showing an advantage over melphalan
alone. The SWOG opened their new trial a few months ago
which compares cisplatinum-adriamycin-cytoxan to the
same combination plus BCG, on the same schedule and to the
best previous arm, AC-BCG.
The GOG is considering a simular study.

I should add that BCG is active in our stem cell assay
reducing ovarian tumor colony formation to about 40 to 50 %
of the control at a concentration of one BCG organism for
every ten tumor cells cultured. Data which will be
published shortly, also indicates that, in ovarian cancer,
macrophages appear to facilitate tumor colony growth.
Either removing the macrophages prior to culture or
treating them with BCG inhibits clonogenicity of the tumor
stem cells. Dr. Buick, in our group, has recently completed
some studies showing that adding back the macrophages from
the patient's malignant effusion, even if separated by a
layer of agar, will reconstitute the proliferation of the
tumor stem cells. This suggests BGC conceivably may be
acting through a feeder-layer effect on the macrophages.

CHAIRMAN: Other comments regarding immunotherapy ?

DR. SMITH: I shouldn't break the seal of confidentiality, but I had a chance to go over all those charts. I was appalled at that study. I have never seen such a terrible study in all my life! Almost 40% of the patients in that study, I wouldn't accept as entered. I was appalled at such notes from the surgeon that all tumor had been removed, and then by ultra-sound the following week a mass had been found. Then the patient had chemotherapy with the mass disappearing one month later; that was called a complete response.

DR. SALMON: I only disagree on one thing, Dr. Smith. I, personally, did not carry out that trial. I'm only reporting a Group trial, as a member of the Group. However, my understanding is that the definition of complete response used in that trial required a second look laparotomy, although many of the patients did not have it. For this reason, the complete response rate has been low.

DR. SMITH: I don't think there have been many second-look operations.

DR. SALMON: You might look to the chapter in the book.

DR. DEMBO: Going back to the subject of single agent versus combination therapy in patients with Stage III and IV with bulky disease, my understanding from the Hexa-CAF L-PAM study was:the benefit of Hexa-CAF was largely confined to patients who had   disease less than 2 centimeters. The proportion of complete responses in patients with the disease greater than 2 centimeters was almost identical in the two-treatment arms.

Do you know whether any other data indicates availability of curative therapies for these patients. It has a lot of implications for physicians in the community who do not have the expertise to use a combination of drugs or the financial resources that we take for granted in North America. Is it criminal not to treat these patients with combination therapy?

CHAIRMAN: Let me respond briefly, because you've mentioned
our data. I think in some sense what you said is true.
The most dramatic effect is seen in the patients with
minimal residual disease. This observation has been made
in other trials as well. I would emphasize that it's a
single and relatively small trial. On analyzing a variety
of sub-groups, one can get into situations where
differences are sometimes significant and sometimes not.
In any sub-group, regardless of the extent of residual
disease, the type of histologic grade, the histologic type,
the age or any other parameter one wishes to look at, the
survival of the group treated with the combination is
better than the group treated with L-PAM alone. The group
you described fares better when treated with a combination
than with a single alkylating agent. You are correct in
saying that in this sub-set of patients the advantage for
the combination is not statistically significant, so the
matter is not completely resolved by our study.

DR. GRIFFITHS: Instead of arguing about it, why not
operate on and then you'll have minimal residual disease.

DR. HOLLAND: Dr. Dembo, the adriamycin-platinum combination
arm shows statistically significant longer survival for
patients with poorly differentiated tumors. The survival
benefits were not limited to those with small tumors,which
has been confirmed in three separate series of patients
with adriamycin-platinum. I think you unnecessarily
emotionally charge the discussion when you ask :
"Is it criminal?" I'd just say, it's ill-advised.

DR. DEMBO: That wasn't exactly the context of the question.
I showed that therapy can affect the survival curves in
two ways. It can either prolong survival without increasing
the number of patients cured, or it can increase the
proportion of survivors. No data has been shown to indicate
if combination therapy is affecting the survival at the
moment. A distinction should be made of clinical
investigation by experienced people from its application
in the community. The same reservations that were made

about applicability or recommendability for radiation in minimal disease should be made on this topic as well.

DR. HOLLAND: The evaluation of the sub-specialties of medical oncology and of gynecologic oncology that now stand with the longer-standing radiotherapy shouldn't give you as much pause about whether there's expertise to administer combination chemotherapy. Indeed, the problems that arise in its administration in the past, in my experience, have arisen because people who weren't qualified to give it have done so. But there are well specialized groups now, in medical and gynecologic oncology, who are quite used to this and I see no reason to think that it will cause more problems than radiotherapy given in the hands of a novice.

CHAIRMAN: We shall not have time to discuss further the duration of treatment or new drugs and approaches.

PART TWO

TESTICULAR CANCER

12 ROLE OF SURGERY IN THE MANAGEMENT OF NONSEMINOMATOUS GERM CELL TUMORS OF THE TESTIS

D. G. Skinner

Dramatic changes have occurred in the management of nonseminomatous germ cell tumors of the testis so that currently these tumors carry the best prognosis of any solid tumor encountered in the adult male. Improved chemotherapy has been largely responsible for the improved survival, but surgery remains the cornerstone in overall management planning. The role of surgery is threefold. First, radical orchiectomy establishes the diagnosis and completely controls the primary tumor, regardless of extent of local tumor growth or various histologic cell types. Secondly, a meticulous retroperitoneal lymph node dissection remains the single most important determinant in selecting the least toxic chemotherapeutic adjuvant, eliminates metastatic retroperitoneal disease, and has obviated the need for postoperative radiation therapy. Third, surgery has become an integral adjuvant to intensive combination chemotherapy for advanced disease inasmuch as it can completely remove massive retroperitoneal disease and the histology derived from such cytoreductive surgery provides important prognostic information and direction for subsequent need for alteration in chemotherapy.

Evidence that radical orchiectomy controls the primary tumor is derived from the fact that scrotal recurrence or subsequent metastases to groin nodes draining the scrotum has not occurred in 175 consecutive patients treated at the UCLA Hospital from 1971. Local growth patterns such as invasion of the cord structures outside the testis have had no prognostic implications on overall survival or the ultimate pathologic stage of disease for this consecutive group of patients. A careful pathologic sampling of the

A.T. van Oosterom et al. (eds.), Therapeutic Progress in Ovarian Cancer, Testicular Cancer and the Sarcomas, pp. 159-172. All rights reserved.
Copyright 1980 by Martinus Nijhoff Publishers, The Hague/Boston/London.

primary tumor does allow accurate classification, but a review of our experience suggests that subgrouping the tumor
other than simply labeling it a nonseminomatous tumor is probably of little clinical significance. If pure choriocarcinoma,
an extremely rare tumor comprising less than 1% of all non-
seminomatous germ cell tumors of the testis (10) is excluded,
experience indicates that survival is not statistically influenced by cell type - this observation includes all
patients with pure embryonal carcinoma, teratocarcinoma,
teratoma and mixtures with seminoma and choriocarcinomatous
elements. Experimental clinical data continues to support
Friedman's contention that germinal tumors of the testis
arise from totipotential primordial germ cells, and that
there is a natural tendency toward maturation or the development of adult teratomatous tissue (8, 9, 10, 19, 20, 31, 32).

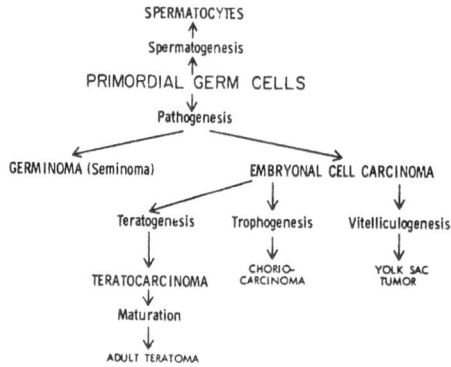

Figure 1. Pathways of differentiation and transformation of
testicular tumors. From Friedman (9)

Thus, it comes as no surprise to clinically find primary
tumors containing a wide variety of cell types as well as
observing different and often more mature histologic
patterns in metastases.

Since 1973 with the report by Samuels and associates
(22) concerning the effect of the combination of vinblastine
sulfate and bleomycin in advanced nonseminomatous germ cell

tumors of the testis, and the addition of cis-platinum in
1977 by Einhorn and Donohue (6), dramatic improvement in the
long term survival for patients with all stages of disease
have been reported so that in 1979 nonseminomatous germ cell
tumors of the testis carry the best prognosis of any solid
tumor encountered in man. Within the past year, three
centers have reported a mean and 97% tumor free survival for
all patients with Stage A and B disease treated since 1973
without exclusion on the basis of extent of disease (7,29,30).

TUMOR FREE SURVIVAL

Series	Stage A	Stage B	Total A+B	Retroperitoneal Recurrence
Staubitz (30)	21/22* 95%	15/16 94%	36/38 95%	0
Donohue (7)	57/57 100%	54/55* 98%	111/112 99%	1
Skinner (29)	42/42 100%	32/35* 91%	74/77 96%	0
TOTAL	120/121* 99%	101/106*95%	221/227 97%	1

Table I. Consecutive patients with pathologic Stage A and B
nonseminomatous germ cell tumors treated since 1974 at three
centers by meticulous retroperitoneal lymphadenectomy and chemotherapy without radiation therapy. (*1 death other cause - not
tumor). There are no exclusions due to extensive retroperitoneal
disease.

Basic to the treatment plan at these centers has been a
careful surgical staging by means of a meticulous retroperitoneal lymph node dissection along with subsequent use
of adjuvant chemotherapy. There is now unequivocal evidence that a meticulous retroperitoneal lymph node dissection
effectively controls local disease with low morbidity and a
mortality rate of less than 0.5%. Only one retroperitoneal
recurrence was observed among the 227 collected patients
including Stage B_3 patients treated for massive retroperitoneal disease (Table I). Pre or postoperative radiation
therapy was not utilized in any of the patients treated at
the three centers. Two of the centers have utilized a consistent, previously reported plan of management (26) utilizing aggressive prophylactic chemotherapy according to
pathologic stage (29, 30). The third center has reserved
aggressive chemotherapy for evidence of failure and then

utilized intensive chemotherapy with the combination of platinum, vinblastine sulfate and bleomycin (5,7).

Despite these results there continue to be reports questioning the need for lymphadenectomy, suggesting that radiation therapy may be equivalent to lymphadenectomy in controlling retroperitoneal disease (1, 2, 16,34,36) or that consideration might be given to a less meticulous node sampling procedure or even withholding lymphadenectomy entirely in patients without evidence of metastases upon presentation relying on improved chemotherapy to salvage those patients that eventually fail (12,37). It seems timely, therefore, for those of us advocating lymph node dissection to reexamine our material in terms of the need for a thorough lymph node dissection, the accuracy of clinical staging utilizing the sensitive radioimmunoassay determinations of the beta subunit of serum human chorionic gonadotrophin (HCG) and alpha fetoprotein (AFP), and lymphangiography. Finally, what data is available to support the use of radiation therapy and does its use compromise subsequent effective chemotherapy?

In regards to clinical staging by means of serum tumor markers, a recent review has revealed striking limitations in the sensitivity of currently available HCG and AFP determinations in the management of patients without advanced

TABLE II

STAGE	# PATIENTS	HCG (%)	AFP (%)	EITHER (%)
A	67	7	9	10
B_1	15	29	33	50
B_2	23	52	43	64
B_3	6	83	75	100
C	31	84	60	93

Frequency of elevated levels in serum samples obtained after orchiectomy, but immediately before any other therapy in 142 patients with nonseminomatous germ cell tumors. HCG = beta subunit human chorionic gonadotropen

AFP = alpha fetoprotein

These figures represent data collected since 1973 from a combined group of patients treated at the Walter Reed Army Medical Center, the National Cancer Institute and the UCLA Hospital. From Skinner and Scardino (20).

disease (25,29). While the incidence of one or both markers being elevated increases with stage of disease, the contrary is also true; patients with minimal retroperitoneal disease have a high incidence of false negative values - 50% for patients with pathologic Stage B_1 disease and 36% for patients with more extensive Stage B_2 disease (29).

Lymphangiography also has difficulty in detecting minimal disease with an overall accuracy which varies considerably according to the criteria of interpretation as well as the experience of the radiologist (3, 11,14,17,21,35). The reported incidence of false positive determinations ranges from 9 to 54% with false negative ranging from 9 to 30%. Those series using strict criteria for positive interpretations, which results in a low incidence of false positives, report the higher incidence of false negatives and vice versa. Within each pathologic substage of disease for patients with positive nodes, there are no reports to indicate the specific false negative incidence but our own data indicates a very high error rate in those patients with micrometastases (Stage B_1).

Experience at our institution also indicates that computerized tomography probably does not substantially improve the accuracy of lymphangiography with most errors occurring in patients with micrometastases. Therefore, if one contemplates therapy based on clinical staging or a limited node sampling procedure designed to preserve ejaculation, such patients will be subjected to the need for extremely close observation, with mental anguish of an unknown prognosis with many more eventually needing intensive chemotherapy utilizing drugs with unknown long term sequelae. The long term effects of the operation and less toxic chemotherapy are known; less than 0.5% operative mortality with low morbidity and infertility due to ejaculatory impotency in approximately 70%. The importance of ejaculatory impotency, however, may be overstated as many of these patients have an anatrophic contralateral testis with markedly abnormal sperm counts prior to undergoing any retroperitoneal surgery.

164

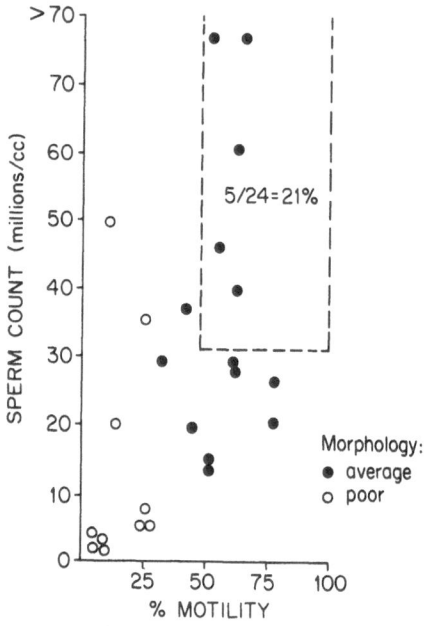

SEMEN ANALYSIS IN 24 PT WITH NSGSTT AFTER
ORCHIECTOMY BUT BEFORE ANY OTHER THERAPY

Figure 2

Figure 2 shows the results of semen analyses in 24 patients
following orchiectomy but before any other therapy. Only
five (21%) had semen of sufficient quantity or quality to
be considered fertile. In these patients semen cryopreser-
vation is available should such patients desire subsequent
insemination of their spouse. We have found no other
alterations in sexual function. Therefore, it should be
emphasized that the results of therapy utilizing a plan of
management based on careful, meticulous surgical staging is
known, has been reproduced in other centers, and has resulted
in the highest cure rate achieved for any solid tumor in man.
Because of this, we feel it seems inappropriate to advocate
more conservative treatment schemes until hard data is forthcoming from a large series of patients managed in another
fashion.

The best results reported utilizing radiation therapy
to the retroperitoneum following orchiectomy as primary

therapy of nonseminomatous tumors has originated from
Holland (36) and England (34). Tyrrell and Peckham (34)
reported an 84% two year disease free rate for 88 Stage A
patients and a 58% disease free rate for 29 patients with
clinical Stage B disease (only 33% survival if the metastatic
nodal deposits were greater than 2 cm. on lymphangiography).
These survival figures following orchiectomy and radiation
therapy differ considerably from the respective tumor free
survival rates of 99% for Stage A patients and 95% for Stage
B patients managed with lymphadenectomy and chemotherapy
without radiation.   Therefore, current evidence does not
support the contention that radiation therapy is equal to
treatment schemes based on lymphadenectomy in the management
of early stage disease.   Furthermore, radiation therapy makes
subsequent use of intensive combination chemotherapy hazardous, particularly the use of effective doses of vinblastine
sulfate.   It comes as no surprise, then, that several major
centers within the United States that have tried radiation
therapy either alone or in combination with lymphadenectomy
have abandoned clinical trials.   Walter Reed Army Medical
Center, which initiated a prospective trial of radiation
therapy alone vs. lymphadenectomy with sandwich radiation
therapy for early stage disease have abandoned radiation
therapy altogether (33), and The San Diego Naval Hospital,
which advocated sandwich radiation therapy before and after
lymphadenectomy, has abandoned radiation therapy (15).   The
only major center still utilizing radiation therapy, the M.
D. Anderson Hospital, has abandoned postoperative radiation
therapy, giving only relatively low doses preoperatively (13).

While it is possible the future may offer a more
limited node sampling procedure in an effort to preserve
fertility, current evidence suggests that it is the patients
with the most limited microscopic disease that benefit most
from the staging and may, thereby, avoid recurrence and the
need for intensive platinum, vinblastine sulfate and bleomycin chemotherapy.   This point should be emphasized in lieu
of the lack of sensitivity of biochemical tumor markers for

minimal disease and our inability to carefully assess and
monitor the retroperitoneal nodes. A meticulous surgical
staging procedure currently allows selection of the least
toxic chemotherapeutic agent or combination tailored to
maximum survival of the individual patient, eliminates retroperitoneal recurrence, and remains the single most important
factor in dictating therapeutic plans. Results of therapy in
1979 based on lymphadenectomy and adjuvant chemotherapy
yield a tumor free survival of 97% for all patients with
clinical Stage A and B disease, results not equaled by any
other form of management.

The role of surgery in the management of advanced
disease is less well defined. Without question improvement
in combination chemotherapy, particularly the combination of
platinum, vinblastine sulfate and bleomycin (4,5,6), has
been so impressive that surgery has become adjunctive to the
primary curative goals of chemotherapy. Patients with widely
disseminated disease with or without bulky retroperitoneal
metastases should be treated initially and vigorously by intensive combination chemotherapy utilizing the Einhorn and
Donohue protocol (6) modified by a reduction in the dosage
of vinblastine sulfate. Nonetheless, surgery plays an important role in the management of these patients by removing
all retroperitoneal disease and providing histologic material
to better assess the effects of the chemotherapy, occasionally
indicating the need to alter drugs. Experience at UCLA
in the treatment of advanced disease by the combination of
platinum, vinblastine sulfate and bleomycin alone has not
been as good as that reported by Einhorn with most failures
occurring in those patients harboring any pulmonary metastases
greater than 2.5 cm. in diameter or initially having bulk
retroperitoneal abdominal disease (23). Some authors have
advocated cytoreductive surgery before chemotherapy with the
hope of diminishing tumor burden, thereby rendering chemotherapy more effective (12,18). Early trials at initial
massive debulking resulted in significant complications in
terms of tumor spill, prolonged postoperative recovery, and
the catabolism of these postoperative patients which delayed

utilization of the needed effective chemotherapy (4). Furthermore, a retroperitoneal resection of large tumor masses does
not lend itself to early control of the vascular pedicle as
in other tumor systems thereby necessitating tumor manipu-
lation. It seemed appropriate, therefore, to treat such
patients preoperatively with chemotherapy. Beginning in the
early 1970s our utilization preoperatively of older, less
effective drugs indicated that combination chemotherapy could
significantly shrink the tumor bulk, produce a thick fibrous
capsule or desmoplastic reaction around the tumor mass, making
resection possible in all cases without tumor spill or leaving
residual tumor. In fact, of our 35 patients with massive
Stage B_3 and C disease treated by a treatment protocol that
did not include cis-platinum, 29 or 83% achieved a complete
response and 26 (74%) of these remain free of tumor 24 to 96
months later (27). Since 1977 all patients have been
managed by the protocol illustrated in Figure 3 utilizing
preoperative platinum, vinblastine sulfate and bleomycin.
Surgery is performed through a thoracoabdominal approach
described previously and wedge resection of persistent ipsilateral pulmonary nodules are performed at the same time
(27,28). If pulmonary disease persists in the contralateral

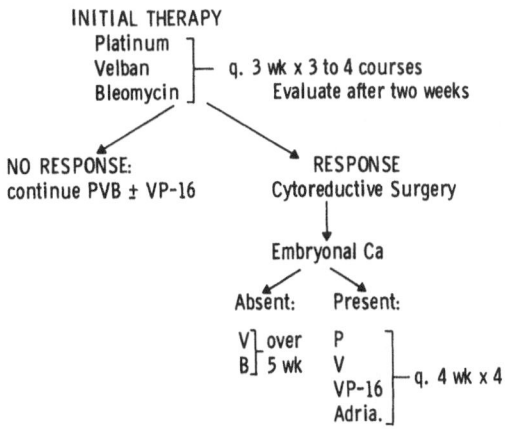

Figure 3

lung and is amenable to surgical resection, a formal contralateral thoracotomy is then performed four to six weeks
later. Histology of the resected tissue has revealed persistent embryonal carcinoma in approximately one third of
these patients, mature teratoma with or without extensive
fibrosis and necrosis in approximately one third, and only
fibrosis without any evidence of cancer in approximately one
third. Of interest, preoperative serum tumor markers have
been unreliable in determining who harbors persistent embryonal carcinoma. Obviously those patients with elevated
markers are found to have embryonal carcinoma, but in most
patients the markers fall to normal during chemotherapy and
a substantial number of patients with normal markers still
have evidence of embryonal carcinoma at operation (25,29).
It continues to be our policy to operate on all patients with
advanced disease following three to four courses of the
platinum, vinblastine sulfate and bleomycin protocol despite
clinical evidence of a complete response by all noninvasive
measurable parameters. Others have recommended surgery for
only those patients with an abnormal CT scan or other evidence
of persistent disease (4). Our reason for recommending surgery for all patients is twofold: first to assure that all
retroperitoneal disease is controlled, thus preventing late
failure in an area extremely difficult to monitor; secondly,
the histology obtained at surgery dictates subsequent chemotherapy. For example, those patients with only mature teratoma and/or fibrosis without evidence of embryonal carcinoma
do well without the need for continuing intensive combination
chemotherapy utilizing platinum. On the other hand, those
patients with persistent embryonal carcinoma clearly need
further intensive chemotherapy. Fewer than 50% of these
patients survive despite additional courses of platinum,
vinblastine sulfate and bleomycin (4). Therefore, we feel
the need to alter subsequent sequential chemotherapy adding
the investigational drug VP-16-213, a Podophyllotoxin derivative, and Adriamycin to platinum and bleomycin.

Another consideration is the extent of cytoreductive
surgery following chemotherapy. Is biopsy only or "lumpec-

tomy" sufficient or should the operation be a meticulous dissection similar to the one we do for Stage A and B disease? Our experience and that of others (4) indicates that the dense desmoplastic reaction around the great vessels and residual tumor bulk as well as the cystic changes that occur following chemotherapy make it impossible to judge by gross inspection just what tissue harbors persistent cancer. Foci of embryonal carcinoma have been found in association with solid fibrosis, cystic or necrotic tissue. Therefore, there seems no feasible method to identify visibly or by palpation what in actuality remains a microscopic diagnosis. Therefore we recommend as complete and meticulous a retroperitoneal lymph node dissection as feasible in each case. The results of an integrated management plan currently yield a complete response rate in excess of 80% for all patients who present with massive abdominal disease (4,29).

In summary, the 1970s have seen dramatic changes in the management of nonseminomatous germ cell tumors of the testis resulting in a tumor free survival of 97% for all patients with Stage A and B disease and a tumor free survival in excess of 70% for patients with advanced disseminated disease. Improved chemotherapy has been largely responsible for this survival, but a meticulous lymphadenectomy remains the most important determinant in selecting the least toxic chemotherapeutic adjuvant, eliminates local retroperitoneal recurrence and obviates the need for radiation therapy.

REFERENCES

1. Blandy, J.P.: Testicular neoplasia. IN Urology, Ed.
    J. Blandy, Oxford, Blackwell, p. 1206, 1976.

2. Caldwell, W.L.: Why retroperitoneal lymphadenectomy for
    testicular tumors? J. Urol., 119:754, 1978.

3. Clements, J.C., McLead, D., Fowler, J.E. Jr. and Stutz-
    man, R.E.: Staging errors in testicular tumors.
    Presented before 1978 Kimbrough Urologic Seminar.
    Reported in Urology Times, May 1979.

4. Donohue, J.P. and Einhorn, L.H.: Cytoreductive surgery
    for metastatic testis cancer: Considerations of timing
    and extent. J. Urol., In press, 1979.

5. Donohue, J.P., Einhorn, L.H. and Perez, J.M.: Improved
    management of nonseminomatous testis tumors. Cancer,
    42:2903, 1978.

6. Einhorn, L.H. and Donohue, J.P.: Improved chemotherapy
    in disseminated testicular cancer. J. Urol., 117:65,
    1977.

7. Einhorn, L.H. and Donohue, J.P. Personal communication,
    1979.

8. Friedman, N.B.: Pathology of testicular tumors. West.
    J.Med., 126:362, 1977.

9. Friedman, N.B.: Pathology of testicular tumors. IN
    Genitourinary Cancer, Ed. Skinner and deKernion,
    Philadelphia, W.B. Saunders Co., p. 430, 1978.

10. Friedman, N.B. and Moore, R.A.: Tumors of the testis:
    a report on 922 cases. Ml. Surgeon, 99:573, 1946.

11. Hussey, D.H., Luk, K.H. and Johnson,D.E.: The role of
    radiation therapy in the treatment of germinal cell
    tumors of the testis other than pure seminomas.
    Radiology, 123:175, 1977.

12. Javadpour, N. and Bergman, S.: Recent advances in
    testicular cancer. Curr. Prob. Surg., 15:1, 1978.

13. Johnson, D.: Personal communication, 1978.

14. Jonsson, K., Ingemansson, S. and Ling, L.: Lymphography
    in patients with testicular tumors. Brit. J. Urol.,
    45:548, 1973.

15. Lynch, D.F. Jr., McLord, L.R., Nicholson, T.C., Richie,
    J.P. and Sargents,C.R.: Sandwich therapy in testis
    tumor: Current experience. J. Urol., 119:612, 1978.

16. Maier, J.G. and Lee,S.N.: Radiation therapy for testicular cancer. Urol. Clin. No. Amer., 4:486, 1977.

17. Maier, J.G. and Schamber, D.T.: The role of lymphangiography in the diagnosis and treatment of malignant testicular tumor. Amer. J. Rad. Ther. Nuc. Med., 114: 482, 1972.

18. Merrin, C., Takita, H., Beckley, S. and Kassis, J.: Treatment of recurrent and widespread testicular tumors by radical reductive surgery and multiple sequential chemotherapy. J. Urol., 117:291, 1977.

19. Pierce,G.B. and Abell, M.R.: Embryonal carcinoma of the testis. IN Sommers, S.C. (Ed): Pathology Annual. New York, Appleton-Century-Crofts, 1970, Vol. 5, 27-60.

20. Price, E.B. Jr., and Mostofi, F.K.: Secondary carcinoma of the testis. Cancer, 10:592, 1957.

21. Safer, M.L., Green J.P., Crews, Q.E. and Hill, D.R.: Lymphangiography accuracy in staging of testicular tumor. Cancer, 35:1603, 1975.

22. Samuels, M.C., Johnson, D.E. and Holoye, P.Y.: The treatment of Stage C metastatic germinal cell neoplasia of the testis with bleomycin combination chemotherapy. Proc. Amer. Assoc. Cancer Res., 14:23, 1973 (Abstract).

23. Sarna, G. and Skinner, D.G.: Cis-platinum diammine dichloride (CDDP) alone and in combination. Submitted for publication, Cancer Treatment Reports, 1979.

24. Scardino, P.T. and Skinner, D.G.: Germ cell tumors of the testis: Improved results in a prospective study using combined modality therapy and biochemical tumor markers. Surgery, 86:86, 1979.

25. Scardino, P.T., Skinner, D.G., McIntire, K.T. and Waldmann,T.A.: Limitations on the sensitivity of serum levels of HCG and AFP in detecting and monitoring germ cell tumors of the testis. Presented before 1979 Annual Meeting AUA, New York. Submitted for publication J. Urol. 1979.

26. Skinner, D.G.: Nonseminomatous testis tumors: A plan of management based on 96 patients to improve survival in all stages by combined therapeutic modalities. J. Urol., 115:65, 1976.

27. Skinner, D.G.: Considerations for management of large retroperitoneal tumors: Use of the modified thoracoabdominal approach. J. Urol., 117:605, 1977.

28. Skinner, D.G. and Leadbetter, W.F.: The Thoracoabdominal
    Radical Retroperitoneal Lymph Node Dissection. Film
    1972. Available AUA Library, ACS Film Library and
    Eaton Medical Film Library.

29. Skinner, D.G. and Scardino, P.T.: Relevance of bio-
    chemical tumor markers and lymphadenectomy in manage-
    ment of nonseminomatous testis tumors: Current per-
    spective. Read before 1979 Annual Meeting Genito-
    urinary Surgeons, Pebble Beach, California. Submitted
    for publication J. Urol. 1979.

30. Staubitz, W.: Personal communication, February 1979.
    Material presented in discussion of Skinner, D.G. and
    Scardino, P.T. Paper "Relevance of Biochemical Tumor
    Markers and Lymphadenectomy in Management of Non-
    seminomatous Testis Tumors: Current perspective."
    For publication Trans. Amer. Assoc. GU Surgeons 1979.

31. Stevens, L.C.: Origin of testicular teratomas from pri-
    mordial germ cells in mice. J. Natl. Cancer Inst., 38:
    549, 1967.

32. Stevens, L.C.: Embryonic potency of embryoid bodies
    derived from a transplantable testicular teratoma of
    the mouse. Develop. Biol., 2:285, 1960.

33. Stutzman, R.: Personal communication, 1978.

34. Tyrrell, C.J. and Peckham, M.J.: The response of lymph
    node metastases of testicular teratoma to radiation
    therapy. Brit. J. Urol., 48:363, 1976.

35. Wallace, S. and Jing, B.S.: Testicular malignancies
    and the lymphatic system. IN Testicular Tumors,
    D. Johnson, Ed., Kimpton Publ., London, p. 71, 1972.

36. Werf-Messing, B. van der: Radiotherapeutic treatment
    of testicular tumors. Int. J. Rad. Oncol. Biol. Phys.,
    1:235, 1976.

37. Whitmore, W.: Personal communicaton, Presented in
    summation of the Second National Symposium on Genito-
    urinary Cancer, Los Angeles, March 1979.

13 ROLE OF RADIOTHERAPY IN THE TREATMENT OF TESTICULAR CANCER

B. H. P. van der Werf-Messing

Since the introduction of megavoltage therapy, radiation therapy as the single treatment modality for non-seminomatous testicular tumours has mainly in British and Dutch centres received special attention. The purpose of this paper is to assess the advantages and shortcomings of radiotherapy as compared with other treatment modalities. Especially with largely improved chemotherapeutic possibilities the future place of radiation therapy in combined modality schedules has to be identified.

In the majority of radiotherapy centres, after hemicastration radiation therapy is given to the regional lymph nodes, i.e. the lumbar lymph nodes and to the homolateral iliac lymph nodes. Some centres prefer including the contralateral iliac lymph nodes as well. The value of elective irradiation of mediastinal and supraclavicular lymph nodes remains debatable. In case of proven or doubtful incomplete removal of the primary, scrotal and homolateral inguinal irradiation has to be added. Similarly, after previous scrotal surgery, e.g. for incomplete testicular descensus, homolateral inguinal nodes have to be considered as regional and hence have to be irradiated.

In the Rotterdam Radiotherapy Institute patients are usually seen after hemicastration. The clinical work-up consisted in the past of physical examination, routine laboratory tests including urinary chorionic gonadotrophins (UCG); IVP; chest X-ray; since 1960 lymphangiography and chest tomography were added. Staging was done according to the UICC-Classification 1968 (N_0M_0: lymphography negative; N_1M_0: lymphography positive; N_2M_0: palpable abdominal mass; any N with M_1: tumour beyond the diaphragm). All patients without evidence of malignancy beyond the diaphragm (M_0) were irradiated to the lumbar region and

A.T. van Oosterom et al. (eds.), Therapeutic Progress in Ovarian Cancer, Testicular Cancer and the Sarcomas, pp. 173-180. All rights reserved.
Copyright 1980 by Martinus Nijhoff Publishers, The Hague/Boston/London.

the homolateral iliac nodes. A dose of 4000 rad in 4 weeks was given by 2 opposing fields in 20 fractions. Elective mediastinal and supraclavicular irradiation was given in case of a palpable abdominal mass (N_2) or in case of per continuity filling of mediastinal lymph nodes during lymphangiography. The same irradiation dose was given as to the subdiaphragmatic areas. The actuarial survival rates are presented in table 1 (1).

Table 1. Actuarial Survival after Radiation Therapy at the Rotterdam Radiotherapy Institute (TNM-Classific. 1968).

Histological Type	Clinical Category	No.	5-y Surv%		10-y Surv%
MTI A	$M_0 + M_1$	53	45		45
(treated by Superv.)	M_0	36	70		70
	M_0N_0	14	100		100
	M_0N_1	13	35		35
MTI A/S	$M_0N_{X,0,1,2}$	17	± 75		± 75
MTI B	$M_0 + M_1$	59	23		23
(treated by Superv.)	M_0	24	50		50
MTI B/S	$M_0 + M_1$	18	± 25		± 25
(treated by Superv.)	M_0	8	± 45		± 45
MTT	$M_0 + M_1$	26	± 25	7-y	± 25
(treated by Superv.)	$M_0N_{X,0,1}$	7	100	7-y	100
All non-Seminomas	N_0M_0	29	± 90	9-y	± 90
	N_1M_0	35	± 45		± 45

Malignant teratoma intermediate A (MTI_A) had a better prognosis than malignant teratoma intermediate B (MTI_B) and malignant teratoma anaplastic (MTA); [the latter two have, according to international rules, during the last years been grouped together as teratoma undifferentiated (MTU)]. In case of combined seminoma and malignant teratoma the non-seminomatous component finally determines prognosis. In case of MTI_A and malignant teratoma tropho-blastic (MTT), lymphographically without evidence of lymph node involvement, survival is 100%. The 5- and 10-year survival of all non-seminomatous malignancies $N_0 M_0$ is about 90%; in case of lymphographically involved lymph nodes (N_1) it drops to 45%. These results are comparable with those reported in literature by other radiothera-peutic centres (table 2).

Table 2. Non-Seminomatous Testicular Tumours. Survival after Radiotherapy (TNM-Classific. 1974).

	Clinical Lymph nodes (Lymphography)	No.	5-y Surv%
Blandy (2)	MTI $\Big\lbrace$ N_0	49	89
	$N_{1,2,3}$	10	33
Maier (3)	N_0	29	86
	$N_{1,2,3}$	11	82
Peckham (4)	N_0	110	$\pm$ 85
	$N_{1,2}$	44	60
Tierie (5)	N_0	34	82
	N_1	13	54

Results after lymphadenectomy with or without radiation therapy, after sandwich therapy and after lymphadenectomy in combination with chemotherapy are presented in table 3. From these data it is evident that results of radiation therapy, surgery with or without radiotherapy, and surgery with or without chemotherapy are comparable if lymphangio-graphy is negative or if the lymph nodes are pathologi-cally not involved. Slight differences can be attributed to the discrepancies between lymphangiography and patho-logical findings (table 4).
In case of positive lymphangiography, it is debatable whether radiation therapy is inferior to the combination of surgery and chemotherapy. In order to compare objec-tively the various treatment modalities it is obligatory

Table 3. Non-Seminomatous Testicular Tumours. Survival
after Surgery (S) + Radiotherapy (X).

	Lymph nodes				
	Ly.graphy / Pathology			No.	5-y surv%
Whitmore (6) (S ± X)	?	+		159	49 } 65
		-		204	80
Walsh (7) (S ± X)	?	+	3-y	20	60 } ±80
		-		44	93
Maier* (8) (S ± X)	N_O	+		160	±40 } 65
		-		154	±76
Staubitz* (9) (S)	?	+	3-y	20	75 } 87
		-		45	93
Schmucki (10) (S)	?	+		45	37 } 68
		-		51	95
Hussey (11) (S ± X)	N_O	+	3-y	14	64 } ±7C
		-		85	74

*Excl. pos. lymph nodes above renal pedicle (± 10%)

Survival after Sandwich Therapy

Earle (12)	?	+	20	48 } 68
		-	12	100
Maier (8)	N_O	+	133	±41 } 58
		-	119	±77
	$N_{1,2}$	+	37	7

Survival after Surgery + Chemotherapy

	Pathological Stage			
	A		B	
	No.	5-y Surv%	No.	5-y Surv%
Donohue (13)	30	100	28	86
Staubitz (14)	22	95	16	94
Skinner (15)	42	100	35	91

Table 4. Non-Seminomatous Testicular Tumours. Correlation between Lymphography and Pathology.

	False Positive (Ly.gr. + Path. -)		False Negative (Ly.gr. - Path. +)	
Hussey (11)	2/18	11%	18/106	17%
Maier (16)	3/35	8.5%	6/24	25%

to compare patients in the same clinical stage, indicating the methods for staging (e.g. including modern assessment of markers in the staging etc.), mentioning exclusions from the type of treatment, comparing the histological types (MTI and MTU).

As the therapeutic problems are not the involved lymph nodes - they can be dealt with equally effectively by surgery and by radiation therapy - but the development of distant metastases, usually pulmonary metastases, which are probably initially present as micrometastases, it is important to assess the indication for adjuvant chemotherapy. The relationship between clinical and/or pathological lymph node involvement and the subsequent development of metastases has been reported by Hussey (11) (table 5).

Table 5. Influence of Nodal Status at Lymphadenectomy on the incidence of Extranodal Metastasis (Stages I, II_A, II_B) (March 1944 - September 1973).

Clinical Stage	Negative Nodes	Positive Nodes
I	10/93 (10.3%)	5/18 (27.8%)
II_A	1/15 (6.7%)	10/21 (47.6%)
II_B	1/2	4/6
Total	12/110 (10.9%)	19/45 (42.2%)

Hence, the evidence of lymph node involvement might be an indication for adjuvant chemotherapy.

Peckham (4) has shown that in case of clinically positive lymph nodes with a diameter not exceeding 2 cm, survival after radiation only is nearly identical to survival in case of clinically negative lymph nodes, hence the indication for adjuvant chemotherapy in this situation is

debatable. Prognosis becomes poor in case of pathological
lymph nodes larger than 2 cm. Apparently in this group
- usually not suitable for curative surgery - radiotherapy
with adjuvant chemotherapy is justified. In case of a
bulky abdominal mass, debulking chemotherapy - which also
might deal effectively with micrometastases elsewhere -
followed by radiotherapy seems a rational approach. A remaining mass - usually a fibrotic lump - can be explored
and eliminated surgically.

If pulmonary metastases are discovered at an early
stage, with whole lung irradiation up to about 3000 rad in
4 weeks followed by a booster to the metastases (additional 3000 to 4000 rad), a cure rate of 40% could be achieved
in the Rotterdam Radiotherapy Institute (17). However,
with the advance of chemotherapy, the whole lung irradiation has been substituted by chemotherapy, which is
followed by a booster to the initially involved lung area.

Based on own data analysis and literature reports the
Rotterdam Radiotherapy Institute and the Royal Marsden
treatment schedule has been developed as presented in
table 6.

Table 6. Non-Seminomatous Testicular Tumours. Treatment
policy acc. to TNM 1974. Royal Marsden (London) and
R.R.T.I. (Rotterdam)

- $N_0 M_0$ [*]	- 4000 / 4 wks
- $N_{1,2}$ ($\emptyset \leq 2$ cm) M_0 [*] (one or more nodes +)	- 4000 / 4 wks + Booster X ($\pm$ Elective Mediast. and Supraclav. X)
- N_2 ($\emptyset > 2$ cm) - N_3 (palp. mass) $\Big] M_0$ - N_4 (supradiaphr. nodes)	- Chemotherapy (Einhorn) + X Booster $\pm$ Surgery
- Any N M_1	

[*]If markers persist or develop after radiotherapy:
chemotherapy.

The emphasis of this treatment approach still lies on
radiotherapy. The main disadvantages of this approach are:
perhaps undertreatment of clinically N_0 cases which might
be microscopically positive; difficult vigorous chemotherapy for subsequently developing metastases; risk of
bowel injury, especially after previous abdominal surgery.
One advantage of radiation therapy over surgery is indis-
putable: the cured young men can have normal children;
more than 40 perfect children have been born to non-seminomatous testicular tumour patients after irradiation at
the Rotterdam Radiotherapy Institute.

REFERENCES

1. Werf-Messing, B. van der. Radiotherapeutic treatment
   of testicular tumors. Int.J.Radiation Oncology Biol.
   Phys., 1, 235-248, 1976.

2. Blandy, J.P., Chapman, R.H., Pollock, D. and Molland,
   E. The management of tumors of the testis. In: Current
   Controversies in Surgery, 489-499, 1976.

3. Maier, J.G. and Mittemeyer, B. Carcinoma of the testis.
   Cancer, 39, 981-986, 1977.

4. Peckham, M.J., Hendry, W., McElwain, T.J. and Calman,
   F.F.M. The multimodality management of testicular
   teratomas. In: Adjuvant therapy of cancer, S.E. Salmon
   and S.E. Jones, eds., Elsevier/North Holland Biomedical Press, Amsterdam, 1977.

5. Tierie, A.H., Battermann, J.J. and Hart, G. Radio-
   therapie van testistumoren. Tijdschrift Kanker, 2, 22-
   23, 1978.

6. Whitmore, W.F., Jr. Germinal tumors of the testis.
   Sixth National Cancer Conference Proceedings,
   Philadelphia, Lippincott, 219-245, 1970.

7. Walsh, P.C., Kaufman, J.J., Coulson, W.F. and Goodwin,
   W.E. Retroperitoneal Lymphadenectomy for Testicular
   Tumors. JAMA, 217, 309-312, 1971.

8. Maier, J.G. and Sulak, M.H. Radiation therapy in malignant testis tumors. Cancer, 32, 1212-1226, 1973.

9. Staubitz, W.J., Early, K.S., Magoss, I.V. and Murphy,
   G.P. Surgical management of testis tumor. J. Urol.,
   111, 205-209, 1974.

10. Schmucki, O., Geroulanos, St., Baumann, Ch. Resultate der retroperitonäalen Lymphknotenausräumung bei Hoden-teratokarzinomen. Helv.chir. Acta, 43, 357-361, 1976.

11. Hussey, D.H., Luk, K.H. and Johnson, D.E. The role of radiation therapy in the treatment of germinal cell tumors of the testis other than pure seminoma. Radiology, 123, 175-180, 1977.

12. Earle, J.D., Bagshaw, M.A. and Kaplan, H.S. Supervolt-age radiation therapy of the testicular tumors. Amer. J. Roentgen., 117, 653-661, 1973.

13. Donohue, J.P., Einhorn, L.H. and Perez, J.M. Improved management of nonseminomatous testis tumors. Cancer, 42, 2903-2908, 1978.

14. Staubitz, W. Personal communication, 1979.

15. Skinner, D.G. and Scardino, P.T. Relevance of bio-chemical tumor markers and lymphadenectomy in manage-ment of non-seminomatous testis tumors: Current per-spective. Read before 1979 annual meeting, Genitouri-nary Surgeons, Pebble Beach. Submitted for publication J. Urol. 1979.

16. Maier, J.G. and Schamber, D.T. The role of lymphangio-graphy in the diagnosis and treatment of malignant testicular tumors. Am.J.Roentgenol., 114, 482-491, 1972.

17. Werf-Messing, B. van der. The treatment of pulmonary metastases of malignant teratoma of the testis. Clin. Radiol., 24, 121-123, 1973.

14 COMBINATION OF CHEMOTHERAPY AND RADIOTHERAPY IN THE TREATMENT OF TESTICULAR CANCER

A. Barrett, W. F. Hendry, T. J. Mc Elwain and M. J. Peckham

INTRODUCTION

Patients with early stage testicular cancer have long been amenable to cure by orchidectomy and local treatment to abdominal lymph nodes whether by surgery or radiotherapy. With the advent of effective drug combinations, chemotherapy has offered the prospect of cure for patients with metastatic disease. There may however be a group of patients with bulky disease in one or more sites who will benefit from a combined therapy approach and this group will be reported here in detail.

STAGING

Patients presenting to the Royal Marsden Hospital undergo staging investigations as shown in Fig. 1

Fig. 1. INVESTIGATIONS

Review Histology

Chest X-ray and whole lung tomography

Lymphogram/IVP

Liver scan

Liver and abdominal ultrasound

EMI scan of abdomen and thorax

Full blood count

Ureum and Electrolytes

Liver function tests

B-HCG

AFP

Hormones

Lung function tests

Sperm testing and banking

EDTA clearance

A detailed comparison of CT scanning with conventional staging procedures has shown that valuable additional information is obtained by scanning (1).
Assessment of mediastinal node involvement is more accurate (Fig. 2) and detection of unsuspected lung metastases is relatively common (Fig. 3).

Fig. 2. TESTICULAR TERATOMA MEDIASTINUM 96 PATIENTS

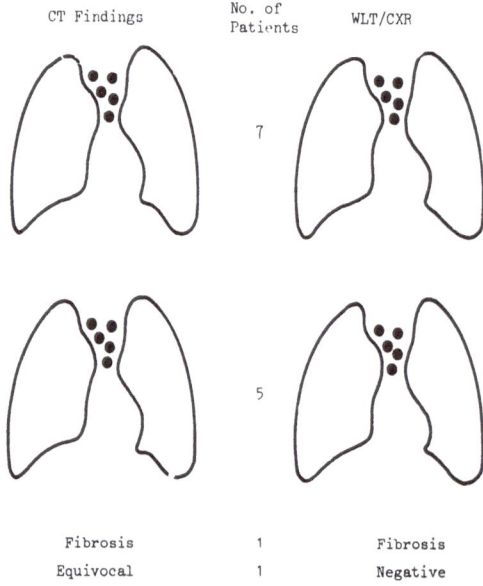

Fig. 3. INCIDENCE OF LUNG METASTASES

Lymphangiography if carefully interpreted is useful at the time of initial staging but less sensitive in the detection of response (Fig. 4a and 4b).

Fig. 4a. COMPARISON OF CT WITH LYMPHOGRAPHY
IN TESTICULAR TERATOMAS - 52 PATIENTS
- GROUP A

LYMPHOGRAM		CT FINDINGS	
	NO. PATIENTS	NEGATIVE	POSITIVE
Negative	18	16	2 *
Positive	31	1	30 *
Equivocal	3	3	-
TOTAL	52	20	32

* Additional information obtained with CT

Fig. 4b. CORRELATION LYMPHOGRAM FOLLOW-UP FILM
WITH CT 41 PATIENTS TESTICULAR TERATOMA

INITIAL LYMPHOGRAM		FOLLOW-UP			
		LG+ CT+	LG+ CT-	LG- CT+	LG- CT-
Positive	15	5	1	9	-
Negative	26	-	-	-	26

Following these investigations the patients are staged as shown in Fig. 5. Evaluation of treatment results suggests that these groupings do have prognostic significance.

Fig. 5. STAGES

I: <u>No disease evident outside testis</u>

II: <u>Infradiaphragmatic nodal disease</u>

    IIA   metastases $\leqslant$ 2 cm diameter

    IIB   metastases $>$ 2 cm, $<$ 5 cm diameter

    IIC   metastases $\geqslant$ 5 cm diameter

III: <u>Supradiaphragmatic nodal disease</u>

    $IIIM_1$ mediastinal mets $\leqslant$ 2 cm diameter

    $IIIM_2$ "   " $>$ 2 cm, $<$ 5 cm diameter

    $IIIM_3$ "   " $\geqslant$ 5 cm diameter

    $IIIN_1$ supraclavicular mets $\leqslant$ 2 cm diameter

    $IIIN_2$ "   " $>$ 2 cm
                                        $<$ 5 cm diameter

    $IIIN_3$ "   " $\geqslant$ 5 cm diameter

IV: <u>Extranodal disease</u>

    IVL_1 pulmonary mets $\leqslant$ 4 in number
                                $\leqslant$ 2 cm diameter

    IVL_2 "   "   more than 4,
                                $\leqslant$ 2 cm diameter

    IVL_3 "   "   more than 4,
                                $>$ 2 cm diameter

    IVH+   hepatic involvement

    Other sites, bone, brain, etc. named.

HISTOLOGY

The histology was classified according to the criteria
of the British Testicular Tumour Panel into one of the
following categories:

Malignant teratoma undifferentiated (MTU)

Malignant teratoma intermediate   (MTI)

Malignant teratoma trophoblastic   (MTT)

(These categories approximate to the classification employed
in the United States as: embryonal carcinoma,
teratocarcinoma and choriocarcinoma respectively.)

TREATMENT OF EARLY STAGE DISEASE

Traditionally, radiotherapy has been the mainstay of
treatment of early stage testicular tumours in England and
our policy has been to treat patients with Stage I disease
with a 'dog leg' field to cover bilateral paraortic and
renal hilar nodes and ipsilateral iliac nodes, and in
patients with Stage II disease to treat the mediastinum and
bilateral supraclavicular nodes in addition using doses of
4000 rads to uninvolved areas and 4500 rads to areas of
disease.

This contrasts with the American approach where surgery
is used both to allow accurate staging and as therapeutic
management (2). However the results obtained by these 2
very different approaches are very similar. Long term survival rates of 80% were obtained in Stage I and II patients
treated between 1964 and 1975 (3). In our most recently
assessed series 28 out of 28 Stage I and IIA patients
treated between January 1976 and March 1978 were alive and
disease free at 13- 37 months (median 23) (Fig. 6).

Three relapsed after irradiation and are so far in
complete remission following chemotherapy. We think that
these results justify the belief that lymphadenectomy is
unnecessary as a routine in early cases. If irradiation
is given optimally, very few sequelae are seen and some of
the side effects of surgery, such as sterility, are avoided.

Fig. 6

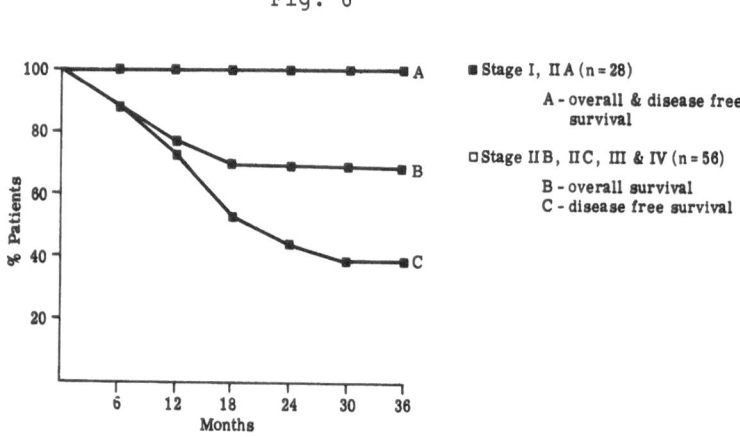

TREATMENT OF ADVANCED DISEASE

In patients with advanced disease with involvement of liver or bone or with large volume lung disease, our policy has been to use chemotherapy alone. Results for this group (L_3H+) are shown in Fig. 7.

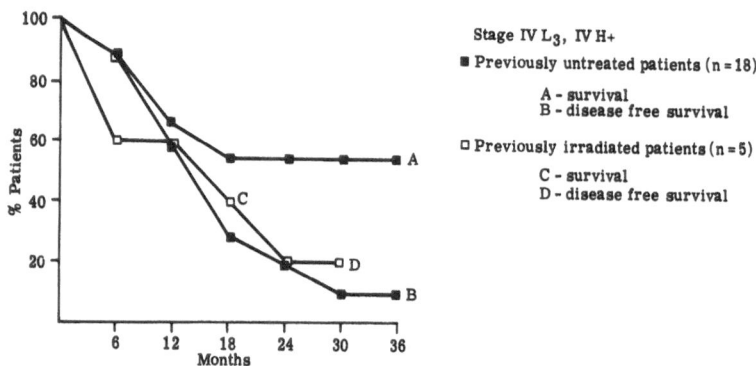

From 1976 to 1978 we used the Samuels' regime (4). More recently we have used Vinblastine, Bleomycin and Platinum in combination as described by Einhorn (5). Results however remain disappointing with complete remission rates of 20% or less.

Following a study in our Unit of VP 16 - 213 as a
single agent in which 3 patients achieved complete remission and 8 partial remission out of a group of 24 previously treated patients with progressive disease (6) (Fig. 8),
we are now using a combination of 4 drugs; Vinblastine,
Bleomycin, Platinum and VP 16 - 213 in these patients to
try to increase the cure rate.

Fig. 8

VP 16- 213 AS A SINGLE-AGENT IN TESTICULAR CANCER

Phase II Study

120 mg/m^2 i.v. daily x 5 repeated 2 - 4 weekly

No. of patients	CR	PR	Improvement	Total resp.
24	3	8	2	46 %

COMBINATION TREATMENT FOR LOCALLY BULKY TUMOUR

From an historical group of patients treated between 1964 and 1975 we had shown clearly that bulky abdominal disease could not be controlled by radiotherapy alone and led to a decreased survival (7).
Other groups have reported the same prognostic significance of bulky disease in patients treated by chemotherapy (8) (9).

In Stages IIB and C and IVC_1 L_1 or L_2 patients we have therefore been carrying out a study of chemotherapy followed by radiotherapy and lymphadenectomy to try to determine the role of each of these factors in the control of bulky disease.

Patients have received 4 - 6 courses of Vinblastine, Bleomycin and Platinum, or before October 1978 of Vinblastine and Bleomycin using the Samuels' regime. One month after completion of chemotherapy full re-staging is carried out. If there is no evidence of progressive local disease or development of new metastases and AFP and HCG levels have returned to normal, radiotherapy is given using an inverted Y field initially. Four thousand rads are given in 4½ weeks by opposing fields using a 6 MeV linear accelerator. A CT planning scan is then performed to define any residual node mass accurately and a further 500 - 1000 rads is given to this area alone with fields designed to spare the spinal cord and kidneys.

One month after completion of radiation, surgery is performed. A CT scan is used to determine whether the tumour is removable or whether there is involvement of the inferior vena cava or other adjacent structures. Definition of the exact location and upper limit of the tumour facilitates the decision as to which surgical approach should be used. Twenty-three patients have been treated by this combined approach and results are shown in Fig. 9.

Fig. 9. ADVANCED MALIGNANT TERATOMA - COMBINED CHEMOTHERAPY -
RADIOTHERAPY ± SURGERY 1976-1978

STAGE	TOTAL PATIENTS	NED	RANGE (months)	MEDIAN (months)	DEAD Tumour	DEAD Post-op	DEAD CT
II III	13	11	6-37	13	1	1	0
IVL_1 IVL_2	9	9	9-36	30	0	0	0
TOTAL	22	20 (90%)			1	1	0

SURGICAL RESULTS

A full surgical analysis of 15 of these patients (Group B)
is presented here

Fig. 10. PATHOLOGY OF PRIMARY TESTICULAR TUMOUR
RELATED TO TREATMENT GROUP

GROUP	NUMBER	PATHOLOGY OF TESTIS TD	PATHOLOGY OF TESTIS MTI	PATHOLOGY OF TESTIS MTU
1. Old series (1968-76)	13	2	10	1
2. Chemotherapy and radio-therapy (protocol)	15*		7	5
3. Chemotherapy only	6		1	5
	34	2	18	11

* including one seminoma with increased markers.

and compared with a group of 13 patients treated between
1968 and 1976 with radiotherapy alone followed by surgery
(Group A) and with 6 patients undergoing surgery after
chemotherapy alone (Group C).

A midline incision was used in 24 cases to approach the mass by the technique of Mallis and Patton (10). In 4 cases a thoraco-abdominal approach was needed (11) whilst a retro-peritoneal loin approach was used in 4 patients (12). The excised tissue was fixed in formalin and stained with haematoxylin and eosin.

The residual tumour was removed completely in all but one case where tumour involved the spinal roots of the femoral nerve and excision was inevitably incomplete.

The anterior midline incision gave good exposure and there were no problems of wound healing even in irradiated patients. Where massive tumours had to be removed the additional exposure provided by the thoraco-abdominal approach was very helpful. The loin incision was much less satisfactory as no posterior plane of cleavage was found and access to the great vessels was limited. In most cases the mass was discrete and could be dissected out from sur-rounding tissues with little difficulty. Dense fibrosis appeared to occur following chemotherapy and/or radiothera-py only in patients with seminomatous lesions but in this group it does present a serious problem and we would now try to avoid surgery if possible.

In 5 cases the ipsilateral kidney had to be removed because it or the ureter was inseparable from the tumour. In 2 patients with right-sided tumours part of the vena cava was resected (with preservation of the left renal vein) when tumour was found extending up through the lumen towards the heart.

The pathological findings are shown in Fig. 11.

Eight out of 13 (61%) of patients in Group I had per-sisting active disease whereas in the combined therapy group only 2 out of 15 showed histology similar to that seen in the primary tumour. Nine showed teratoma differentiated and 4 necrosis or fibrosis only. In the chemotherapy only group 4 out of 6 cases showed persisting disease.

Fig. 11. PATHOLOGICAL FINDINGS IN EXCISED LYMPH NODES
(COMPARE WITH Fig. 10)

| GROUP | NUMBER | PATHOLOGY OF NODES | | | |
		NEM	TD	MTI	MTU
1. Old series	13	1	4	5	3
2. Chemotherapy and radio- therapy (protocol)	15	4	9	1	1
3. Chemotherapy only	6	1	1	1	3

One patient died post-operative of secondary
haemorrhage giving a mortality rate of 3%. In retrospect he
should have been considered inoperable because of tumour
infiltration into the intervertebral foramina.
All patients complained of backache for 2 - 3 months
following surgery and of ejaculatory impotence.
Transient mild hydronephrosis was occasionally observed.

Two patients with active disease developed lung metastases immediately after abdominal surgery. In one the
disease was rapidly progressive and fatal. The other survives at 12 months with lung metastases which remain static
during continuing treatment with VP 16.

RADIOTHERAPY FOR LUNG METASTASES

It was initially our policy to treat solitary lung
metastases with radiotherapy following chemotherapy using
a 'postage stamp' field. However, the radiation following
after Bleomycin administration led to dense fibrosis which
was indistinguishable on chest radiographs from tumour and
made follow-up assessment very difficult. We are not now
using this approach but some of our patients have since
undergone thoracotomy when X-ray suggested persisting
disease after chemotherapy.

SURVIVAL RATES

The overall survival for these groups is shown in
Fig. 12

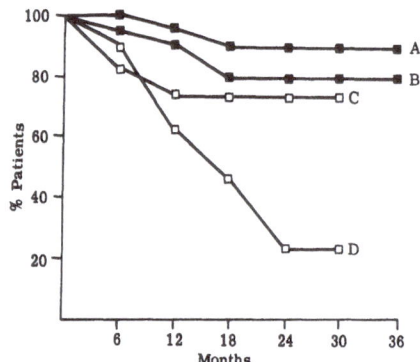

Stage IIB, IIC, III, IV L_1, L_2 (n = 21)

■ Previously untreated (n = 21)

    A - overall survival
    B - diseases free survival

□ Previously irradiated (n = 12)

    C - overall survival
    D - disease free survival

CONCLUSIONS

As far as the management of the early stage patient is
concerned, our policy of orchidectomy and radiotherapy
alone is producing encouraging results. All patients in
this group who have relapsed have had raised markers after
orchidectomy and have developed lung metastases soon after
completion of radiotherapy. This may therefore represent
a subgroup of patients in whom chemotherapy is required for
cure. We now feel that supradiaphragmatic radiation for
Stage IIA disease should be avoided as toxicity of any
subsequently required chemotherapy is greatly enhanced by
wide field treatment.

Seventy per cent of patients in the combined treatment
protocol are tumour free. The disease free survival for
previously untreated patients was significantly better than
that obtained in previously irradiated patients (Fig. 9)
and this underlines the need to make the optimal
therapeutic choice at the outset.

This difference may be due to chemotherapy being compromised by impaired haematological tolerance in the irradiated patient or to the fact that only previously untreated patients were eligible for planned combined chemotherapy - radiotherapy.

It is not yet possible to evaluate the relative contribution of radiotherapy and surgery in the management of advanced disease in our patients as the numbers are too small and the follow-up time too short. They are encouraging enough for us to undertake a prospective randomised study of chemotherapy and surgery versus chemotherapy, radiation and surgery. Our findings suggest that neither chemotherapy alone, nor radiation following chemotherapy are sufficient to control all bulky disease, but the reduction in tumour volume obtained and the greater differentiation observed may lead to better cure rates from surgery.

REFERENCES

1. Husband, J.E., Barret, A. and Peckham, M.J.
   Evaluation of computed tomography in the management of
   testicular teratoma.
   Clin. Radiol., 30: 243-252, 1979.

2. Skinner, D.G.
   Non-seminomatous testis tumours: a plan of management
   based on 96 patients to improve survival in all stages
   by combined therapeutic modalities.
   Journal of Urology, 115: 65-69, 1976.

3. Peckham, M.J. Hendry, W.F., McElwain, T.J. and Calman,
   F.M.B.
   In Adjuvant Therapy of Cancer, pp 305-320.
   Proceedings of the International Conference on the
   Adjuvant Therapy of Cancer held in Tucson, Arizone, U.S.A.
   March 2-5-1979. Ed. Salmon, S.E. and Jones, S.E. Publ.
   North-Holland Publishing Company, Amsterdam, Oxford and
   New York, 1979.

4. Samuels, M.L., Holoye, P.Y. and Johnson, D.E.
   Bleomycin combination chemotherapy in the management
   of testicular neoplasia.
   Cancer 36, 318-326, 1975.

5. Einhorn, L.H. and Donohue, J.P.
   Cisdiamminedichloroplatinum, Vinblastine and Bleomycin
   combination chemotherapy in disseminated testicular
   cancer.
   Annals of Int. Med. 87, 293-298, 1977.

6. Fitzharris, B., Kay, S.B., Muttu, S., Newlands, E.S.,
   Peckham, M.J. Barrett, A. and McElwain, T.J.
   VP 16-213 as a single agent in advanced testicular
   teratoma tumours.
   European Journal of Cancer (in press)

7. Tyrrell, C.J. and Peckham, M.J.
   The response of lymphnode metastases of testicular
   teratomas to radiation therapy.
   British Journal of Urology 48, 363-370, 1976.

8. Stoter, G., Sleijfer, D.T., Vendrik, C.P.J., Koops, H.S.,
   Struyvenberg, A., Van Oosterom, A.T., Brouwers, T.M.,
   and Pinedo, H.M.
   Combination chemotherapy with cisdiammino-
   dichloroplatinum, vinblastine, and bleomycin in advanced
   testicular non-seminomas.
   Lancet, 1: 941-945, 1979.

9. Einhorn, L.H. and Donohue, J.P.
   Improved management of non-seminomatous testis tumors.
   Journal of Urology, 177: 65-69, 1977.

10. Mallis, N. and Patton, J.F.
    Transperitoneal bilateral lymphadenectomy in testis
    tumor.
    Journal of Urology, 80: 501-503 1958.

11. Skinner, D.G. and Leadbetter, W.F.
    The surgical management of testis tumors.
    Journal of Urology, 106: 84-93, 1971.

12. Hinman, F., Gibson, T.E. and Kutzmann, A.A.
    The radical operation for teratoma testis. An analysis
    of 79 cases, 10 of which are personal.
    Surgery, Gynecology and Obstetrics, 37: 429-451, 1923.

15 TESTICULAR CANCER: THE INDIANA UNIVERSITY EXPERIENCE

S. D. Williams, L. H. Einhorn and J. P. Donohue

1 Introduction

Dramatic advances in the therapy of disseminated germinal neoplasms
have been made in the 1970's. All patients, even those with far
advanced disease, are potentially curable (1,2). The development
of effective systemic therapy has raised major questions with regard
to its relationship with surgery, both for patients with advanced
disease and for those with tumor confined to the primary and
regional lymphatics. New active single agents are being studied,
and the biology and natural history of testicular neoplasia is
better understood. This report will summarize 5 years of experience
with testicular cancer at Indiana University.

2 Disseminated Disease

Our first generation study was composed of 50 patients (47 evaluable)
treated between 1974 and 1976. They were treated with cis-platinum
(DDP) + vinblastine (Vlb) + bleomycin (PVB). The rationale for
this regimen has described previously (1), as have the patient population and earlier results (1,3). The treatment regimen is shown
in Table 1. Of particular note, all patients received maintenance
Vlb and only 3 courses of DDP were required for those patients
attaining complete remission (CR).

TABLE 1: TREATMENT REGIMEN

DDP 20 mg/M^2 IV daily x 5

Vlb 0.4 mg/kg IV push day 1

Bleomycin 30 units IV push days 1, 8, 15

Repeat above every 21 days for total of

3-4 courses (see text)

Given with continuous infusion of normal saline

Table 2 shows results of induction therapy and current status. It
must be emphasized that the last relapse from CR we have seen was

17 months after initiation of chemotherapy; this was the only relapse beyond 9 months. As follow-up of the 28 patients free of disease (NED) is from 3-5 years, all of them almost certainly can be considered cured.

TABLE 2: RESULTS - PVB

Complete remission	33/47 (70%)
Partial remission	14/47 (30%)
NED after surgery	5/47 (11%)
Presently NED (3-5 years)	28/47 (60%)

The acute toxicity of induction for these 50 patients was described in an earlier publication (1). In brief, by far the major difficulty experienced was myelosuppression from Vlb. In general, this was limited to granulocytopenia, except in patients who had received prior radiation therapy in whom severe thrombocytopenia and anemia were commonly seen. Eighteen patients (38%) required emergency hospitalization for granulocytopenia and fever and 7 (15%) had documented serious bacterial infection. We were quite pleased with the therapeutic results seen but concerned about the magnitude of hematologic toxicity.

During this same time period, we had the opportunity to treat 10 patients with far advanced disease who had progressed on prior Vlb + bleomycin before referral. We chose to treat these patients with DDP + Adriamycin (ADR). The rationale, patient population, treatment regimen, and results have been published previously (4). Although only 1 patient attained CR, which was not durable, we were impressed with the dramatic responses obtained in view of the magnitude of disease of these patients. Thus, ADR seemed worthy of incorporation into initial treatment regimens.

Accordingly, our second generation study was initiated in 1976 and continued until June, 1978. This study involved randomization between 3 different induction regimens. The first was identical to the initial program. The second was also the same except the Vlb dosage was reduced to 0.3 mg/kg in an effort to reduce hematologic toxicity. The third arm included ADR (50 mg/M^2); the Vlb dose was 0.2 mg/kg. Once again, only 3 courses of DDP were required and all patients received maintenance Vlb.

Table 3 shows the results of this study; follow-up is from 1-3 years. Results of all 3 arms are identical and strikingly similar to that seen in the initial study. The groups were comparable with regard to histology, extent of disease, and prior therapy.

TABLE 3:   RESULTS - PVB + ADR

	PVB (0.4)	PVB (0.3)	PVBA	Total
Number	26	27	25	78
Complete remission	18 (69%)	17 (63%)	18 (72%)	53 (68%)
Partial remission	8 (31%)	10 (37%)	5 (20%)	23 (30%)
NED with surgery	5 (19%)	4 (15%)	2 (8%)	11 (14%)
Continuously NED	18 (69%)	18 (67%)	17 (68%)	53 (68%)

Table 4 outlines the hematologic toxicity of the 3 arms. As can be seen, reducing the dosage of Vlb considerably reduced the incidence of granulocytopenic fever and infection. Thus, we no longer recommend the higher dosage of Vlb.

However, it was felt that further evaluation of the 3-drug versus 4-drug combination was necessary. Thus, we embarked on our third and currently active study, which is a group wide study of the Southeastern Cancer Study Group. Induction therapy is a randomization between the latter 2 arms of the previous protocol with the exception that all patients receive a mandatory fourth course of DDP. Complete responders at 12 weeks are allocated at random to receive maintenance Vlb versus no further therapy. No firm conclusions can be drawn yet from this study.

TABLE 4:   TOXICITY - PVB + ADR

	Granulocytopenic fever	Infection
PVB (0.4)	9 (35%)	3 (12%)
PVB (0.3)	4 (15%)	0
PVBA	6 (24%)	1 (4%)

We currently have 164 patients evaluable for response to induction chemotherapy. Table 5 shows the complete response rate (chemotherapy ± surgery) according to histologic type. It is apparent that patients with embryonal carcinoma have a considerably higher CR rate. To a certain degree, however, this may be related to extent of disease because patients with other cell types tend to present with bulky tumor.

TABLE 5: COMPLETE RESPONSE RATE BY HISTOLOGY

	Total	NED (%)
Seminoma	19	13 (68)
Embryonal	88	78 (89)
Teratoma	3	2 (67)
Teratocarcinoma	40	27 (68)
Choriocarcinoma	12	6 (50)
Yolk sac	2	2 (100)

Table 6 gives the same information according to extent of disease. The criteria used are that of Samuels (2). Of patients with "minimal" disease at initiation of chemotherapy (Groups A, C, and E), 95.4% attained disease-free status. We believe this has profound implications for adjuvant studies, which will be discussed in a subsequent section.

TABLE 6: COMPLETE RESPONSE BY EXTENT OF DISEASE

		Total	NED (%)
A.	Minimal pulmonary	30	28 (93)
B.	Advanced pulmonary	38	26 (66)
C.	Minimal abdominal + pulmonary	24	23 (96)
D.	Advanced abdominal	54	35 (65)
E.	Elevated marker only	11	11 (100)
	Other	7	6 (86)
	Total	164	128 (78)

Table 7 related CR rate to prior therapy. Patients who have received prior irradiation are only modestly less likely to have a complete response. This is contrary to our earlier experience and is due to a change in our treatment philosophy. Initial doses of myelosuppressive drugs are reduced by 25%. Nonetheless, severe and prolonged granulocytopenia almost invariably will ensue. Formerly, treatment courses were frequently delayed until marrow recovery. We now give courses of schedule regardless of the granulocyte count. Obviously, facilities for supportive care must be available.

TABLE 7: COMPLETE RESPONSE BY PRIOR THERAPY

	Total	NED (%)
Surgery alone	102	81 (79)
Prior chemotherapy	38	29 (76)
Prior radiotherapy	30	21 (70)

3 PVB Toxicity

Hematologic toxicity was discussed previously. Another major
concern formerly was DDP-induced renal failure. Detailed analysis
of our experience with the renal toxicity of PVB is beyond the
scope of this publication. However, several facts have emerged.
An occasional patient in our initial series developed major distur-
bances in renal function, and in one instance, acute renal failure.
It appeared that the major risk factor was the use of aminoglycoside
antibiotics and we now scrupulously avoid these. In addition,
dehydration seemed to play a major role. Consequently, all patients
receive continuous intravenous hydration. By these techniques,
significant renal damage is extremely rare and virtually all patients
complete induction chemotherapy with normal or near-normal renal
function. In addition, with follow-up to 5 years no patient has
developed progressive renal disease.

Bleomycin-induced pulmonary fibrosis is another major potential
problem. It is more likely to occur in older patients or those
who have had radiotherapy to the chest. In our experience, the most
reliable indicator of early pulmonary fibrosis is changes on physical
examination of the chest. We discontinue bleomycin for patients who
develop a lag of expansion of a hemithorax or unexplained rales.

No long-term toxicity has yet been identified and patients
after completing induction therapy, rapidly return to normal performance status. We have seen no second malignancies. The effects
on fertility are unknown and need further study. However, 3 of
our patients have fathered healthy children.

4 Adjuvant Therapy

During this same time period, we have had the opportunity to care
for a large number of patients with Stage I (tumor limited to the
testis) and Stage II (testis + retroperitoneal node involvement)

disease. All patients received an inguinal orchiectomy followed
by retroperitoneal lymphadenectomy (bilateral in most). Subsequently,
they received adjuvant therapy as described below and were followed
by monthly serum marker determinations and chest x-rays for one
year and every other month studies for the second year. They were
treated promptly at relapse with PVB $\pm$ ADR.

There were 57 Stage I patients, 33 having been followed for 2
years and 50 for 1 year. Four relapsed, and all were treated with
PVB and currently all 57 remain disease-free. None received adjuvant
therapy.

From 1973-1977, 31 patients with pathologic and resected Stage II
disease received 2 years of adjuvant therapy with Actinomycin-D.
Relapse was seen in 15, and these patients were treated with
PVB $\pm$ ADR. One died and 30/31 are now disease-free.

In 1977 in a small pilot study 7 patients with Stage II
disease received 6 weeks of PVB (2 courses of DDP; 6 weeks of
bleomycin). All have been followed for 2 years and all remain NED.

More recently, our treatment philosophy has been to use no
adjuvant therapy for Stage II disease. There have been 24 such
patients (2 year follow-up in 12; 1 year in 21). Seven relapsed
and all entered CR with PVB $\pm$ ADR. An additional patient died of
unrelated causes.

Thus, in our experience, virtually all patients with loco-
regional disease only will be cured with or without adjuvant therapy.
Those who relapse will be detected early and treated early because
their follow-up is meticulous. We have already shown that patients
with "minimal" metastatic disease virtually always can be rendered
NED with chemotherapy. Thus, it could well be that adjuvant therapy
is unnecessary. The ultimate answer to this question will require
a random prospective study; such a study is in progress.

5 Future Directions

About 60% of patients with disseminated germinal neoplasms can expect
to be cured of their disease by modern therapy, as can virtually all
of those with Stage I or II disease. This is most gratifying but
much remains to be done. There are many avenues for future
investigation. More effective initial chemotherapy and "salvage"
regimens can be defined (for example, using VP-16-213) and toxicity
reduced (for example: better anti-emetics). The necessity, if any,

of maintenance therapy for metastatic disease and adjuvant therapy for Stage II patients can be evaluated in prospective clinical trials. Long-term toxicity will be defined. Particularly exciting is the possibility of defining a subset of patients clinically who can be successfully treated by orchiectomy alone. Nonetheless, without doubt the future is bright for all patients with testicular cancer.

REFERENCES

1. Einhorn LH and Donohue JP: Cis-diamminedichloroplatinum, vinblastine, and bleomycin combination chemotherapy in disseminated testicular cancer. Ann Int Med 87:293-298, 1977.

2. Samuels ML, Lanzotti VJ, Holoye PY, et al.: Combination chemotherapy in germinal cell tumors. Cancer Treat Rev 3:185-204, 1976.

3. Einhorn LH and Donohue JP: Combination chemotherapy in disseminated testicular cancer - The Indiana University experience. Sem Oncol 6:87-93, 1979.

4. Einhorn LH and Williams SD: Combination chemotherapy with cis-diamminedichloroplatinum and Adriamycin in testicular cancer refractory to vinblastine plus bleomycin. Cancer Treat Rep 62:1351-53, 1978.

16 THE VAB SCHEMES OF TREATMENT FOR GERM CELL TUMORS

R. B. Golbey

Germ Cell Tumors are rare. They most frequently arise in the testicle and are the leading cause of cancer deaths in men from 25-34 years of age, but occasionally are seen primary in the ovary, retroperitoneum, and mediastinum. The lessons learned from the study of testicular tumors are applicable to those tumors arising from germ cells in other sites.

Many of these tumors can be effectively controlled, while they are still confined to the primary site and the regional nodes, by surgery and/or radiation therapy. Once they are disseminated however death from disease in less than one year can be reliably predicted unless systemic chemotherapy is effectively employed.

The possibility of "cure" of this tumor, even after dissemination has been recognized since the late 1950's when complete responses and prolongation of disease-free survival were first described.[1]. The treatment used then was a combination of Actinomycin-D, Chlorambucil, and Methotrexate. This was the first effective drug combination used. The use of this "triple" regimen produced results that were better than those achievable with any one of the drugs used alone.

Methotrexate was used because of its known activity against gestational trophoblastic tumors.[2]. Actinomycin-D was used because of demonstrated activity in phase II studies, and Chlorambucil was used because of the possibility that a "radiometic drug" would enhance the activity of the Actinomycin. The addition of this drug did in fact seem to prolong the duration of the antitumor effect achievable with Actinomycin alone.

With this combination one in two patients showed some effect, one in five had complete disappearance of disease, but less than one in ten had prolonged control of the disease and possible cure.[3]. As time passed and the

duration of disease-free survival increased the possibility of cure of a solid tumor other than the "transplanted"
placental choriocarcinoma became applied.

No additional improvement in response rates was seen until
the efficacy of Vinblastine and Bleomycin as single-agents,
and in combination, was observed.[4]. This combination, as
originally reported, produced an overall response rate of
76% at the cost of significant morbidity and occasional
mortality.

The activity of the combination led us in 1972 to incorpo-
rate Vinblastine and Bleomycin at a somewhat reduced dosage into a combination with Actinomycin-D (VAB-I). The
three drugs were given as pulse doses twice in the first
week and once weekly thereafter as tolerated. The program
was well tolerated initially but pulmonary toxicity was
seen with continued administration of Bleomycin. At this
time, the VAB I data show an overall response rate of 47%
(32/68) and a CR rate of 22% (15/68). Six of the fifteen
patients with a CR have relapsed leaving nine patients, or
13%, as long-term free of evidence of disease and potential cures.[5].

During this period, 16 of the failures to this simple
pulse dose regimen were treated with a combination of
Bleomycin by continuous infusion plus a pulse dose of
cis-Platinum. Sixty-eight percent (11/16) of these patients
had partial remissions (PR) with a median duration of
2½ months. [6].

A protocol, subsequently called VAB II, was then designed
in 1974 to replace the original VAB. Vinblastine and
Actinomycin-D on day 1 were followed by a continuous infusion of Bleomycin for 1 week and a pulse dose of 1.2
mg/kg of cis-Platinum on day 8. This induction was followed
by a consolidation phase using the first three drugs weekly, with substitution of cis-Platinum for Actinomycin-D
every third week. The induction program was repeated 4
months after beginning therapy. Following this reinduction,
maintenance therapy was begun with Chlorambucil daily plus
Vinblastine and Actinomycin D intravenously every 3 weeks,
all continuing for 2 to 3 years. Fifty patients have been

treated with VAB II, all of whom had measurable metastatic
disease. The CR rate was 50% (25/50), with a CR rate of
60% (15/25) in patients not previously treated with drugs.
Eleven patients remain alive and free of evidence of disease at this time; a potential cure rate of 22%.[7].
While this protocol was being studied, the problem of the
dose-limiting nephrotoxicity of cis-Platinum was confronted.
This was important because cis-Platinum is probably the
most active single-agent yet studied against this group
of diseases. A technique involving prehydration and
mannitol induced diuresis was developed after animal studies.[8]. Patients who had failed VAB II were then treated with high- dose cis-Platinum (120 mg/m^2). There were
5 PRs and 1 minor remission (MR) in 9 adequately treated
patients, all of whom had become resistant to cis-Platinum
at doses of 1.2 mg/kg. Nephrotoxicity was less severe,
and was reversible in most cases. Again, remissions were
short-lived but encouraging since they occurred in previous treatment failures.

VAB III was then designed in 1975 to include high dose
cis-Platinum.[9]. A pulse dose of Cyclophosphamide was
added during induction since, used as a single-agent, the
drug had caused 3 PRs in 5 patients with testicular cancer,[9] and we had noted 4 MRs in 7 patients with testicular cancer who had failed other chemotherapy. The consolidation phase was made less intensive by the deletion of
Bleomycin and the addition of Chlorambucil, and by giving
the intravenous drugs every 3 weeks instead of weekly.
Adriamycin was added to the consolidation phase because
it had been active as a single-agent in 14 of 20 patients
with testicular cancer treated in another trial.[11].
The reinduction at about 5 months was retained, as was the
subsequent maintenance program.

VAB III was given to 92 patients with metastatic testicular
cancer, with 89 of them adequately treated. The CR rate
was 62% (55/89). Of these 55, 15 have subsequently relapsed, for a 27% CR relapse rate. Forty of 89 patients are
still free of evidence of disease for a potential cure
rate of 45%. In the previously untreated group of 45 pa-

tients, 24 are still alive without evidence of disease; a rate of 54%.

In the previously treated group of 44 patients, 16 are still alive without evidence of disease; a rate of 36%. This degree of difference in disease-free survival between patients previously treated with chemotherapy and previously untreated is a consistent observation thoughout our studies. The PR rate was 22% (20/89) and the MR rate was 11% (10/89). Only 4 of 89 adequately treated patients had no objective response to the VAB III protocol[12]. Since most relapses on VAB III occurred in the first 6 to 8 months of chemotherapy, the VAB IV protocol was designed in 1976. The induction was almost identical to VAB III, but a reinduction without Bleomycin was introduced at 16 weeks after the initiation of therapy, followed by a full reinduction with Bleomycin at 32 weeks. The subsequent maintenance program was the same as on VAB III.[13]. Fifty-five patients have been entered on this treatment program. Of these 29 achieved CR after chemotherapy alone. An additional 11 patients were free of evidence of disease after surgical removal of residual tumor after some response to chemotherapy. The histology of the residual tumor after chemotherapy was mature teratoma (five), necrotic tumor (one), and residual tumor (five). The relapses after CR on chemotherapy alone (5/29 17%) and after chemotherapy plus adjuvant surgery (2/11 18%) are the same. The total CR rate is 73% (40/55) with 60% (33/55) continuing free of evidence of disease at this time.[12-13]. When the protocols are compared after equal time of follow-up VAB IV has about the same rate of induction of CRs as did VAB III but has a lower relapse rate. The end results are improved by the use of surgery to remove residual foci of tumor.

In the course of these studies risk factors were identified which influence the likelihood of obtaining a complete response and a potential cure. Adverse factors are: (1) prior chemotherapy and resistance to one or more of the agents in the combination; (2) histology: embryonal

carcinoma is more sensitive than teratocarcinoma which
in turn is much more sensitive than is pure choriocarcinoma. Foci of choriocarcinoma in a mixed tumor have only
a minor impact on prognosis; (3) bulk of tumor: the greater the cell burden the less the expectation of achieving
cure.

VAB V was designed specifically for those patients with
adverse risk factors. It intensified and prolonged the
induction phase of the treatment. Toxicity was more severe but the goal of the treatment does not appear to
have been achieved. The results are currently being
analysed in detail.

VAB VI is the protocol currently under study. It employs
the same induction as VAB III and VAB IV except that the
dose of Bleomycin in each induction has been reduced to
a priming dose and three days of continuous infusion.
The full course is repeated twice at monthly intervals,
and a third time without Bleomycin. Occasionally, a fourth
course is given, without Bleomycin, to patients in whom
tumor regression is incomplete but continuing. After the
completion of this induction program, if necessary and
if feasible, any foci of residual tumor are surgically
resected. After resection of residual , viable, malignant
tumor two additional induction courses are administered.
If the tumor was all mature teratoma, or scar tissue no
further inductions are given. In either case after the
last induction, maintainance therapy with Actinomycin-D
and Velban every three weeks is given. The entire period
of therapy is one year. It is too early to evaluate the
results of this treatment schedule but more complete remissions are being seen.

Because of the significant impact of chemotherapy on
metastatic germ cell tumors the question naturally arose
as to whether chemotherapy could more easily and more
effectively cure patients by being used in the adjuvant
setting at a time when the patient had no evidence of
macrometastases. The VAB I protocol was used in the adjuvant setting. [14]. Sixty-two patients with Stage II
disease in whom all evidence of disease was resected were

treated with pulse doses of Velban 0.06 mg/kg., Actinomycin-D 0.02 mg/kg, and Bleomycin 0.05 mg per kilogram
each given weekly times six followed after a two week
interval by Actinomycin-D 0.02 mg/kg, and Chlorambucil
p.o. 0.1 mg/kg. times seven each given every fourteen
days for one year. During the second year the interval
was increased to every twenty-one days. Of the sixty-two
patients treated, nine recurred in less than eighteen
months and one recurred at eighteen months. The remaining
83% continue free of evidence of disease. This result is
better than the expected result in Stage II patients
treated with surgery alone, but the degree of benefit
cannot be quantitated because of the known variability
of bulk of disease in this stage. Prognostic differences
between patients with microscopic disease and patients
with barely resectable disease exist, but have not been
adequately defined in any reported surgical series.
Retrospectively in this group of 62 patients we identified
a good risk and a poor risk group. The good risk had
negative tumor markers, fewer than five nodes involved,
and the largest node was 2 cm or less in diameter.
More disease than this worsened the prognosis.
There were 33 patients in the good prognosis group, all
of whom are free of evidence of disease, with a median
follow up exceeding two years. Of the 29 poor prognosis
patients 10 have recurred within the two years with
most of the metastases manifesting themselves within
6-8 months after surgery. This group therefore has 65%
surviving free of evidence of disease. While this is
probably an improvement over the results with surgery
alone it is not good enough.
Since 1975 we have stopped giving adjuvant chemotherapy
to the good risk group. They are carefully followed and
will be treated only if they recur. The poor risk group
have been treated with VAB III in exactly the same fashion
as were patients with advanced disease. To date 22 patients have been entered and followed for a median of
10 months with no recurrences. It will be at least
another year before firm conclusions can be drawn. [14]

Conclusion

Stepwise progress has been made in the treatment of germ
cell tumors. More effective treatments for advanced
disease are evolving. The judicious selection of
poor risk patients for adjuvant chemotherapy early in
their disease and the use of therapy known to be the
most effective in advanced disease will go a long way
toward achieving the attainable goal of 100% cures in
this disease.

REFERENCES

1. Li, M.C., Whitmore, W.F., Golbey, R.B., et al.
   Effects of combined drug therapy on metastatic cancer
   of the testis.
   JAMA 174, 1291-1299, 1960.

2. Li, M.C., Hertz, R., Bergenstal, D.M.
   Therapy of choriocarcinoma and related trophoblastic
   tumors with folic acid and purine antagonists.
   N. Engl. J. Med. 259, 66-74, 1958.

3. Kaufman, R.J.
   Testicular carcinoma in Cancer Chemotherapy.
   Ed. Elkerbout, F., Thomas, P., Zwavelinq, A.
   Leiden University Press, 215-225, 1971.

4. Samuels, M.L., Lanzotti, V.J. Holoye, P.Y., et al.
   Combination chemotherapy in germinal cell tumors.
   Cancer Treat. Rev. 3, 185-204, 1976.

5. Wittes R.E., Yagoda, A., Silvay, O., et al.
   Chemotherapy of germ cell tumors of the testis I.
   Induction of remissions with Vinblastine, Actinomycin-
   D, and Bleomycin.
   Cancer 37, 637-645, 1976.

6. Cvitkovic, E., Currie, V., Krakoff, I.H., et al.
   Bleomycin infusion with cis-Platinum diammine dichlori-
   de as secondary chemotherapy for germinal cell tumors.
   Proc. Am. Soc. Clin. Oncol. 16, 1208, 1975.

7. Cheng, E., Cvitkovic, E., Wittes, R.E., et al.
   Germ cell tumors (II): VAB II in metastatic testicular cancer.
   Cancer 42, 2162-2168, 1978.

8. Hayes, D.M., Cvitkovic, E., Golbey, R.B., et al.
   High-dose cis-Platinum diammine dichloride: amelioration of renal toxicity by mannitol diuresis.
   Cancer 39, 1372-1381, 1977.

9. Cvitkovic, E., Hayes, D., Golbey, R.B.
   Primary combination chemotherapy (VAB III) for metastatic or unresectable germ cell tumors.
   Proc. Am. Soc. Clin. Oncol. 17, C-237, 1976.

10. Buckner, C.D., Rudolph, R.H., Fefer, A., et al.
    High-dose Cyclophosphamide therapy for malignant disease.
    Cancer 29, 357-365, 1972.

11. Monfardini, S., Bajetta, E., Musumeci, R., et al.
    Clinical use of Adriamycin in advanced testicular cancer.
    J. Urol. 108, 293-296, 1972.

12. Golbey, R.B., Reynolds, T., Vugrin, D.
    Chemotherapy of metastatic germ cell tumors.
    Sem. in Oncology 6, 82-85, 1979.

13. Vugrin, D., Cvitkovic, E., Cheng, E., et al.
    Chemotherapy of testicular carcinoma with VAB IV.
    Proc. Am. Soc. Clin. Oncol. 20, C-192, 1979.

14. Vugrin, D., Cvitkovic, E., Whitmore, W.F., Golbey, R.B.
    Adjuvant chemotherapy in germ cell tumors.
    Sem. in Oncology, 6, 94-98, 1979.

17 COMBINATION OF CHEMOTHERAPY AND DEBULKING SURGERY

C. Merrin

INTRODUCTION

In 1973 we first developed a therapeutic strategy combining multiple drugs chemotherapy with reductive surgery for the treatment of advanced non seminomatous testicular tumors. (1)

We have used this approach during the past 6 years. Our experience is reported herein.

MATERIALS AND METHODS

Seventy seven patients with advanced Stage II (6 patients) and Stage III (71 patients) testicular carcinoma were entered in this study and followed from November 1973 to February 1979. Their ages varied from 15 to 58 years with an average of 27 years. Histologically there were 28 embryonal carcinomas, 26 teratocarcinomas and 23 mixed tumors containing cytotrophoblastic elements.

The patients were evaluated by physical examination, excretory urography (IVP), bilateral pedal lymphography, chest tomography, liver and brain scan, metastatic radiologic survey, aortography, inferior venacavography, audiograms, and pulmonary function tests, serum studies included (beta sub unit fraction) of human chorionic gonadotrophin and alpha fetoprotein determinations as well as routine biochemical and hematological studies.

The patients were treated with a combination of Cis-Platinum, Vincristine, Bleomycin, Prednisone and Actinomycin D (77 patients). (Table 1) Ten patients received the same combination of drugs with Vinblastine previously (Vinblastine 0.05 mg/kg/day IV for 2 days). It was later replaced by Vincristine because of serious toxicity.

Patients who achieved a complete clinical response within the first 3 months continued chemotherapy for a total period of 2 years. Patients who achieved a partial response only in the first 3 months were submitted to surgery to excise residual tumor. After surgery they continued chemotherapy until relapse or a total period of 2 years. (Table II)

Table I

Chemotherapy Schedule For Advanced Testicular Tumor

Remission Induction (6 Weeks)

Bleomycin (Weeks 1 and 3)
Cis-Diamminedichloroplatinum and
   Vincristine (Weeks 1 to 6)
Prednisone (Weeks 1 to 4)

Consolidation (9 Weeks)

Actinomycin D (Weeks 7 and 13)
Cis-Diamminedichloroplatinum and
   Vincristine (Weeks 7, 10, 13)

Maintenance (2 Years)

Actinomycin D (q 6 Weeks)
Cis-Diamminedichloroplatinum (q 3 Weeks)

Bleomycin - 30 units/day infused in 5 hours
Cis-Diamminedichloroplatinum - 1 mg/kg
Vincristine - 2 mg
Prednisone - 10 mg BID
Actinomycin D - 0.5 mg/day/5 days

Table II

Treatment Program For Advanced Non Seminomatous Testicular Tumors

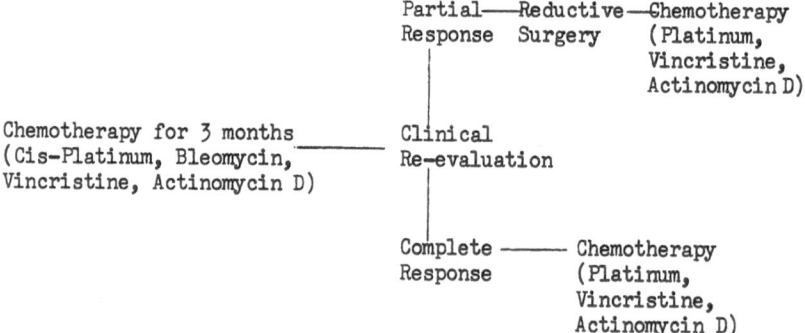

Partial——Reductive—Chemotherapy
Response Surgery (Platinum,
                Vincristine,
                Actinomycin D)

Chemotherapy for 3 months   Clinical
(Cis-Platinum, Bleomycin,   Re-evaluation
Vincristine, Actinomycin D)

Complete —————— Chemotherapy
Response   (Platinum,
                Vincristine,
                Actinomycin D)

Total Chemotherapy Time: 2 Years.

Fourteen patients were treated with chemotherapy alone, 22 patients underwent a simultaneous excision of metastases in the abdomen and the chest. Ten patients underwent resection of metastases in the abdomen and the chest in two separate operative procedures. Twenty five patients had resection of abdominal and retroperitoneal metastases and 6 patients had resection of thoracic metastases.

SURGICAL TECHNIQUES

A. Large Retroperitoneal Masses

Large masses in the retroperitoneum adhere to or invade the vena cava, aorta, renal vessels, duodeum, pancreas and the small and large bowel. The techniques of resection was variable according to the organs which were involved. The anterior approach was used through a midline transperitoneal incision going from the symphisis pubis to the xyphoid process. As in the classical retroperitoneal lymphadenectomy the posterior parietal peritoneum was entered through an incision going from the angle of Treitz down to and around the cecum. The right colon was mobilized. When the vena cava was invaded venacavectomy was performed (3 patients).Fig 1.When kidney (3 patients) or bowels were invaded (6 patients), nephrectomy and or bowel resection was performed. In the presence of circumscribed liver metastases partial hepatectomy was performed (1 patient). (When necessary the abdominal incision can be extended along the left side of the sternum by transsection of the costo-chondral junction to allow better access to the postero-superior part of the retroperitoneum. The incision can also be extended along the 10th intercostal space.)

B. Surgical Approach to the Metastases in the Mediastinum and Lungs

(2) (Figure 2) Metastases to the lungs are most often bilateral. It is therefore necessary to explore both sides and the mediastinum to be sure not to miss any lesion. The only approach suitable for the purpose is the midline transternal approach. The mediastinum is exposed. Both pleuras are opened exposing the lungs. The pericardium is incised to explore the superior vena cava, the aorta and the trachea. Tissues surrounding these structures are excised because they are often the site of occult metastases. The lungs are palpated and metastases are excised, taking care to remove only a small rim of normal tissue. This is a local excision rather than a wedge resection, because it is important to preserve as much normal lung parenchyma as possible. The lungs are then sutured with continous 3-zero sutures.

214

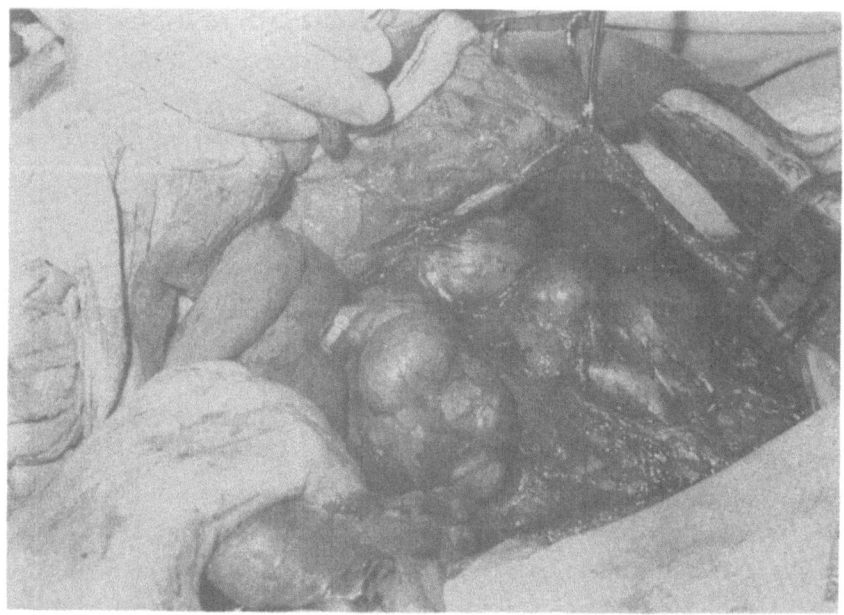

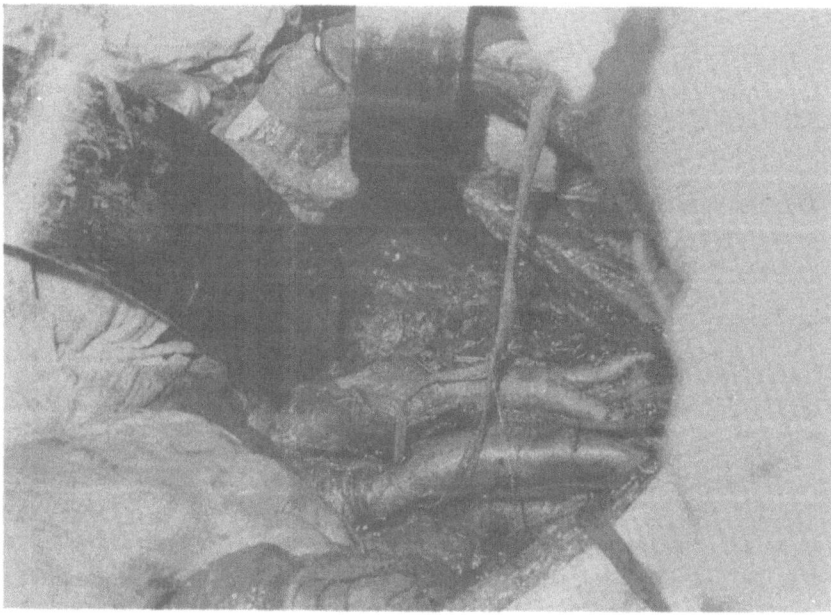

<u>Figure I</u>

A. Large retroperitoneal masses adherent to the vena cava and the
aorta. These masses have the cystic appearance which is characteristic of mature teratomas.

B. After reductive surgery most of the tumor has been excised. Some
tumor is still present on the anterolateral aspect of the aorta. A
partial resection(longitudinal) of the vena cava has been performed.

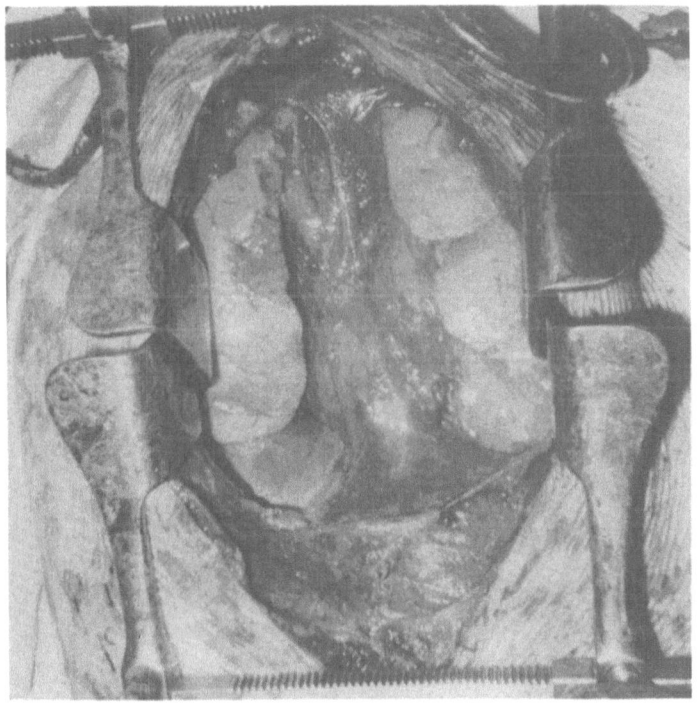

Figure 2

Midline transternal approach to the chest with good exposure of the
mediastinum and both lungs.

In this fashion up to 60 metastases were excised with no dangerous decrease of the functional pulmonary capacity. This approach allowed
resection of mediastinal masses, pulmonary lobectomy (2 patients) and
even pneumonectomy (1 patient). The parietal pleura can be visualized
and pleural metastases were excised (3 patients).

This technique has been used successfully for the excision of lung
metastases from tumors other than testis. (3)

C. Simultaneous Excision of Metastases in the Abdomen and the Chest

(Figure 3) When metastases exist at the same time in the retroperitoneum (2) the abdomen and the chest it is necessary to excise all the
lesions in a simultaneous fashion.

If the operations were done in sequence, first the abdominal then the
thoracic part , by the time the patient recovered the non operated
lesions may have increased in size and new metastases may have developed.

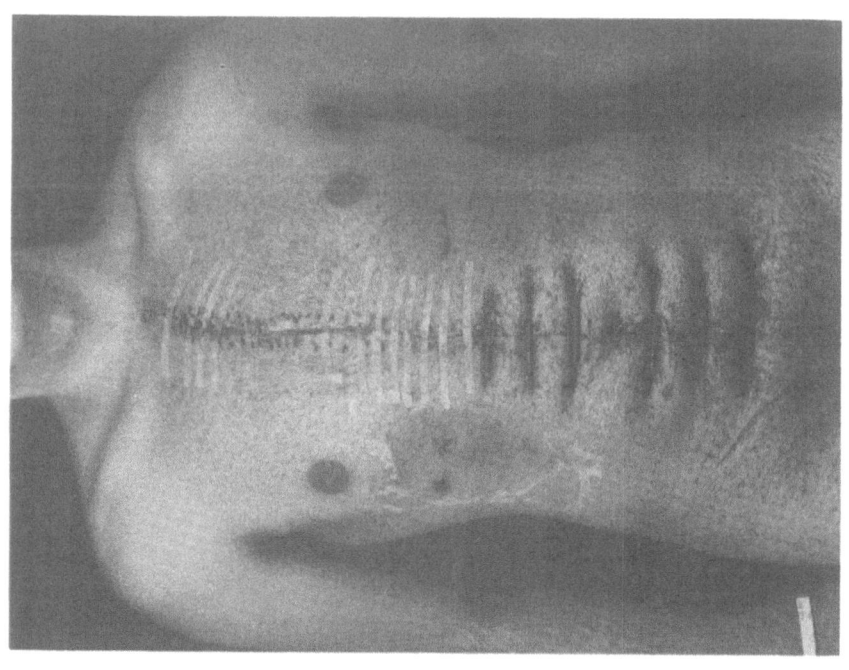

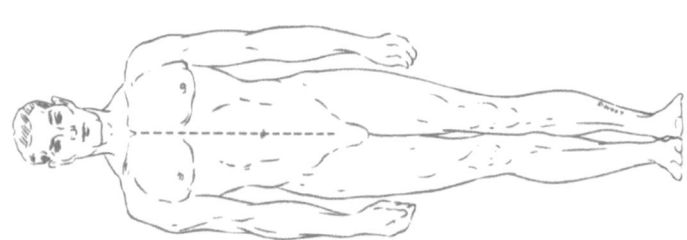

Figure 3
A. Incision used for the simultaneous excision
of metastases in the abdomen and the chest.
B. Postoperative view of the same incision.

The abdominal part is performed first. The abdomen is opened through a midline incision going from the symphysis pubis to the xyphoid process in the manner previously described for the excision of large retroperitoneal masses. After resection of the intra-abdominal and retroperitoneal lesions the abdomen is closed and the midline incision is extended to the base of the neck entering the chest through a midline transsternal approach in the manner described previously for the resection of lung and mediastinal metastases.

RESULTS

Sixty four patients (83%) achieved a complete clinical remission. Of these, 17 patients (22%) recurred within 6 months to 1 year. Forty seven patients (61%) have remained in complete clinical remission for 14 to 48 months. Of these 30 patients have been free of disease for more than 2 years. Eleven patients have been free of disease for more than 18 months, and 6 patients have been free of disease for more than 12 months.

A partial clinical response was achieved in the remaining 13 patients which lasted 2 to 30 months. All of these patients, as well as the patients who recurred after an initial complete response received a modified therapeutic regimen including Cyclophosphamide, Mithramycin and Adriamycin, but later died from the progression of their disease.

Surgery was effective in transforming 24 partial responders into lasting complete responses. (51% of all the lasting complete responders.) Of the 63 patients who underwent surgery, 51 were considered to have a complete resection of their residual disease and therefore were considered complete responders. Twenty four of these patients showed partial or complete transformation of the tumor into mature (histologically benign) teratoma (18 complete; 6 partials). (Figure 1A). Sixteen patients exhibited complete necrosis of the tumor (Figure 4A), and 11 patients had residual malignant tumor.

The 12 remaining patients underwent only partial resection of their residual tumors. All of them showed malignant residual disease. Eleven patients with residual malignant tumor who underwent complete resection recurred.

All the patients who recurred or in whom complete resection was impossible, exhibited the same type of residual tumor: A modified

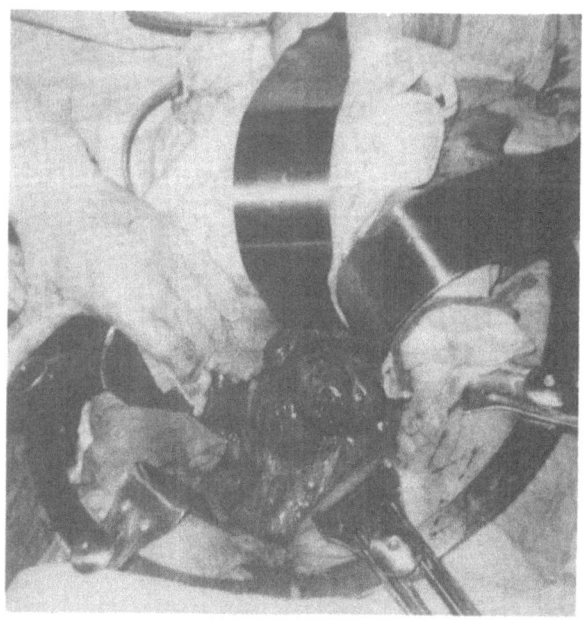

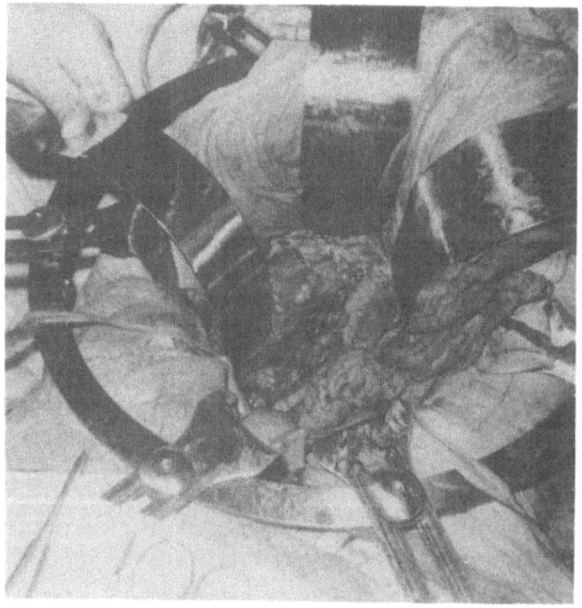

Figure 4

A. Complete necrosis of retroperineal metastases after chemotherapy.
B. The same area after resection of the tumor. An inferior veno-
cavectomy has been performed.

embryonal cell carcinoma with increased fibrous stroma which grossly infiltrated the surrounding structures (very much like an inflammatory carcinoma). This tumor could not be dissected free from healthy tissues.

Thirty three patients presented with this type of tumor. Of these 8 patients had residual cytotrophoblastic elements in addition to the embryonal cell carcinoma.

The 16 patients who had complete necrosis of the residual tumor should be interpreted as chemotherapeutic complete responders. Therefore the total number of complete responders to chemotherapy alone should be 30 patients (39%).

CHEMOTHERAPEUTIC TOXICITY (Table III)

All of the patients had varing degrees of nausea and vomiting. The intensity of these symptoms were not constant. Some patients had minimal or no nausea and no vomiting at that time. Mild to moderate renal toxicity expressed by increase in serum creatinine and BUN was seen in 2 patients (2.5%). Mild auditory toxicity was seen in 2 patients (2.5%). Mild leukopenia was seen in 2 patients (2.5%). Thrombocytopenia was present in 19 patients (25%). Alopecia was observed in all patients, mild mucositis was seen in 15 patients (19%). Ten patients developed allergy to Cis-Platinum and 1 patient had seizures after Platinum administration without evidence of brain metastases. No lung fibrosis was observed.

Table III

Chemotherapy Toxicity after Treatment of Advanced Testicular Tumors
With Cis-Platinum, Bleomycin, Vincristine and Actinomycin D

Vomiting	77	100%
Nausea	77	100%
Nephrotoxicity (Mild)	2	2.5%
Auditory (Mild)	2	2.5%
Leukopenia (Mild)	2	2.5%
Thrombocytopenia (Mild)	19	25%
Alopecia	77	100%
Neurotoxicity	0	0%
Seizures	1	1.3%
Allergy	10	13%
Mucositis (Mild)	15	19.5%
Lung Fibrosis	0	0%

POSTOPERATIVE COMPLICATIONS

The patients who were submitted to resection of their abdominal and/ or retroperitoneal metastases (25 patients), the patients who underwent resection of metastases in the abdomen and the chest (in two different operations) (10 patients) and the patients who had resection of metastases in the chest (6 patients), had no major postoperative complications. No death was observed, and all the patients in these 3 categories were completely recovered by 2 weeks.

The group of patients treated by simultaneous excision of metastases in the abdomen and the chest (22 patients) developed the following postoperative complications; one patient (who had been treated previously with IV push Bleomycin) died in the postoperative period. Post mortem examination revealed lung fibrosis secondary to Bleomycin toxicity. Three patients developed postoperative respiratory failure which required the use of respirators for 2 to 4 weeks. They all recovered. No major complications were observed in the remaining 18 patients in this category. Some of the minor complications were; fever (8 patients) transient paroxysmal tachycardia (1 patient). All the 18 patients were ambulated in the first postoperative day. Their chest tubes were removed between the 5th to 8th day. All the 18 patients were completely ambulatory by the 10th postoperative day.

DISCUSSION

The necessity to perform tumor reduction by surgery prompted us to reassess and modify the traditional approach to cancer surgery. We were confronted with patients having large masses of tumors with multiorgan metastases, very often present simultaneously in the abdomen and the chest. In the past such lesions were considered unresectable. Was it possible to establish new principles for a methodic and rational excision of these lesions?

The first problem was to determine operability. How large should a tumor be to be unresectable? How many metastases would preclude intervention? How to define "unresectable" lesions? As such an experience did not exist previously, we decided to use a pragmatic approach, and considered "a priori", that no mass was unresectable on theorectical grounds. The number of metastases present in different organs did not contraindicate surgery whenever it was technically possible and the condition of the patients could allow it.

Another consideration was the timing of the surgery in relation to chemotherapy. Should it be done before or after? Initially we thought that surgery before chemotherapy was more rational because by decreasing the tumor mass it would permit a better distribution and efficacy of antineoplastic drugs. (4)

An early experience in some patients operated before receiving chemotherapy when their tumor had a short doubling time showed that new metastases appeared often before chemotherapy could be started. It then became clear that reductive surgery could not be performed unless the tumor was at rest and the doubling time had been slowed down to allow for enough time for surgery and recovery without the danger of tumor dissemination.

Some patients who could not tolerate surgery initially received chemotherapy first, post chemotherapy surgery was found to be less difficult because of a significant decrease in vascularization and tumor size. In addition some patients had no residual disease.

We therefore concluded that reductive surgery should be done after chemotherapy because: A.) Some patients could achieve a complete clinical response with drugs only (in this study 39% of all the complete responders). B.) The tumor should be at rest when surgery is performed to allow for adequate recovery time without the development of new metastases. C.) Chemotherapy by decreasing tumor size and vascularization may facilitate surgery. Surgery should not be delayed because fibrosis occurs and resections of residual lesions may become very difficult. The optimum time in our opinion is after 2 to 3 months of chemotherapy.

We have previously reported on the benign transformation of malignant testicular tumors after chemotherapy. (1-5) In this study, 24 patients who initially had embryonal carcinomas or/and teratocarcinomas showed a partial or complete transformation into histologically benign teratoma. Two explanations are possible for this phenomenon: A.) Chemotherapy destroys only the immature malignant cells, leaving intact the mature benign cells. B.) Chemotherapy by altering cell kinetics pushes the totipotential malignant cell toward differentiation into mature teratoma. Several facts seem to indicate that the second hypothesis is the most probable. Some patients had initially embryonal cell carcinoma in which it was not possible to find mature cells. Therefore the possibility of destroying only the mature cells sparing the well differentiated cells could not occur. (One of such patients had a large pelvic mass which was initially excised showing only embryonal cells. After 45 days of chemotherapy the mass reoccured and was reexcised. It was composed entirely of mature teratoma.)

This second hypothesis appears also to be in agreement with the totipotential germ cell theory of Dixon and Moore. (6) In addition the same phenomenon occurs spontaneously in this tumor (7) and in others. (Neuroblastoma) (8-9)

Some investigators will object to the "benign" denomination because "benign" metastases have been observed. This observation does not contradict our interpretation of the phenomenon and can be explained as follows. Totipotential malignant cells metastasize and become transformed after the metastatic process has transformed into histologically benign mature teratoma. In our previous experience we have seen that such mature teratomas do not respond to chemotherapy or/and radiotherapy and that they grow and invade locally. They become clinically malignant as they destroy neighboring organs. (Two of our patients died. One of benign teratomatosis of the abdomen with invasion of the liver and pancreas and the other of "benign" mediastinal teratomatosis invading lungs and heart.)

Therefore mature teratomas should be excised surgically at a time when they are still small. In our experience, benign transformation occurs in 2 to 3 months of chemotherapy, surgery should be performed at that time.

The prognostic meaning of benign transformation into mature teratoma is excellent and all the patients in our series who displayed such a transformation and underwent surgery achieved and remained in complete clinical remission.

It is interesting to speculate on which drug has the ability to produce such a transformation. Chronologically we have observed this phenomenon since we started to use large doses of Bleomycin. There is also experimental evidence that Bleomycin can transform"in vitro"malignant Friend leukemic cells into benign cells. (10)

Therefore Bleomycin may play an important role in this transformation"in vivo." Other drugs probably also have the same action. (We have also observed such a transformation after radiotherapy.)

Previously we combined Cis-Platinum with Bleomycin, Vinblastine and Actinomycin D. The therapeutic results were good but severe mylodepression was observed. When we used Bleomycin in single bolus IV injections , we observed severe mucositis, fever and several cases of lung fibrosis. As a result treatments had to be interupted during long periods of time during which the tumor grew and spread, (2 patients).

It became apparent that serious toxicity should be avoided during the induction period of the chemotherapy in order to obtain, without delays a complete clinical remission. We therefore decided to modify our protocol and combine the drugs in a way that could minimize toxicity and maximize therapeutic efficacy.

We replaced Vinblastine by Vincristine to avoid myelodepression. We used Bleomycin in slow infusion (5 hours) combined to Prednisone to avoid fever and mucosis and decrease lung fibrosis. Cis-Platinum was used in slow infusion with Mannitol to decrease renal and auditory toxicity to a minimum by maintaining a low level of circulating Platinum and thus remaining below the toxic tissue threshold. The slow infusion had also the advantage of increasing the half life of the drug and thus (in theory) increased therapeutic effectiveness. Mannitol by reversing the osmotic gradient in the renal tubules (11) blocked reabsorption of Na, water and Cis-Platinum contained in the glomerular filtrate, inhibiting the penetration of Cis-Platinum into the tubular cells and therefore preventing renal toxicity. As the result of these modifications we observed no more mylodepression, no more lung fibrosis and minimal renal and auditory toxicity.

The therapeutic efficacy of this combination appears to be comparable to other regimes which are much more toxic. (12)

IN CONCLUSION

We have developed a systematic approach to the treatment of advanced non seminomatous testicular tumors. This approach is based on the careful integration of multimodal therapies, requiring a precise evaluation of each patient and an individualization of the therapeutic problems to solve.

The inappropriate use of an inadequate therapy at the wrong time may destroy the only chance of cure for these patients.

REFERENCES

1. Merrin, C., Takita, H., Weber, R., Wajsman, Z., Baumgartner, G.,
   Murphy, G.
   Combination Radical Surgery and Multiple Sequential Chemotherapy
   for the Treatment of Advanced Carcinoma of the Testes (Stage III)
   Cancer 37 1 Jan 1976 20-29

2. Merrin, C., Takita, H.
   Cancer Reductive Surgery - Report on the Simultaneous Excision of
   Abdominal and Thoracic Metastases From Widespread Testicular Tumor
   Cancer 42 #2 August 1978 495-501

3. Takita, H., Merrin, C., Didolkar, M., Douglass, H., Edgerton, F.
   The Surgical Management of Multiple Lung Metastases
   Annals of Thoracic Surgery 24 #4 Oct 1977 359-364

4. Carter, S.K., Soper, W.T.
   Integration of Chemotherapy with Combined Modality Treatment of
   Solid Tumors
   Cancer Treatment Rev 1: 1-13 1974

5. Merrin, C., Baumgartner, J., Wajsman, Z.
   Benign Transformation of Testicular Carcinoma by Chemotherapy
   (letter)
   Lancet 1:43 1975

6. Dixon, F.J., Moore, R.A.
   Tumors of the Male Sex Organs
   "Atlas of Tumors Pathology" Vol 8 Washington D.C. Armed Forces
   Institute of Pathology 1952 31b-32

7. Willis, G.W., Hajdu, S.I.
   Histologically Benign Teratoid Metastases of Testicular Embryonal
   Carcinoma - Report in Five Cases
   Am. J. Clin. Pathol. 59 338-342 1973

8. Cole, W.H., Emerson, T.C.
   Spontaneous Regression of Cancer
   Philadelphia W.B. Saunders 1963

9. Cushing, H., Walback, S.B.
   The Transformation of a Malignant Sympathicoblastoma into Benign
   Ganglioneuroma
   Am. J. Pathol. 3: 203 1927

10. Sugano, H., Funisawa, M., Kawaguchii, T., Ikawa, Y.
    Enhancement of Erythrocytic Maturation of Friend Virus Induced
    Leukemia Cells "In Vitro"
    Unifying Concepts of Leukemia
    Bilb. Haemat #39 Editors R.M. Dutcher, L. Chieco-Bianchi 943-954
    Karger Publis. Basel 1973

11. Berger, E.Y., Farber, S.J., Earle, D.P.
    Renal Excretion of Mannitol
    Proc Soc Exp Biol Med 66:62 1947

12. Einhorn, L.H., Donohue, J.P.
    Chemotherapy for Disseminated Testicular Cancer
    Urol. Clin. N. Amer. 4:407 1977

18 NEW LEADS FROM THE LABORATORY FOR TREATING TESTICULAR CANCER

D. D. von Hoff

Introduction

As demonstrated elsewhere in this volume there have been great accomplishments in the treatment of even patients with advanced testicular cancer particularly in terms of disease free survival. However, there are still a few patients who fail induction therapy and some who relapse despite an early remission. For the 40% of patients who do not go into or remain in remission additional therapy is needed. Perhaps the laboratory has a few clues which might be used in the future for treatment of testicular cancer. In this paper we will cover the following points. First, a few little known facts about testicular cancer models will be presented. Next, one particular system, the human tumor stem cell assay system (1-4) will be discussed including the methodology of the system and confirmatory evidence which proves tumor is growing rather than fibroblasts. Finally, some clinical applications of the system will be discussed with a particular emphasis on testicular cancer.

Testicular Cancer Models

Testicular cancer is a relatively rare tumor in man affecting 2.2 males per 100,000. Therefore, to study the tumor a good laboratory model is needed. Table 1 lists some of the available laboratory models.

Supported in part by BRSG grant 507 BR-5654 awarded by Biochemical Research Support Grant Program. Division of Research Resources. National Institutes of Health and American Cancer Society Institutional Grant, IN. 116 B.

Table 1: Laboratory Models for Testicular Cancer

1. Experimental teratoma in the fowl induced by zinc or copper

2. Teratocarcinoma cell lines from mice

3. Human embryonal carcinoma transplanted to cheek pouch of cortisone treated golden hamster

4. Human testicular cancer Xenograft in nude mice

5. Large animal models
   Swine (crypotochid testis-autosomal recessive)
   Horse (heavy horses)
   Dog (boxer most frequent)

The first model devised was the experimental teratoma in the fowl (rooster or duck). Teratomas could be induced in the testes of domestic fowls by injecting metal salts of zinc or copper. The induction of teratomas was only possible during the seasonal gonadal growth that occurs during the late winter and early spring months (5). This model is of extreme interest when one remembers that when patients are treated with platinum-containing combinations there are occasional reversions of the tumors to benign teratomas. It would be interesting to see if cis-platinum would induce teratomas in the testes of domestic fowls. The mechanism of teratoma induction in the fowl by the zinc and copper is not known.

Cell lines of teratocarcinomas derived from mice have been a favorite model to study differentiation of that tumor type but have as yet not been relevant to the human situation.

Human testicular tumor transplanted into the cheek pouch of the hamster or as a xenograft in nude mice have been developed. The nude mouse xenograft was only recently reported by Lee, Giovanella and coworkers (6) and was reported to regress with treatment by high dose thymidine. These results need to be confirmed.

There are at least three large animal models for testicular cancer. The swine is a good animal because the cryptorchid testes is autosomally recessively inherited (7). Big heavy horses have a very high incidence of testicular cancer but are hard to keep in the lab . Of all of the dogs the boxer has the highest incidence of testicular cancer (8, 9). One can see that the ideal laboratory model for studying testicular cancer has not yet been found.

Human Tumor Stem Cell Assay System

The human tumor stem cell assay system is an in vitro soft agar technique developed by Hamburger and Salmon (1, 2) which purportedly allows growth of human tumor progenitor or stem cells. This in vitro system has the potential for helping select the appropriate chemotherapy for an individual patients tumor much like the method we now have for choosing an antibiotic for a particular infection. Briefly the methodology we used is as follows: A single cell suspension is made from the malignant effusion, marrow or solid tumor and this suspension is incubated with and without various drugs at clinically achievable concentrations for one hour at 37° centigrade. The cells are then washed twice to remove the drug and are then resuspended in CMRL 1066 enriched media. Agar is added to the cells in the media and the mixture is placed as a top layer over an underlayer of McCoys 5A media plus agar. The plates are incubated in a 7% CO_2 atmosphere and examined for colony growth at weekly intervals. This method is essentially the same as that described by Drs. Hamburger and Salmon (1, 2, 3), except we have not used conditioned media in the bottom layer of agar (4).

As shown in figure 1, multiple colonies grow in the culture plates by day 10 - 15. These colonies are counted on a counting grid. Colony counts on drug-treated plates are compared to control plate counts (not exposed to drugs) and the percent of colonies surviving can be calculated.

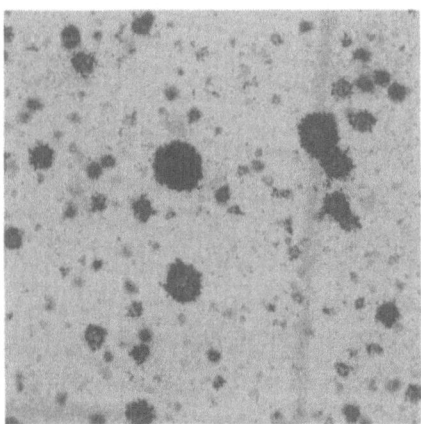

Figure 1: Human testicular cancer colonies growing in soft agar culture. Day 12 of culture (30 x inverted microscope).

Our first years experience with the more common tumor types is summarized in Table 2.

Table 2: Growth of Tumor Stem Cell Colonies
From Various Human Neoplasms

Type of Tumor	Number of Patients With + Cultures/Total Tested
Ovarian	54/70
Neuroblastoma	42/52
Breast	14/19
Melanoma	20/32
Colorectal	14/20
Lung Cancer	
Oat	22/28
Squamous	24/26
Adenocarcinoma	22/24
Head and Neck	14/32
Testicular	15/21
Multiple Myeloma	6/10
Osteogenic Sarcoma	6/10
Rhabdomyosarcoma	6/12
Endometrial	6/6
Pancreatic	3/3
Cervical	6/6
Ewings Sarcoma	4/4
Renal	4/6
Hepatoma	4/4
Prostate	6/10
Thyroid	2/4
Wilms	1/2
Normal Marrow	0/38

We now have over 510 specimen cultures. The most extensive experience is with ovarian cancer where 54 of 70 tumors have formed colonies in culture. Neuroblastoma has grown exceptionally well and breast cancer, melanoma, colorectal, lung cancer and head and neck cancer can be grown in a respectable percentage of cases.

We have limited but encouraging experience with testicular cancer where 15 of 21 tumors cultured have formed colonies in the soft agar culture system. In summary, of 510 tumors put into culture 372 of the tumors formed colonies. The overall percent of tumors which formed colonies in culture was 73%.

Confirmational Studies That Tumor is Growing

One major problem is to prove the colonies growing in culture are indeed tumor cell colonies and not just fibroblasts or granulocyte macrophage colonies. Confirmational studies to prove the colonies are malignant and representative of the tumor in the patient include histologic studies, a search for tumor markers, chromosomal analysis or injection of cells from the colonies into nude mice to see if tumors would develop in the mice.

Light and electron microscopy studies of colonies growing from testicular cancer specimens have shown pictures consistent with epithelial tumors. Pathologists could not specifically say these tumor cells were testicular in origin. This information led to looking for tumor markers. Testicular cancer is ideal because it frequently secretes tumor markers. The first marker looked for was the Beta subunit of Human Chorionic Gonadotropin (HCG) (See figure 2). A choriocarcinoma which was secreting HCG in the patient was cultured in soft agar and the levels of HCG rose with time as compared to a control plate growing ovarian cancer.

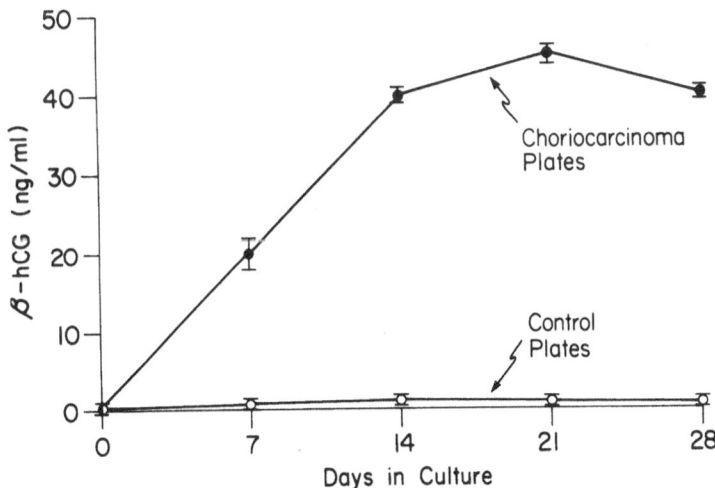

Figure 2: Levels of βHCG in culture plates growing colonies of choriocarcinoma of the testis . Note increasing levels with increasing time in culture.

A similar experiment with an embryonal carcinoma specimen which was secreting alph-feto protein in the patient showed increasing levels of that marker in the culture plate with time in cultures. (See figure 3)

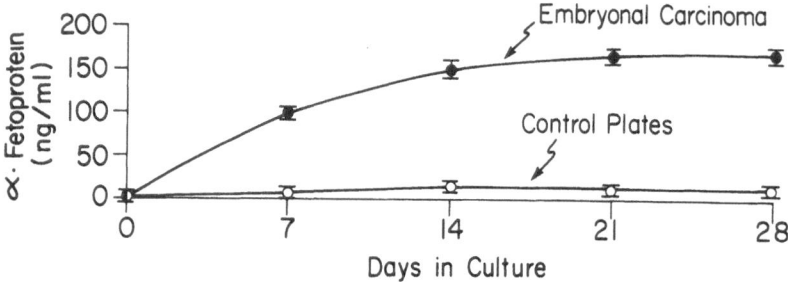

Figure 3: Levels of alpha-feto protein in culture plates growing embryonal cell carcinoma of the testis.

Both of these markers are consistent with the tumor "breeding true" in the culture plate since the blood from each of these patients contained elevated HCG levels and alpha seto progein levels respectively. This marker secretion has been well documented for other tumors growing in the human tumor stem cell assay system (4).

Early chromosomal studies on metaphase spreads of cells from the testicular cancer colonies have demonstrated modal chromosome counts of 52-58 suggesting the cells in the colony are malignant. When 200 of the testicular cancer colonies are injected into one nude mouse a tumor did not form after 4-5 weeks. This work is being repeated.

Overall, then we feel these histology, markers, and chromosome studies offer some confirmatory evidence that the cells growing in the plate are similar to the tumor cells growing in the patients.

Clinical Applications of Stem Cell System

To date a number of clinical applications of the stem cell system have been attempted. These will be covered with particular emphasis on testicular cancer. Certainly the most important aspect of the system is to try to find out if it is truly predictive for response of an individual patient's tumor to chemotherapy. To obtain drug sensitivity information all one does is count the number of colonies that appear on control plates and compare this to the number of colonies that survive on drug treated plates. With these two numbers the percent of tumor kill by the drug can be calculated.

Over the past six months we have cultured 415 patients' tumors. Only 105 of the tumors had enough cells in the specimen to perform drug sensitivity tests. Two-thirds of the patients had failed prior chemotherapy and one-third had had no prior chemotherapy.

In these 105 patients there were 151 times the drugs tried in the plate were tried in the patient. Seven times we said the tumor was sensitive to a drug in the plate and the patient responded to that drug (these were true positive). There were eight times the tumor was sensitive in the plate but the patient did not respond. Three times the patient's tumor was resistant in the plate but the patient responded (these were false negatives) and 133 times the tumor was resistant in the plate and the patient did not respond (true negative. (See Table 3)

Table 3: In Vitro-In Vivo Correlations

No. of Patients	Sensitive In Vitro and In Vivo	Sensitive In Vitro/ Resistant In Vivo	Resistant In Vitro/ Sensitive In Vivo	Resistant In Vitro and In Vivo	No. of Corre- lations
105	7	8*	3+	133	151

*False positives
+False negative

In summary, the accuracy for a positive prediction (sensitivity) by the system was 0.7 while the accuracy for a negative prediction (specificity) was 0.94.

With testicular cancer growing in the stem cell system we find the following: Twenty-one testicular cancer specimens have been received. Fifteen of the specimens have formed colonies in culture. Plating efficiencies (# of colonies/# of nucleated cells plated) ranged from 0.008 to 0.01% (median 0.01). Overall, 71% of the testicular cancer specimens received formed colonies in soft agar. With the exception of one malignant ascites specimen, all specimens received were solid tumors. As far as chemosensitivity studies on these specimens 12 of the 15 specimens which grew had enough cells provided in the original specimen to do drug sensitivities. Eight of the patients were previously untreated while four had failed primary 3 - 6 drug chemotherapy.
As can be seen in Table 4 the tumors were sensitive (sensitivity defined as equal to or greater than a 70% kill of colonies) to a number of the drugs clinically.

Table 4: Chemosensitivity of 12 Testicular Cancers
in Human Tumor Stem Cell Assay

Drug tested	No. of times sensitive* in vitro/ No. of times tested
Cisplatinum	5/9
Vinblastine	4/9
Bleomycin	3/9
Adriamycin	1/9
Actinomycin D	4/9
Chlorambucil	3/9
VP-16	2/6
Dihydroxyanthracenedione	1/6
Diglycoaldehyde	1/2
m-AMSA	0/2
Methyl GAG	0/2
Interferon (human leukocyte)	0/2

*sensitive is defined as ≥70% decrease in number of
colonies

Because of small numbers of tumor specimens we have not had a great deal of opportunity to investigate new agents. However, the new drug anthracenedione with which we have just completed a phase I trial showed some activity as did diglycoaldehyde a purine nucleoside derivative which has been temporarily shelved because of renal toxicity even though there was a complete remission noted in a patient with seminoma in the phase I trial with the drug. The stem cell system is ideal for looking at both new and old agents without having to perform the phase II trials in the patients. There are increasingly fewer patients and with expensive drugs like interferon the leads can be obtained in vitro before committing patients and funds to a phase II trial.

Conclusions

In conclusion, there is a paucity of experimental models for testicular carcinoma. We have demonstrated that testicular carcinoma will form colonies in the human tumor stem cell assay system. Histology, tumor markers, and karyology support the concept the human tumor stem cell assay system reflects the in vivo situation.

The human tumor stem cell assay can be used to: (1) determine the chemosensitivity of an individual patient's tumor, (2) to screen for new agents active in testicular cancer, and (3) to study the biology of radioresistance and differentiation of testicular cancer.

REFERENCES

1. Hamburger, A.W., and Salmon, S.E. Primary bioassay of human tumor stem cells. Science 197: 461-463, 1977.

2. Hamburger, A.W., and Salmon, S.E. Primary bioassay of human myeloma stem cells. J Clin Invest 60: 846-854, 1977.

3. Salmon, S.E., Hamburger, A.W., Soehnlen, B., Durie, B.G., Alberts, D.S., Moon, T.E. Quantitation of differential sensitivity of human-tumor stem cells to anticancer drugs. N Engl J Med 298: 1321-1327, 1978.

4. Von Hoff, D.D., Johnson, G.E. Secretion of tumor markers in the human tumor stem cell assay system. Proc Am Assoc Cancer Res and ASCO 22: 51, 1979.

5. Falin, L.T. Experimental teratoma testis in the fowl. Am J Cancer 38: 199-211, 1979.

6. Lee, S.S., Giovanella, B.C., Stehlin, J.S., Brunn J.C. Regression of established human tumors in nude mice induced by continuous infusion of thymidine (TdR). Proc Am Assoc Cancer Res 19: 103, 1978.

7. Cotchin, P. Spontaneous tumors in young animals. Proc Roy Soc Med 68: 653-655, 1975.

8. Brudey, R.S. Canine and feline neoplasmas. Advances in Veterinary Science and Comparative Medicine 14: 309-354, 1970.

9. Pendergress, T.W., Hayes, H.C. Cryptorchism and related defects in dogs: Epidemiologic comparisons with man. Teratology 12: 51-55, 1975.

19 NEW DRUGS IN THE TREATMENT OF TESTICULAR CANCER

F. M. Muggia

The chemotherapy of testicular cancer has undergone
substantial changes in the past few years (1) and an entire new set of questions regarding the management of these
patients has been introduced. During the 1960s limited
(about 10%) long-term success was achieved with the triple
therapy introduced by Li (2) and its various modifications
(1). Samuels in the 1970s introduced combinations of
Vinblastine (V) and Bleomycin (B) that proved to be considerably more effective (3). The addition of cisplatin
(P) to this latter regimen increased even further the
efficacy of chemotherapy in advanced germ cell tumors
(4). This PVB combination first reported by Einhorn and
Donohue (4), and the VAB series, which have also included
cyclophosphamide and actinomycin D (A) during induction,
developed independently by Golbey and co-workers (5)
have become established as the standard regimens for testicular cancer of the non-seminomatous type. All other
treatments must be compared in efficacy to these regimens
which have had wide clinical application. Seminomas are
also, according to the experience of Einhorn (6), sensitive
to the PVB regimen. In spite of the therapeutic successes
achieved, the major challenges continue to be failure to
achieve complete remission, (at least in 40% of patients)
and eventual relapse from complete remission, (at least in
20%). In order to improve results, one may consider two
new areas for clinical investigation: 1) integration of
established active drug into current combinations or sequences and 2) search for new agents and/or combinations
effective after progression or following treatment with
the initial chemotherapy. In the same vein, however, it
is important to stress that treatment failures often result from careless follow up permitting the development of
very advanced states, or from poorly applied therapeutic measures. Major inroads can be made now in the

A.T. van Oosterom et al. (eds.), Therapeutic Progress in Ovarian Cancer,
Testicular Cancer and the Sarcomas, pp. 235-246. All rights reserved.
Copyright 1980 by Martinus Nijhoff Publishers, The Hague/Boston/London.

treatment of patients with testicular cancer by proper referral to centers with experience in the management of
this disease.

1. Integration of established active drugs into primary
    combinations

The development of the PVB regimen by Einhorn and
Donohue (4) represents an example of including a new,
active drug, cisplatin, to the most active regimens available at the time - the VB regimens established by Samuels
(3). There is some question, at least raised by the
latter author, whether cisplatin does in fact have .to be
added in all circumstances of disseminated testicular
carcinoma. Samuels has expressed a preference for using
VB alone in circumstances where it is nearly always successful (7). Most researchers, however, believe that the
major current questions to be asked in studies evaluating
chemotherapy are: 1) What dosage of cisplatin is optimal?
2) How many courses of cisplatin-containing regimens must
be given? 3) What drugs should be added as maintenance or
consolidation? Table 1 indicates how studies by institutions and cooperative groups have raised and attempted to
answer some of these questions. Finally, Adriamycin and
more recently VP-16-213 have been added to the basic VPB
regimen (with some reduction in Vinblastine dosage) in a
randomized study and in pilot protocol, respectively. The
VAB series based on studies by Golbey and co-workers have
addressed very much the same issues, i.e. the optimal
amount of cisplatin. However new drugs cannot be easily
incorporated into this regimen, since it already contains
5 drugs during induction and an additional two during the
maintenance phase.

The testing of VP-16-213 is based on relatively
scanty data, but nevertheless reporting a high response
rate in a small number of patients (16,17,18). Preliminary experience of this drug in combinations which include
all induction drugs of the PVB regimen except Vinblastine

TABLE 1

TESTICULAR CANCER:

EVOLUTION OF THREE CHEMOTHERAPEUTIC STRATEGIES

Study Group (Ref.)	Acronym	Description and Comments
A. Samuels et al (7) M.D. Anderson	VB-1	V 0.4 mg/kg total d 1 + 2 monthly
		B 30 u im biw x 10
	VB-2	B given by infusion preceding V
	VB-3	B given after V ; some higher V dose
	VB-3 + P	Adds P 100 mg/m^2 x 3
Einhorn (4) Indiana	VB-1 + P	See below: PVB regimen
Swiss group (8)	VB/AP	Modified VB-3 followed by AP x 2 courses 60 mg/m^2 each
Seeber et al (9) Essen	VB/AP versus AP/VB	Randomized study of above
B. Einhorn (10) and SEG 78G4240	PVB versus modified PVB and PVB + A	See above: VB-1 + P x 3 courses V decreased to 0.3 mg/kg V decreased to 0.2 mg/kg A; 50 mg/m^2
Samson SWOG (11) 7610	VBP	Modified PVB, P 15 mg/m^2 x 5 maintenance Cb-AcD/V
Samson SWOG (11) 7817	VB low P versus VB-high P	Maintenance C-ActD/A/V
PAHO/NCI ARG 78-06	VBP + VP 16-213	Adds VP16 60 mg/m^2 d 15,17,19 of every 4 week cycle
C. Memorial (12) Sloan Kettering Cancer Center (13)	VAB-I VAB-II VAB-III VAB-IV	V, Act D, and B C and P added, latter at 40 mg/m^2 B by infusion, P at 120 mg/m^2 maintenance Cb-Act D/Cb-A + low P P intensified
Merrin (14) Roswell Park	Modified VAB-II	Includes Prednisone, Vincristine
DeWys (15) ECOG 1877	Modified VAB-III	Randomizes low P (40 m^2) d 1 + versus high P (120/m^2) d 1

Abbreviations: V = Vinblastine P = Cisplatin Cb = Chlorambucil
B = Bleomycin   C = Cyclophosphamide
Act D = Dactinomycin   SEG = Southeastern Group
ECOG = Eastern Cooperative Oncology Group
SWOG = Southwestern Oncology Group
PAHO = Pan American Health Organization

indicates a very favorable response rate for those patients
which have received such treatment after relapsing on the
Vinblastine maintenance phase.

Adriamycin has better established effectiveness as a
single agent (19) and has also formed part of effective
combination regimens (1). Its contribution to current
induction regimens is being evaluated in a randomized
study by the SEG. A preliminary evaluation by Einhorn and
colleagues was not particularly encouraging (10).

Other active agents which could be considered for introduction into the PVB regimen include cyclophosphamide,
dactinomycin or mithramycin. The former two are, in fact,
part of some or all of the VAB regimens. These drugs have
not been demonstrated to impart a greater effectiveness
to this regimen over that of PVB; however, no direct comparison of the two regimens has been carried out. Mithramycin, on the other hand, has a narrow therapeutic index
and is generally regarded as not suitable for combinations.
Nevertheless, one combination including this agent has
reported favorable results in abstract form with 100% responses out of 11 patients; only two, however, manifested
complete remissions (20).

Finally, it is important to note that the PVB regimen
may be almost 100% effective in achieving cures in the
presence of low tumor burdens. The Indiana experience with
this regimen in patients with surgically-staged Stages I
and II who relapsed during follow up with monthly X-rays
and markers has been universally favorable, although longer
follow up is needed to know whether all patients rendered
disease-free with PVB will remain so (21). This and other
experience point out, however, that "debulking" with surgery or with radiotherapy must be considered as alternatives to the testing of more complex combination schemes.
Such alternatives must be considered in patients presenting
with high tumor burden since their failure rate on chemotherapy remains considerable.

2. Search for new agents

The search for new active drugs logically proceeds in patients who have failed the primary combinations. Table 2 indicates those regimens in use upon treatment failure. The activity of cisplatin was easily recognized under these circumstances. It is more difficult to interpret results obtained with combinations administered upon failure of maintenance programs and which also include some or all of the drugs given during the induction phase.

TABLE 2

TESTICULAR CANCER: CHEMOTHERAPY FOR FAILURE OF INDUCTION

Drug	Preceding Regimen	Comments (Ref.)
Cisplatin	Various	60% response, pooled series (16)
B-COMF	VB-1	Also used as consolidation (7)
VP 16-213 versus Ifosfamide	VB/AP or AP/VB	Ongoing study by Seeber et al (9)
P + A + VP 16-213 + B	V after PVB induction	Ongoing study by Indiana (16), SEG (16)

Abbreviations: see Table 1
O = Vincristine (Oncovin) F = 5-Fluorouracil

As previously noted, before investigative chemotherapy treatment is initiated, one must consider: 1) surgical resection of metastatic foci and 2) treatment with different dose-schedules of agents already utilized during induction. Some have, in fact, expressed the conviction that cisplatin at higher doses may be effective when lower doses have failed. However, when one repeats a course of chemotherapy with a combination of agents to which partial resistance has been demonstrable, one risks that the result may be excessive toxicity without dramatic therapeutic gains.

Data with new single agents is not available and extensive data on single agents as was obtained in the past is unlikely to be obtained except through coordinated efforts involving major Cancer Centers and Cooperative groups. Agents which have been considered of established value must also be reassessed in the context of current new drug trials; that is, following failure of multiple drug chemotherapy. Such agents could include alkylating drugs in non-seminomatous tumors, 5-Fluorouracil, actinomycin D and mithramycin, particularly following failure of PVB. A master protocol design for single agent drug testing in testicular cancer is being adopted by the EORTC as has been done for other diseases where induction chemotherapy is quite effective, but where data on new agents may be productive and therefore must be efficiently sought. The master protocol format ensures a standard for eligibility criteria and assessment of response that imparts a certain measured reliability to the data accrued. Relevant prognostic factors to be considered in protocols for new drug evaluation are shown in Table 3.

TABLE 3

TESTICULAR CANCER: PROGNOSTIC FACTORS IN NEW DRUG EVALUATION

1. Histologic type (seminoma, embryonal, terato-, chorio-, mixed)

2. Prior radiotherapy

3. Classification of bulk disease (minimal or major pulmonary, abdominal)

4. Liver versus no liver involvement

5. CNS versus no CNS involvement

6. Markers (hCG, AFP, LDH)

The following must be considered for investigation in disseminated testicular cancer when other measures fail:

A. Alteration in dose schedules of established drugs.
One must consider the efficacy of certain drugs, such as
adriamycin, when given by continuous infusion. Exploration of high doses of cisplatin has been mentioned as a
logical step when lower doses fail. Intravenous melphalan
is another possible agent to consider. Moderate dose
methotrexate with folinic acid rescue, on the other hand,
has been used in combination, with little success (22).

B. Analogs of established drugs. Ifosfamide has been
effective alone and in combinations in testicular cancer
(23). Analogs of cisplatin are of highest priority for
future testing. Only the malonato 1,2 diaminocyclohexane
derivative is currently actively receiving clinical trial
(24). Interest in this compound has been heightened by
objective regression in two instances of cisplatin-resis-
tant germ cell tumors. Analogs of anthracyclines present
other interesting possibilities, as does the new bleomycin,
pepleomycin and the new vinca alkaloid, vindesine (25).
Some activity was reported with this agent, although
comparative data relative to vinblastine will be required
to advance this drug further in the management of testicular cancer. Similarly, with other analogs lack of absolute
cross-resistance, comparative efficacy data, or distinct
indication of amelioration of toxicities will be required
to integrate them into current treatment regimens.

C. Other potential drugs for investigation. The activity
of methotrexate in gestational choriocarcinoma and to a
lesser extent in other germ cell tumors, makes other dihydrofolate reductase inhibitors such as Baker's antifol
and DDMP of potential interest. The glutamine antagonist,
diazo-oxo-norleucine (DON), had already shown activity
in choriocarcinoma during early clinical experience and is
currently being restudied (26). The DNA-intercalating
agents, m-AMSA and the anthracenediones, represent other
drugs that need testing. A number of drugs with activity
in other tumor types such as hexamethylmelamine and the

hexitol, dibromodulcitol, are other logical targets for
study. Gallium nitrate is also of interest because of
the activity of other metallic compounds such as platinum.
Table 4 summarizes the type of drugs which are considered
highest priority for investigation in testicular cancer.

TABLE 4

TESTICULAR CANCER: CATEGORIES OF NEW DRUGS FOR EVALUATION

I. Established Drugs, New Dose Schedules
    cisplatin, high dose (> 100 mg/m^2)
    adriamycin, continuous infusion
    melphalan, iv
    vinblastine, continuous infusion

II. Analogs of Established Drugs
    ifosfamide
    malonate 1,2 diaminocyclohexane-platinum
    aclacinomycin A; AD-32
    pepleomycin
    vindesine

III. Miscellaneous Investigational Drugs
    Baker's antifol; DDMP
    diazo-oxo-norleucine
    hexamethylmelamine
    dibromodulcitol
    gallium nitrate
    m-AMSA

Finally, it is important to reemphasize the value of
testing new drugs even in diseases where chemotherapy is
relatively successful and few patients enter Phase II
(efficacy) investigational trials. The observation of a
dramatic regression in a patient with testicular cancer
kindled the interest in cisplatin (1). Such patient would
not have been eligible for treatment if one were to re-
strict drug testing to specific diseases as designated
by the "clinical panel" (cancer of breast, colon, lung,
melanoma, leukemia and lymphoma) of the Division of Cancer
Treatment (27). In diseases of relatively low prevalence
such as, testicular cancer, suitable new drugs for testing
might be selected by giving priority to otherwise active
drugs and/or supplemented by drug sensitivity assays as
illustrated by Salmon and Von Hoff elsewhere in this
volume.

REFERENCES

1. Jacobs, E.M., Muggia, F.M., and Rozencweig, M. Chemotherapy of testicular cancer: from Palliation to curative adjuvant therapy. Sem. Oncol. 6: 3-13, 1979.

2. Li, M.C., Whitmore, W.F. Jr., Golbey, R.B., Grabstal, H. Effects of combined drug therapy in metastatic carcinoma of the testis. JAMA 174: 1291-1299, 1960.

3. Samuels, M.L., Johnson, D.E. and Holoye, P.Y. Continuous intravenous bleomycin (NSC 125066) therapy with vinblastine (NSC 49842) in state III testicular neoplasia. Cancer Treat. Rep. 59: 563-570, 1975.

4. Einhorn, L.H., and Donohue, J.P. Cis-diammine-dichloroplatinum, vinblastine, and bleomycin combination chemotherapy in disseminated testicular cancer. Ann. Intern. Med. 87: 293-298, 1977.

5. Cheng, E., Cvitkovic, E., Wittes, R., et al.: Germ cell tumors. II. VAB II in metastatic testicular cancer. Cancer 42: 2162-2168, 1978.

6. Einhorn, L.H. Chemotherapy of metastatic seminoma. Proc. AACR and ASCO 20 (Abstract 24), 1979.

7. Samuels, M.L., Johnson, D.E., Brown, B., Bracken, R.B., Moran, M.E. and Von Eschenbach, A.: Velban plus continuous infusion bleomycin (V-3) in stage III advanced testicular cancer: results in 99 patients with a note on high-dose velban and sequential cis-platinum. in: Cancer of the Genitourinary Tract.D.E. Johnson and M.L. Samuels (eds) Raven Press, New York, 1979.

8. Sonntag, R.W., Senn, H.J. and Cavalli, F.: Treatment of metastatic non-seminomatous testicular cancer: a preliminary report of induction chemotherapy followed by maintenance chemotherapy or radiotherapy. Cancer Treat. Rep. 63: 1669-1674, 1979.

9. Seeber, S., et al. Testicular cancer. In: current status and new developments with Cis-platin, edited by S. T. Crooke and S.K. Carter, Academic Press, 1980.

10. Einhorn, L.H., and Williams, J.D. Cis-diammine dichloroplatinum (P) + Vinblastine (V) + Bleomycin (B) + Adriamycin (A) in disseminated testicular cancer. Proc. AACR and ASCO 20 (Abstract C-19), 1979.

11. Samson, M.K., Stephens, R.L., Rivkin, S., Opipari, M., Maloney, T., Groppe, C.W., Fisher, R. Vinblastine, Bleomycin and cis-diamminedichloroplatinum (II) in disseminated testicular cancer: preliminary report of a Southwest Oncology Group Study. Cancer Treat. Rep. 63, 1663-1668, 1979.

12. Muggia, F.M. and Jacobs, E.M. Chemotherapy of testicular cancer: impact on curability. In: Advances in Cancer Chemotherapy. Umezawa, H. et al. (eds.) Japan Science Society Press, Tokyo, University Park Press, Baltimore, pp. 437-452, 1978.

13. Cvitkovic, E., Cheng, E., Whitmore, W. et al. Germ cell tumor chemotherapy update. Proc. AACR and ASCO (Abstract 18) 324, 1977.

14. Merrin, C. Multimodal treatment of advanced testicular tumor with cis-diamminedichloroplatinum (CPDD), bleomycin (Bloe), vinblastine (VLB), vincristine (VCC), and actinomycin D (Act D). Proc. AACR and ASCO 18: 298, 1977.

15. DeWys, W., Begg, C., Slayton, R., Hahn, R.G. and Brodsky, I. Chemotherapy for advanced germinal cell neoplasms. Preliminary report of an Eastern Coop. Group Study. Cancer Treat. Rep. 63, 1675-1680, 1979.

16. Williams, S.D., Einhorn, L.H., Greco, A., Oldham, R., Fletcher, R., and Bond, W.H. VP 16-213: An active drug in germinal neoplasms. Proc. AACR and ASCO 20 (Abstract 29), 1979.

17. EORTC Clinical Screening Group. Epipodophyllotoxin VP-16-213 in the treatment of acute leukemias, hematosarcomas and solid tumors. Brit. Med. J. 3:199-202, 1973.

18. Newlands, E.S. and Bagshawe, K.D. Epipodophyllin derivative (VP 16-213) in malignant teratomas and choriocarcinomas. Lancet ii:87, 1977.

19. Monfardini, S., Bajetta, E., Musemeci, C. Clinical use of adriamycin in advanced testicular cancer. J. Urol. 109:293-298, 1972.

20. Israel, L., DePierre, A. and Aguilera, J. Treatment of the polmonary metastases of testicular cancers by a combination of platinum diammine dichloride (PD), mithramycin (MTM), vinblastine (VLB) and bleomycin (BLM). Cancer Immunology and Immunotherapy 3:28, 1977 (suppl).

21. Einhorn, L.H. and Donohue, J. Adjuvant chemotherapy for testicular cancer: Is it necessary? In: Adjuvant Therapy of Cancer II. S.E. Jones and S.E. Salmon (eds.) Grune and Stratton, pp. 329-335, 1979.

22. McElwain, J.J. and Peckham, M.J. Combination chemotherapy for testicular tumours. Proc. Roy. Soc. Med. 67:297-300, 1974.

23. Schmoll, H.J., Rhomberg, W. and Diehl, V. Ifosfamide (NSC 109724) activity in testicular cancer: mono and combination chemotherapy. Abstracts of 10th International Congress on Chemotherapy, Zurich (Abstract 556), 1977.

24. Muggia, F.M., Wolpert, M.K., Ribaud, P. and Mathe, G. Clinical results with cisplatin analogs. In current status and new developments with cis-platin. Ed:S.T. Crooke and S.K. Carter. Academic Press, 1980.

25. Reynolds, T.F., Vugrin, D., Cvitkovic, E., Gralla, R.J., Young, C.W. and Golbey, R.B. Phase II trial of vindesine in patients with germ-cell tumors. Cancer Treat. Rep. 83:1399-1408, 1979.

26. Muggia, F.M., Catane, R., Douros, J. and Cooney, D. Amino acid manipulations in cancer treatment: a perspective from the NCI workshop. Cancer Treat. Rep. 63:1137-1138, 1979.

27. Muggia, F.M. Rozencweig, M., Chiuten, D.F., et al. Phase II trials: use of a clinical tumor panel and overview of current resources and studies. Cancer Treat. Rep. (to be published).

20 AN UPDATE OF THE DUTCH MULTICENTER PVB-STUDY IN DISSEMINATED TESTICULAR NON-SEMINOMAS

G. Stoter, C. P. J. Vendrik, A. Struyvenberg, Th. M. Brouwers, D. Th. Sleyfer, H. Schraffordt Koops, A. T. van Oosterom and H. M. Pinedo

Since 1976, 71 patients with disseminated testicular non-seminomas have been treated with combination chemotherapy comprising Cis-platinum, Vinblastine and Bleomycin, according to Einhorn[1], usually comprising 4 cycles.
This series includes 40 patients previously reported[2].
Forty-one of 71 patients (58%) achieved a complete remission.

Table 1
Results of the chemotherapy according to the histology

Histology[+]	patients	CR	PR	Toxic Death	Progres
TD	1	-	1	-	-
MTI	13	8	5	-	-
MTU	48	29	14	4	1
MTT	9	4	4	-	1
Total	71	41 (58%)	24 (34%)	4	2

[+] TD = Teratoma differentiated;
MTI = Malignant teratoma intermediate;
MTU = Malignant teratoma undifferentiated;
MTT = Malignant teratoma trophoblastic.

One patient achieved a complete remission during the year of maintenance chemotherapy. Four patients were rendered free of disease by surgery after the completion of the remission induction therapy. Thus, a total of 46 patients (65%) has become free of tumor. Of the 41 patients who achieved a complete remission by induction chemotherapy alone, 2 patients subsequently relapsed after a period of 7 and 13 months, respectively.

A.T. van Oosterom et al. (eds.), Therapeutic Progress in Ovarian Cancer, Testicular Cancer and the Sarcomas, pp. 247-252. All rights reserved.
Copyright 1980 by Martinus Nijhoff Publishers, The Hague/Boston/London.

The latter patient developed brain metastases. A third
patient died of a non-therapy related myocardial infarction after a complete remission duration of 6 months.
Thus, 38 of 41 complete responders are still free of disease after a follow up period of 2-40 months (average 16
months, median 18 months).
Twenty-two complete responders are off therapy for a duration of 3-21 months, an average duration of 8 months and
a median duration of 7 months. Twenty-four patients (34%)
achieved a partial remission. Seventeen out of 24 had progression after 3-8 months while 7 are still in partial remission for 2-12$^+$ months. Four of 71 patients (6%) died of
toxicity; two of Bleomycin induced pneumonitis, one of
agranulocytic sepsis and one of myocardial infarction during hemodialysis for renal failure due to Cis-platinum.
Two of 71 patients showed progression of the disease after
an initial response.
In 29 patients the response to treatment has been histologically verified. It was striking to find necrosis and
fibrosis in 11 of these cases. More mature differentiation
of the malignant tumor was found in eleven patients.
The differentiation into teratoma differentiated did not
lead to inclusion in the complete remission status.

Table 2
Histologically verified response to chemotherapy

Type of Surgery	Patients	Normal Archi- tecture	Ne- crosis	Fi- brosis	More mature hist.	progr.
Supraclav.	1	-	-	1	-	-
Thoracotomy	4	1	-	-	3	-
Laparotomy	24	4	4	6	8	2
Total	29	5	4	7	11	2

The side effects of the chemotherapy were markedly more
severe in those patients who had previously been treated
with radiotherapy (table 3).

Table 3
Side effects of the chemother. according to previous ther

	pretreatment		no pretreatment
	radio ± chemo	chemo	
side effects	18	11	42
Granulocytopenia 500/mm^3, 5 days	13 (72%)	4 (36%)	12 (30%)
Thrombocytopenia 50.000/mm^3, 5 days	10 (56%)	-	5 (12%)
Sepsis	8 (44%)	4 (36%)	2 (5%)
Renal failure	9 (50%)	4 (36%)	5 (12%)

In the non-pretreated patients the response to chemotherapy was better as compared to that in pretreated patients.

Table 4
Relationship between previous treatment and complete remission rate

	Patients	CR (%)
No pretreatment	42	26 (62%)
Chemotherapy	11	6 (55%)
Radiotherapy ± chemotherapy	18	9 (50%)

Patients with advanced abdominal disease- according to
Samuels' criteria[3]- responded less well.
Advanced abdominal disease combined with pulmonary di-
sease was even more resistant to PVB chemotherapy (table 5)
This observation has also been reported by Peckham[4].

Table 5
Results of the chemotherapy according to the extent of
the disease

	patients	CR (%)
Minimal pulmonary tumor	6	5 (83%)
Advanced pulmonary tumor	17	12 (70%)
Advanced abdominal tumor	21	13 (62%)
Minim. abd. + pulm. tumor	10	9 (90%)
Advanced abd. + pulm. tumor	16	1 (6%)
B-HCG as the sole parameter	1	1

It is of interest to note that two out of four patients
who had previously been treated with Samuels' regimen[5]
including Vinblastine and Bleomycin yet achieved a complete
remission by PVB chemotherapy. They are both free of disease for a period of 22[+] months and off maintenance therapy for a period of 13 months. The other two patients
achieved a partial remission of 3 months duration.
In conclusion it appears that the described chemotherapeutic regimen is highly effective even though our patient
population contains a high proportion of pretreated patients. Also in patients who have previously been treated
with VB, the PVB combination may be curative.
We feel that most of the patients achieving a complete
remission, verified by surgery after the chemotherapy,
will actually be cured.

REFERENCES

1. Einhorn, L.H., Donohue, J.,
   Cis-Diammine-Dichloro-Platinum, Vinblastine and
   Bleomycin combination therapy in disseminated
   testicular cancer.
   Annals of Int. Med. 87, 293-298, 1977.

2. Stoter, G., Vendrik, C.F.J., Struyvenberg, A.,
   Brouwers, Th.M., Sleijfer, D.Th., Schraffordt-Koops,
   H., van Oosterom, A.T., Pinedo, H.M.
   Combination chemotherapy with Cis-Diammine-Dichloro-
   Platinum, Vinblastine, and Bleomycin in advanced
   Testicular non-seminoma.
   Lancet 1, 941, 1979.

3. Samuels, M.L., Lanzotti, V.J., Holoye, P.Y.,
   Eamon Boyle, L., Smith, T.L., Johnson, D.E.
   Combination chemotherapy in germinal cell tumors.
   Cancer Treatment Rev. 3, 185-204, 1976.

4. Peckham, M.J., Barrett, A., McElwain, T.J., Hendry,
   W.F.
   Combined management of malignant teratoma of the tes-
   tis.
   Lancet, 2, 267, 1979.

5. Samuels, M.L., Johnson, D.E., Holoye, P.Y.
   Continuous intravenous Bleomycin Therapy with
   Vinblastin in stage III testicular neoplasia.
   Cancer Chem. Rep. 59, 563+570, 1975.

Authors addresses:
H.M.Pinedo and en G.Stoter, Department of Oncology,
   Free University Hospital, Amsterdam.
A.Struyvenberg and C.P.J.Vendrik, Oncology Unit, Department
   of Internal Medicine, University Hospital, Utrecht.
Th.M.Brouwers, H.Schraffordt Koops and D.Th.Sleyfer,
   Department of Internal Medicine and Oncological Surgery,
   University Hospital, Groningen.
A.T. van Oosterom, Department of Radiotherapy and Medical
   Oncology, University Hospital, Leiden.

21 CHEMOTHERAPY OF ADVANCED MALIGNANT TERATOMAS

E. S. Newlands, R. H. Begent, S. B. Kaye, G. J. Rustin and
K. D. Bagshawe

Since Li et al (1960) reported a 10% complete
remission rate using Actinomycin D, methotrexate and
chlorambucil in malignant teratomas, there has been
a substantial improvement in the chemotherapy for this
disease. At present the report by Einhorn and Donohue
(1977) with an initial complete response rate of 32
(64%) out of 50 patients is the most successful series
reported so far. Up to 1979, 28 (56%) of these original
50 patients were still in complete remission (Einhorn
and Williams 1979). Stoter et al (1979) using the same
drug combination as Einhorn and Donohue, obtained a
complete remission rate of 24 (60%) out of 40 patients.

Between 1977 and 1979 we have treated 43 male
patients with malignant teratoma (aged 16-64 years,
mean 28 years). There were 38 testicular primaries,
2 mediastinal primaries and 3 patients with para-aortic
disease and no identified primary in the testis.
The clinical stage of these patients was:

Stage   I :   1

Stage   II :   4

Stage III :   4

Stage   IV :   34

The incidence of the tumour markers, human chorionic
gonadotrophin (hCG) and α-foetoprotein (AFP) was as
follows: hCG alone: 8 patients

AFP alone: 9 patients

both hCG
and AFP : 24 patients

non-marker
producers: 2 patients.

We have also treated 10 patients with malignant ovarian teratomas (age 5-31 years, mean 18 years). Nine of these patients also had elevated tumour markers (hCG alone: 2 patients , AFP alone: 4 patients, both hCG and AFP: 3 patients).

Patients who were referred with clear-cut drug resistance to some of the drugs on the Protocol, were excluded from this study. The chemotherapy schedules, which were partly based on previous reports (Newlands 1976 and Newlands and Bagshawe 1977), were:

TREATMENT A:

Day 1   : Vincristine 1.0 mg/m^2 I.V. 10.00 a.m.;
               methotrexate 100 mg/m^2 I.V. stat 3.00 p.m.,
followed by methotrexate 200 mg/m^2 I.V. as a 12hr
               infusion.

Day 2   : Bleomycin 15 mg given as a 24hr infusion.
               Folinic acid rescue started at 3.00 p.m.
               in a dose of 15 mg twelve hourly for four
               doses.

Day 3   : Bleomycin infusion 15 mg by 24hr infusion.

Day 4   : Forced diuresis with mannitol and hydration
               at the rate of 1 litre hourly was given
               for 3 hours prior to
               Cis-Platinum 120 mg/m^2 by a short I.V.
               infusion, and the diuresis was continued
               at 1 litre hourly for a further 3 hours
               with mannitol. Hydration was continued
               until the patient stopped vomiting.

TREATMENT B:

VP16-213   100 mg/m^2 I.V. Days 1 - 5
Actinomycin -D   0,5 mg   I.V. Days 3, 4 and 5
Cyclophosphamide 500 mg/m^2 I.V. Day 5

TREATMENT C:

Hydroxyurea   500 mg q.d.s., p.o., Days 1 and 2
Vinblastine   5 mg/m^2 I.V. Day 3
Chlorambucil 10 mg b.d., p.o., Days 3, 4 and 5

TREATMENT D:

Day 1   : Vincristine   1,0 mg/m^2 I.V. at 10.00 a.m.
Methotrexate 100 mg/m^2 I.V. start at 3.00
p.m. followed by
Methotrexate 200 mg/m^2 I.V. as a 12hr
infusion.

Day 2   : Bleomycin 15 mg by 24hr infusion.
Folinic acid rescue started at 3.00 p.m.
in a dose of 15 mg twelve hourly for
four doses.

Day 3   : Bleomycin 15 mg by a 24hr infusion.

The sequence of the treatment schedules was:
1) Treatment A, 2) A, 3) B, 4) C, 5) D, and 6) B.
The courses were continued in sequence B, C and D,
unless there was evidence of drug-resistance. When this
occurred, the in-appropriate treatment schedule was
omitted.

A Complete Response required complete disappearance of
clinical, biochemical and C.T. scanning evidence of
disease, and necrotic tissue on biopsy of any residual
lesions where these were present.

Partial Responses were divided into three:

1) partial response with unresectable differentiated
   teratoma and negative tumour markers, referred to
   as P.R.D.,

2) partial response with static residual nodules on
   C.T. scanning and negative tumour markers referred
   to as P.R.C.T. and

3) partial response with evidence of disease activity
   referred to as P.R.A.

No maintenance therapy was given once a complete
response P.R.D. or P.R.C.T., had been obtained for 3
to 4 months.

The results in the 43 male patients, excluding
the 10 patients who are still on treatment and responding from initial therapy, show that 22 (67%) of the
initial 33 patients are off treatment for a range of
1 - 20 months (mean 9.5 months). There have been 19
(57%) complete responses: 1 (3%) P.R.D., 2 (6%) P.R.C.T.
Only 1 (3%) patient, who is on treatment, has a P.R.A.
In figure I a life-table analysis of the 33 patients
who have been on treatment for more than six months,
projects a survival figure of 73%. When analysed by
the sites and initial bulk of tumour (Peckham et al
1979) at presentation, there has been 1 (7%) death
out of 13 patients with non-bulky disease. 9 (30%)
out of 30 patients with bulky disease have died.
There were 6 deaths from resistant malignant teratoma
following an initial response. The other causes of
death were: initial extent of disease, 1, massive pulmonary embolus 1, septicemia due to neutropenia 1, pulmonary oedema while off treatment 1.

Life-table analysis of the 10 patients with
malignant ovarian teratomas is shown in Figure II,
and 9 out of 10 patients are alive with 1 P.R.D. and
1 P.R.A. It appears from this small number of patients,
that ovarian teratomas behave in much the same way
as male teratomas.

The toxicity encountered with this chemotherapy
is relatively mild and less than our previous experience
using high-dose vinblastine containing regimes.
Myelosuppression was manageable with leukopenia
(WBC < 2,000) occurring in 41 (77%) out of 53 patients.
Thrombocytopenia (platelet count < 50,000) occurred in
10 (19%) out of 53 patients. Febrile episodes
associated with neutropenia and given antibiotic cover
occurred in 13 (24%) out of 53 patients.

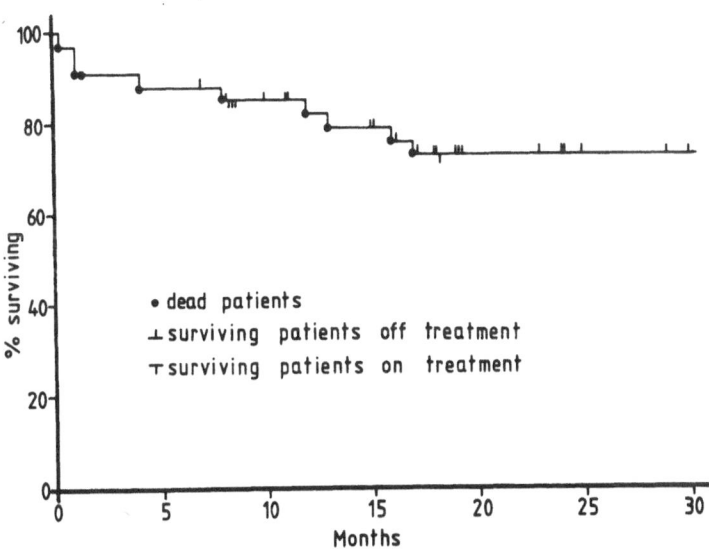

Figure I

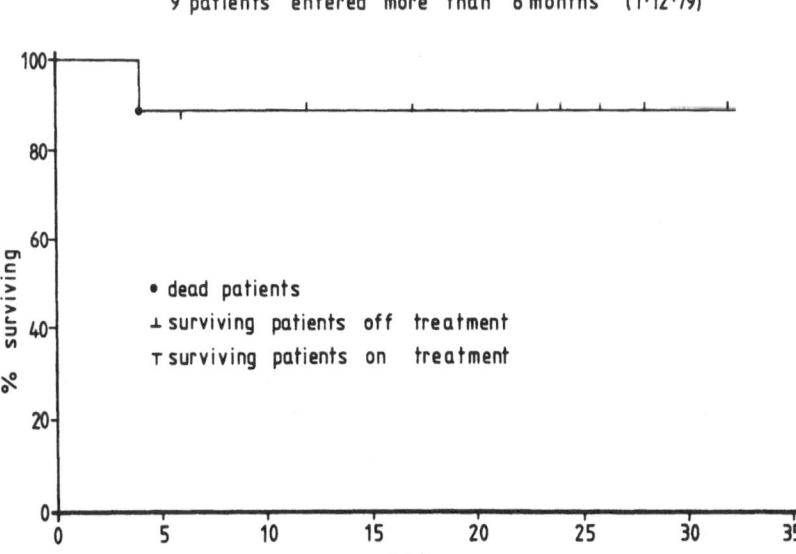

Figure II.

Transiently-raised creatinine levels (> 120 micro mols/ litre) were seen in 19 (36%) of the 53 patients.

In so far as one can compare different series of rare tumours treated in different centres, it would appear that the response rate and remission rate that we have obtained in advanced and bulky teratomas (30 (70%) out of 42 male patients fall into this group) is comparable to the best reported series, although the follow-up period is shorter. There are still problems in eliminating all tumour in patients presenting with very large volumes of malignant teratoma.

REFERENCES

1) Einhorn, L.H., and Donohue, J.   Cis-diammine-dichloroplatinum, vinblastine and bleomycin combination chemotherapy in disseminated testicular cancer.
Annals of Internal Medicine, 87, 293, 1977.

2) Einhorn, L.H., and Williams, S.D.   Cis-diamminedichloroplatinum (P) and Vinblastine (V) and Bleomycin (B) ± Adriamycin (A) in disseminated testicular cancer.
Proceedings of American Society of Clinical Oncology, Abstract C-19, 1979.

3) Li, M.C., Whitmore, W.F., Golbey, R., and Grabstal, H.   Effect of combined drug therapy on metastatic cancer of the testis.
Journal of the American Medical Association, 147, 145, 1960.

4) Newlands, E.S.   Chemotherapy of Testicular Tumours in "Bleomycin in the Treatment of Malignant Diseases". Second London International Symposium, Edited by J.M. Simister, Page 103, 1976.

5) Newlands, E.S., and Bagshawe, K.D.   Epipodophyllin derivative (VP16-213) in malignant teratomas and choriocarcinoma.
Lancet, 2, 87, 1977.

6) Peckham, M.J., McElwain, T.J., Barrett, A., and Hendry, W.F.   Combined management of teratoma of the testis.
Lancet, 2, 267, 1979.

7) Stoter, G., Sleijfer, D.T., Vendrik, C.P.J., Koops, H.S., Struyvenberg, A., Van Oosterom, A.T., Brouwers, T.M., and Pinedo, H.M.
Combination chemotherapy with cis-diamminedichloro-platinum, vinblastine and bleomycin in advanced testicular non-seminomas.
Lancet I, page 941, 1979.

22 CURRENT AND FUTURE MANAGEMENT OF TESTICULAR CANCER
Panel Discussion, held on December 7th, 1979

Chairman: F. M. Muggia (New York)
Panel members: A. Barrett (London), R. B. Golbey (New York),
D. D. von Hoff (San Antonio), C. Merrin (Chicago),
D. G. Skinner (Los Angeles),
B. H. P. van der Werf-Messing (Rotterdam),
S. D. Williams (Indianapolis)

CHAIRMAN:

This panel will cover five basic topics:

1) staging

2) treatment policies of the early stages

3) the sequence of modalities in advanced disease

4) the optimal chemotherapeutic regimen

5) new areas under investigation

1. Staging in testicular cancer

What I would like to do is begin with staging and get a comment on the relative importance of staging on the selection
of treatment of testicular cancer.

DR.VAN DER WERF -MESSING: I should like to emphasize the
need for an international clinical classification of
patients with testicular tumor. There has been an international classification agreed upon, in Europe, Japan
and the United States. The majority of centers think that
their own classification is the best. However, it is
impossible to compare results of treatment. Clinical
staging is a little less reliable than pathological
staging but, for comparison of results, you have to do
a clinical staging as well. You can later subdivide your
patients according to pathological findings. In this
manner you have the possibility to compare results. If
there is a negative lymphography, or if the pathologist
doesn't find pathology in the lymph nodes after surgery,
results are about the same all over the world. With good
surgery or good radiotherapy, and good chemotherapy, you

A.T. van Oosterom et al. (eds.), Therapeutic Progress in Ovarian Cancer,
Testicular Cancer and the Sarcomas, pp. 261-282. All rights reserved.
Copyright 1980 by Martinus Nijhoff Publishers, The Hague/Boston/London.

approach nearly 100% cure. That's established, and nobody
will doubt it. It therefore doesn't matter what you do,
but perhaps the patient could influence the decision on
treatment, based on lymphography, CT-scan, or presence
of markers. If there is no clinical evidence of metastasis,
the patient could select surgery, radiation therapy, or
chemotherapy. And it should not just depend on the "hobby"
of the therapist, but also on the available clinical
facilities in the area where the patient lives or where he
can be referred to.

If you find extensive lymph node involvement - it's only
by clinical trials that you will find out what the best
results will be. Common clinical staging including subsequent histology review is needed to compare later results.
Another important aspect concerns false negative
lymphography in about 20%. However,we have found that
results of radiotherapy are good when lymphography is
negative. If there are doubtful lymph nodes, you can perform
trans-abdominal cytology. This is a possibility which has
been developed in Scandinavia and should perhaps be more
often applied instead of surgery. International panels
should be appointed both for the assessment of histology and
lymphography to facilitate trials and comparison of results.

CHAIRMAN: I was reminded by your answer of the differences
with ovarian cancer staging. There, we see that the
difficulty in comparing trials concerns the application
and sensitivity of the methods used. Whereas here in
testicular cancer we still have a very serious language
difficulty between trials done in different centers.
However, I do know that there are some panel members who
have a divergent opinion as to the importance of staging.

DR.SKINNER: I don't think this is worth making a major
issue of. If one looks at the "T"classification, in
particular, it may possibly turn out that an involvement of
the cord may be predictive of a failure later on. However,
at present, it doesn't seem to correlate at all, because so
many of the patients in the Stage I and II category are

being cured. When you talk about a 95% cure rate of all
Stage I and II tumors, clinical staging is not very
meaningful.

The cost of medical care in the United States is becoming
a tremendous problem. Therefore we should only apply these
staging techniques that will alter or change the therapy.
If you're not going to change your therapy as based on the
staging techniques, then it doesn't make a lot of sense to
spend the money to do this. The big problem that I have
with clinical staging is in small disease. There is no
question that the bulk disease can be determined with a
great deal of accuracy. Nobody knows what the error rate is
in lymphangiography or CT-scanning for the micro-metastases,
in stages B-1 or B-2. There is still a tremendous variation
and it will be difficult to reach agreement on comparable
stages. If you take the A and B's together, and you find
that you have only one tumor death in 80 consecutive
patients, it's not too important to spend a lot of money
and a lot of time in trying to determine who is clinically
N-0 or N-1 or N-2, because they all end up doing the same.

DR.VAN DER WERF -MESSING: The major point, however, is that
the patient may choose not to have surgery.

CHAIRMAN: We'll cover some of this as we get more into the
treatment aspect. It is important to point out that a lot
of the staging classifications have been confusing, because
they have not distinguished between clinical and surgical
pathologic staging - it is important to make this distinction. There is some divergence over how much of an effort
should be put in to develop this equivalence between
clinical and surgical-pathologic staging. I would like now
to elicit some comments on whether markers should be used
for staging and how should they be used.

DR.GOLBEY: I think the problem of markers is very simple.
They have one drawback: they're not positive in 100% of the
patients. When they are positive, they are the most
important help that we can get. They may not have the status

of yet enabling us to make an initial diagnosis - although
when they're positive, it certainly gives you a strong clue
as to cell type. But in advanced disease, for following
your effective therapy, they are absolute. I think this
has to be clearly recognized. The fact that they have
limitations doesn't rule out the fact that they have an
extraordinary usefulness. Markers should be drawn before
the first therapeutic endeavour They should be followed
thereafter. If they are positive initially, the fact that
they become negative is of extreme importance. If they
change, you have something you can hang your hat on. I
attribute a great deal of the progress that has been made
in the treatment of this disease, as opposed to other solid
tumors, to the fact that right from the beginning there
has been a marker available. We're much better off now.
We've got at least three markers.

CHAIRMAN: So, your stress is on the markers for follow-up,
but not necessarily in altering the initial staging.

DR.GOLBEY: No, not really. If you have a patient who has a
positive marker and does not become negative after
orchiectomy, you know you've got residual disease. And
you'd better cope with it. You may not be able to stage
that patient II or III, because the IIs can put out hormones
just as well as the IIIs can. But you know you've got
positive disease and you'd better be prepared to deal with
it. May be it doesn't help for staging in the sense of putting
it into those Roman numerals but it sure tells you something
about the status of the patient.

CHAIRMAN: Could we just have one brief comment on the value
of CT-scans and lymphangiography in staging from Dr.
Barrett.

DR.BARRETT: Concerning markers:patients with raised markers
with no evidence of disease on clinical staging have all
developed disease. We wouldn't hesitate now to treat people
on the basis of raised markers alone.

As far as CT scanning goes, it provides the best method of

detecting disease and following up of patients by groups
who are going to treat patients without surgery. In our
experience, there is an enormous difference in the amount
of information you get from CT scanning and from any other
sort of conventional radiography - even bearing in mind the
technical problems of interpretation. We have seen very
few patients in which the CT scan data has been misleading.

We have had some patients where we've seen things that we
haven't understood, which have subsequently become clear
and, with greater experience, the problems are becoming
less. Anybody starting with CT scanning will run into
problems in interpretation. But it's a method that, with
experience, gives a lot of very valuable information.

CHAIRMAN: Questions from the audience in this particular
aspect?

DR.OLIVER (London): Marker positive after orchiectomy: how
long do you wait for it to go back to normal? Are you in fact
losing time in waiting, because it may take up to a month,
if it's falling at the half life of alpha-feto protein?

DR.GOLBEY: The rate of decay is known for each marker.
Depending on the initial elevation, you can, with frequent
enough determinations, get the slope of the line and
determine whether it continues to fall at that rate. The
minute it's not falling at that rate, the minute it stops
falling, you know you've failed to obliterate the disease.
I don't think that we lose anything -at least in the
routine cases that I can think of - by waiting to find out
what the status of the patient is.

DR.OLIVER: If it's fairly high after orchiectomy, it may
be a month before you can start your radiation or your
lymphadenectomy.

DR.GOLBEY: If you're in a programmed protocol which calls
for steps, despite what the marker shows, you should go
ahead with it. But I don't think you should ignore the

positive evidence of markers.

DR.SKINNER: It should also clearly be stated that in 1979 the established protocols for treating these tumors are set and the expected survival is exceedingly high. There is no data right now to support the suggestion of treatment at this stage, on the basis of markers or lymphangiograms. Until that data is forthcoming in a large number of pa-tients I think that should not be considered.

DR.SALMON: Did any of the panelists discuss the reversion of markers in patients thought to be clinically and pathologically Stage II, after surgical resection. What is the frequency with which marker-positive Stage II patients revert to negative markers subsequent to surgery?

DR.SKINNER: They all should revert, or they're Stage III.

DR.SALMON: By definition, you're changing the stage based on the marker. If those patients who are thought to be Stage II with markers don't revert, then perhaps they could be spared surgery.

DR.GOLBEY: We have not agreed on the set of definitions that enable us to compare stages with and without markers. Each time we have to explain what we mean. If Dr.van der Werf -Messing's suggestions were taken- and I think it was the most important thing we've said today- we've got to have a standard set of notations to make further progress.

DR. SALMON: I'm asking the question right now. If you have a series of patients who would be classified histo-patholo-gically, based on surgical staging, as Stage II, independent of marker information, what proportion of those patients, if they had a positive marker, would revert to negative after surgical procedure?

CHAIRMAN: The NCI data of Javadpour,published from the Adjuvant Treatment of Cancer meeting in Tucson, 1979 indicates that most of the clinical Stage II patients undergoing retroperitoneal node dissection, who were

marker positive initially fell to normal. If such a fall
does not occur it should not change the anatomic classification even though technically they are Stage IIIs.

DR.SKINNER: In my experience, also those that are marker
positive, after node dissection, have all gone to marker
negative provided lung tomograms were negative. A certain
number will become marker positive in the future, with
pulmonary metastases. They still remain Stage II; they
recur as Stage III and they're not reclassified.

2.Treatment policies of the early stages

2) CHAIRMAN: We should go on to discuss the treatment
of Stage I be it clinical or pathological. What is, in the
opinion of the panel, satisfactory treatment for this
stage? What is the purpose of retroperitoneal node
dissection in this connection?

DR.MERRIN: In Stage I, the purpose of retroperitoneal
node dissection is purely staging. The question is:
are we dealing with local disease, or are we dealing with
systemic disease? The answer will direct all further type
of treatment. Therefore, when all the clinical studies
are negative, the only answer to this question lies in the
retroperitoneal lymph node. This is the purpose of the
retroperitoneal lymphadenectomy. Microscopic disease
being present means systemic disease. Certainly the
prognosis is better when you have a minimal amount of
disease. It is immaterial if we have a Stage II, IIA or
Stage IIB or Stage IIC or Stage IIZ; in reality we are
interested in the biological staging. Is it: local
disease or systemic disease? Is it systemic disease with
a small or a large tumor mass? The patients who have a
large tumor mass don't do as well,no matter where the
tumor mass is located.

CHAIRMAN: Other panelists, do you agree with that view
of retroperitoneal lymphnode dissection?

DR.SKINNER: It does tell you exactly the prognosis of that
individual. In three major centers that I indicated today,

there has not been one tumor death in that group of
patients. It's a procedure that carries a very low
morbidity to assure 100% tumor-free survival.I'd like to
see that kind of survival shown in a substantial number
of patients, in other ways of treatment.

DR.VAN DER WERF -MESSING: I'm probably repeating what I
already said: If lymphangiography is negative, in the
major radiotherapy centers you also have a cure rate of
95 to 100%. This means that with radiotherapy you can
eradicate the micrometastases. That will occur in about
20%. I still would like to propagate clinical work-up,
since the patient can choose whether he wants surgery
or radiation therapy. It's his body. I think if the
results are the same in both types of therapy, he should
have a choice.

CHAIRMAN: Is that true in both MTU and MTI?

DR.VAN DER WERF -MESSING: According to the latest results
of the Royal Marsden Hospital study it's the same.

CHAIRMAN: In how many patients?

DR.BARRETT: Twenty eight were involved in that study.

DR.VAN DER WERF -MESSING: And they included Stage IIA.
We had the same in Malignant Teratoma Intermediate and
MTT, although I must admit:we didn't consistently use the
markers.

CHAIRMAN: Could we hear from Dr. Barrett? You're actually
running a trial of whether radiotherapy is necessary
under that circumstance.

DR.BARRETT: In the early-stage disease, the benefit to
the patient from surgery is largely, as Dr.Merrin said,
to determine the prognosis. If the prognosis is excellent,
whatever treatment is applied it seems to me that to
continue with radiation is perfectly satisfactory.
What you won't be able to do if you continue with

irradiation for Stage I disease, is answer such questions
as: is there a place for adjuvant chemotherapy in this
group? Because you won't have the basic data on which to
subdivide the patients.

But, if our experience is confirmed in a larger number
of patients and if we can, by clinical stage, identify
the group of patients who are at risk for disseminating
disease, we will have answered the question in a different
way. There will always be a difference between clinical
and surgical staging . What each of us has to do is to
determine from our staging , in Stage I patients, whether
any additional treatment is necessary.

CHAIRMAN: That leads actually to a very relevant question,
for this early group of patients: Is chemotherapy required
from the beginning in either clinical or pathological
Stage I? I have here a question from Dr. Thomas to Dr.
Skinner. One of your slides shows an improvement of
results from 79% to 95% by adding post-operative chemotherapy. Do you consider it appropriate to treat 80% of
patients who will not benefit from the treatment with
adjuvant chemotherapy?

DR.SKINNER: That slide related to Stage B or patients
with positive nodes. As far as patients with negative
nodes is concerned, it's been our policy to give
actinomycin D during immediate post-operative period and
one course two months later. Our recurrence rate in Stage A
relapsing with pulmonary metastasis is less than 3%.
In Dr.Williams' data it is about 8 to 10 by not using
chemotherapy at all. It's strictly a matter of whether
you want to give very low-risk type of minimal therapy
to everybody in order to reduce your recurrence rate, or
treat no one and accept a higher recurrence rate and a
higher need to subsequently use intensive chemotherapy
upon relapse.

CHAIRMAN: Could we have other views?

DR.WILLIAMS: I don't necessarily want to take another

view. I would just say that in our Stage I patients, we
have 4 of 57 recurrences of people with pathologic Stage I
disease. We have given them no chemotherapy. All 4 are in
complete remission of platinum -velban-bleomycin. All are
alive with no evidence of disease.

Let us reiterate that virtually everybody with Stage I or
Stage II disease should be cured. The only way to solve
this question is a well-designed prospective clinical trial
which is in progress as an NCI Intergroup study.

Other aspects need to be emphasized. Adjuvant therapy
requires several things: a compliant patient, a technically
good retroperitoneal lymphadenectomy and lastly giving an
effective systemic therapy at the time of relapse.

CHAIRMAN: You actually raise the question of the treatment
for the patients with minimal residual or microscopic disease on retroperitoneal node dissection. What is the optimal
treatment for this particular group? As mentioned there is
a national study ongoing which is comparing the effect of
immediate VAB or PVB chemotherapy versus delayed upon
recurrence. We will have to wait for the results of this
study to decide which is the most satisfactory way of
managing these patients.

DR.GOLBEY: Three or four times you said treatment is
satisfactory and I don't know what that means. I would say
at the moment there are at least 10 satisfactory forms of
treatment which give excellent results: 80% to 85% cures.
The relevant question is: can we make this 100%.

CHAIRMAN: Not only good long-term results but also less
morbidity is what we are focusing on.

3. *The sequence of modalities in advanced disease*

I would like to go on to the more advanced group of patients, the ones that have more than 2-centimeter lesions.
It's actually rare to have lesions between 2- and 5 centi-
meter in the retroperitoneal area. Is there some discussion
on using chemotherapy first for bulky disease.

DR.VAN DER WERF -MESSING: Again, there are many approaches.
The E.O.R.T.C. Urological Group has proposed a trial of
chemotherapy, radiation therapy and surgery, in various
combinations.

CHAIRMAN: Comparing which modalities? Comparing using
chemotherapy first.....

DR.VAN DER WERFF-MESSING: There are to be various
comparisons. First surgery, then chemotherapy or first
chemotherapy then surgery or radiation therapy with chemotherapy.

DR.SKINNER: In the United States, there have been two
centers that have looked at pre-operative radiation
therapy and surgery. Pre-operative radiotherapy has clearly increased the morbidity of the operation to the point
that both centers, Walter Reed and San Diego Naval Hospital
have abandoned it in favor of chemotherapy first followed
by surgery. We have tried this and we've given it up because
it hasn't produced as good results. Dr.Merrin indicated
that surgery first for bulk disease is not considered
optimal by surgeons. Tumors often have fairly necrotic and
thin capsules, so incomplete removal, or possibly spill of
the tumor may result in a catabolic patient that can't be
treated for a period of time. The conclusion must be that
bulk disease must be treated with your best things first.
Those are now platinum, velban and bleo in some combination.
Cytoreductive surgery should be performed afterwards.

CHAIRMAN: Dr.Barrett, would you like to comment on your
experience using chemotherapy first and then radiation
therapy.

DR.BARRETT: We've only small numbers of patients who are
treated with different sequences, that is surgery first
followed by radiotherapy or radiation therapy followed by
surgery alone. But, in all cases, the morbidity has been
much greater with any other approach than with chemotherapy, radiotherapy, surgery. And I don't think radio-

therapy is an option after surgery or chemotherapy and surgery combination after radiotherapy. As we said before, you must make the optimal decision at the start of the patient's management.

We tried to answer the question: Does radiation produce any additional benefit over the combination of surgery and chemotherapy? From looking at the presented data we have an indication that it can produce a benefit, although the figures are obviously small and the follow-up times are short. We have found that the histology at the time of surgery shows fibrosis in 43% of the patients, differentiated teratoma in 47% of the patients and active tumor in 8% of the patients. Dr.Merrin found 25% fibrosis, 28% TD and 36% active tumor. The Indiana data show 36% fibrosis, 32% teratoma differentiated and 32% activive tumor. If Dr. Williams is right that the finding of teratoma differentiated is a good prognostic sign, then the higher incidence in the post-radiation surgery group may be a good sign. It would be premature to draw definite conclusions, but in spite of our differing approaches we may be able to combine our data to answer this question.

DR.SKINNER: The percentages of benign teratoma, fibrosis and residual embryonal carcinoma depend on the amount of prior treatment, and one must not necessarily attribute it to the sequence.

DR.BARRETT: Ours has been a very rigid protocol, with only marker negative patients and no evidence of progressive disease after 4 or 6 courses of chemotherapy, being eligible for subsequent radiotherapy and surgery.

CHAIRMAN: At this point, it might be worthwhile to get a comment from Dr. Newlands on his experience with chemotherapy of various germ cell and trophoblastic tumors.

DR.NEWLANDS (London): In bulky disease patients we have not used radiotherapy because our approach has been chemotherapy to shrink it down. Residual disease shown on the CT-scan has been operated upon. We've had all three findings mentioned by Dr.Barrett: active teratoma, fibrosis and differentiated teratoma. We have not seen a response to radiotherapy in residual disease resistant to chemotherapy. We prefer chemotherapy followed by surgery for any residual lesion. Surgical findings may provide information on the effect of chemotherapy on tumor growth and biology.

DR.BARRETT: We also don't use radiotherapy for disease that isn't responding to chemotherapy. The effect of the two different sequences of treatment are being assessed by histology.

CHAIRMAN: We look forward to hearing about the progress of these studies to see the role of radiotherapy after chemotherapy in this bulky disease.Questions?

KLEEBERG (Hamburg, Fed.Rep. of Germany): What is the treatment strategy of the non-gestational (ovarian) choriocarcinoma of the young female? Is it similar to that of the testicular cancer?

DR.NEWLANDS: We've treated 10 patients.Two of them were histologically pure choriocarcinoma. So far 9 out of 10 of our patients are alive, although one has active disease and will probably die. It seems to respond very much like the male counterpart.

CHAIRMAN: This is certainly a much better experience than with the previous chemotherapeutic regimens.

DR.GOLBEY: This does not prove that there is a difference between gestational choriocarcinoma and ovarian choriocarcinoma. Gestational choriocarcinoma will respond to these combinations too. It's not used in every case, because it may be a matter of over-kill. Patients, who do not respond to simple therapy at Memorial go straight on to the VAB program and response is usually anticipated. This holds for both gestational or ovarian choriocarcinoma.

CHAIRMAN: However, the previous experience in ovarian choriocarcinoma with single agents like methotrexate or even with a triple regimen including actinomycin D and alkylating agents was quite poor. This is a documentation that the additional cisplatinum, vinblastine and bleomycin may be much more effective.

DR.GOLBEY: The important fact is that germ-cell tumors respond, in both males and females, regardless of site of origin.

HOSSFELD (Essen, Fed.Rep.of Germany): Dr.Skinner, you stated that in your material you could not see a correlation between histology and results of chemotherapy. However, the speakers following you did find such a correlation. Could you explain this difference?

DR.SKINNER: The correlation was primarily in the radiotherapy-treated groups. The difference in survival was in the MTI, MTU groups that were reported by the radiotherapist. From a surgically treated and chemotherapeutically-treated point of view, we can find no difference in overall survival, with the exception of the pure choriocarcinomas. But choriocarcinomatous foci in other tumors as well as mixtures, with or without seminoma, have behaved the same way. The exception is massive disease, in which case failures are usually in teratocarcinoma rather than in embryonal carcinoma. Drs. Williams and Golbey have the same experience. In the earlier-stage diseases, cell type makes no difference.

DR.WILLIAMS: In the disseminated disease there are differences in complete remission rates according to cell type with embryonal carcinoma patients having a higher rate.

DR.SKINNER: If you believe in the overall primordial germ-cell theory, there really shouldn't be any difference, because they all come from the same cell type.

4. *The optimal chemotherapeutic regimen*

CHAIRMAN: The next issue is, what is the optimal chemotherapy regimen. One question relates to the toxicity of the regimens and long-term consequences. It might be worthwhile, at this point, to hear a comment from Dr. Stoter from the Dutch multi-center trial that has employed the PVB regimen in quite a wide experience.

DR. STOTER:Our cisplatinum experience dates back to 1976. In a Dutch trial, we have up to now treated 71 patients with disseminated testicular teratomas with the Einhorn regimen employing high dose Velban (0,4 mg/kg) usually for 4 cycles. Of those, 60% achieved a complete remission and, in 29 of those patients, we have evaluated the response by surgery. Only 2 patients of the whole series subsequently relapsed. There are 39 patients free of disease for a period of 2 to 40 months, with an average follow-up period of 18 months.

We have given maintenance chemotherapy to complete responders, with a regimen of cisplatinum, 50 milligrams per m2 once every six weeks, and vinblastin,0,2 milligrams per kilogram every three weeks. The toxicity during the maintenance chemotherapy is not very impressive. The harm to the kidneys has been done during the remission induction treatment. In most patients the creatinine clearance falls by 25 to 50% and it stays like that during one year of treatment on maintenance therapy. Twenty-two patients are off all maintenance therapy now. Only 2 cases have relapsed after a period of 5 and 7 months of remission induction treatment. Toxicity during the maintenance phases included cisplatinum allergy in 4 cases. In 2 this was anaphylactic shock, in one repeated dermatitis at every cisplatin dose and in the fourth case there was skin rash with wheezing and facial edema.

CHAIRMAN: Thank you, Dr. Stoter. I think that's an excellent confirmatory trial of Dr.Einhorn's preliminary experience.

There was the suggestion made by Dr.Merrin that we should look at less intensive chemotherapy. I would like to have some opinions expressed by the panel.

Dr. WILLIAMS: I've never been totally convinced that less intensive chemotherapy regimens have yielded as good results. The people who used our treatment regimen like the people in The Netherlands have done very well. They had the misfortune of treating a lot of people with prior radiotherapy, so they had a great deal of hematologic toxicity. We have been criticized for toxicity. The first series of patients from '74 to '76 had some nephro-toxicity before we used routine hydration and before we omitted aminoglycosides. Most people have relatively normal renal function by the time they finish their induction therapy. Bleomycin pulmonary fibrosis should not be a common problem. Since the first 50 patients, we've had one death from bleomycin pulmonary fibrosis. So, what we're talking about is hematologic toxicity. I'm not convinced regimens with less hematologic toxicity are as efficacious.

DR.MERRIN: I was not talking of less intensive chemo-therapy but of a different chemotherapy. There are ways to use drugs in a more or less toxic fashion. In relation to the platinum, there is mounting evidence that when you use the slow-infusion method, there is less acute and cumulative toxicity. The same can be said about bleomycin. Now, there is already preliminary evidence that other drugs like adriamycin, when used in a slow infusion, can be less toxic.
My point was to have a very intensive type of chemotherapy, but to put a great emphasis in minimizing the toxicity.
My criticism of the Einhorn regimen was not of the drugs but more of the method of administration.
I grant Dr.Williams that I may have over-operated a certain number of patients, but there is a dilemma because there is an optimal time to operate. If you misjudge the timing, the patient may lose the opportunity to be cured.Several

things may happen: the tumor is transformed into a mature
teratoma, or there is a complete necrosis of the tumor. In
both instances timing is not important.
But, if there is a residual malignant tumor, then this is
a modified tumor with intense fibrosis and the more you
wait, the more fibrosis develops. Subsequently when you
try to operate on these patients, you generally fail.
The optimal time to operate in my opinion, is between
2 and 3 months of intensive chemotherapy. I therefore
think that I have over-operated at least 16 patients. If I
would have waited, the masses may have disappeared because
they were completely necrotic.

CHAIRMAN: Dr.Merrin, you did not present your results with
chemotherapy alone with your regimen.

DR.MERRIN: I had 14 patients who had chemotherapy alone.
And if you add the 16 patients who had complete necrosis
at the time of surgery, the complete remission rate may
be considered to be 40%.
An interesting problem is the high incidence of transformation in mature teratoma. Those mature teratomas express
themselves as residual tumor. If we don't operate them
relatively fast,they may grow locally. A vicious circle
of more chemotherapy and higher-dose toxicity may be
initiated. Ater that the surgery is much more difficult
because all this chemotherapy certainly increases fibrosis
in the tissue as well as debilitate the patient.

CHAIRMAN: You're citing perhaps an extreme example, but
let's hear from other members of the panel.

DR.GOLBEY: In 1970, we recognized the activity of Dr.
Samuels' program, but found the toxicity led to unacceptable
mortality and morbidity. We tried to modify it by reducing
the dose and then substituting other drugs. For 7 years
now, I have been talking about exactly that. But as I
travel around the world, I find people using the Indiana
schedule and accepting a 5% mortality as "something that

Heaven sent and there's not much we can do about it". There
is a great deal you can do about a 5% mortality from drugs.
And not only the mortality, but also the suffering of many
others. There are ways to get around it and I don't
understand why people stick their heads under a rock
and don't pay attention.

DR.WILLIAMS: First of all the continuous infusion of
bleomycin was done not to decrease toxicity but to increase
the therapeutic efficacy based on some animal studies
and mechanisms of action. I have no experience with
continuously infused platinum. However many claim that
it does not decrease nausea and vomiting. Second the
problem with our regimen is:myelosuppression. This is
particularly prominent following prior radiotherapy.
The toxicity of our regimen, with careful management, is
acceptable.

CHAIRMAN: What is your current experience with the
PVB regimen with a lower dose of velban?

DR.WILLIAMS: We have a high incidence of hospitalization
for granulocytopenic fever.We have had 39 patients in the
most recent study and one drug-related death. This patient
had a bleomycin-induced pulmonary fibrosis, and,
interestingly, also congestive heart failure, Marfan's
syndrome and prior radiation therapy to the mediastinum.

5. New areas under investigation

CHAIRMAN: We ought to touch on new areas of investigation.

DR. SALMON: I really was interested to hear the
applications of the drug assay that Dr. von Hoff
described and indicate that some of the questions that
the speakers have been discussing back and forth now
perhaps could be more suitably answered.One could first
get evidence of equivalent activity of drugs such as
vincristine and vinblastine in vitro prior to altering
currently effective regimens. On the other hand, I wanted

to comment on Dr.Muggia's discussion of the five signal
tumors. If that program had been firmly in place at the
time that platinum came into clinical trial, it may
have never entered testicular cancer management.
We need something more than a small clinical panel for
phase II testing to determine activity and we were
lucky that we didn't have such strict rules at the time.
Now, there are obviously other techniques, because
activity could be picked up with in vitro assay.

CHAIRMAN: The five tumor panel is required, but is not
meant to be restrictive of trials in other diseases, which
are always encouraged. Any other comments?

DR. HOSSFELD (Essen): Dr. Muggia, I would like to
know whether there is more than an empirical
basis for including adriamycin in the treatment of
testicular cancer?

DR.GOLBEY: Dr.Holland's group conducted a trial of
adriamycin and it is active. It didn't seem to add
anything to the combination as we used it. I was interested
in Dr.von Hoff's data, that one out of nine responded
to adriamycin, four out of nine responded to actinomycin-D.
In this system actinomycin happens to be a more active
agent. It may also pick up the patients who will respond
to adriamycin and therefore it may be ineffective to use
them both in the same regimen.

DR.OLIVER: I'd like to come back to the problem of
radiotherapy and the absence of any data on its activity
as a single agent in this disease, and return to the data
that Professor van der Werf -Messing presented, who
reported a 40% 5-year cure with radiotherapy to metastatic
disease in the lung. In her original data, she also shows
that MTI is better than MTU for Stage I.Is that also true
for metastatic disease?

DR.VAN DER WERF -MESSING: The MTI had a better prognosis
in cases of clinically negative lymph nodes. It was 100%

MTI-A and it was roughly 80% MTI-B. And MTI-B now is
included under MTU. But that doesn't apply to patients
with diffuse metastases.

DR.ROZENCWEIG (Brussels): A question to Dr. Williams or Dr.
Stoter. Is there any correlation between the bleomycin toxicity
and the platinum-induced renal toxicity?

DR.WILLIAMS: I can't give you hard numbers. Before using
IV hydration, patients had worse renal function and we
saw a lot more bleomycin mucositis. Pulmonary fibrosis
was always rare.

CHAIRMAN: I'd like to make a statement about chemotherapy. It's important to have a chemotherapy package
to work with, for use in combined modality treatments and
also in advanced disease. Any modifications of this
particular chemotherapy should be evaluated in
prospective trials.

DR.MERRIN: I've been accused of replacing velban by
vincristine although it is not as active as vinblastine.
I've also added actinomycin D. The success of the chemotherapy is related to the time it is given.
If we get very serious toxicity in the induction period,
our sequence of treatment is altered because we have to
wait for a long period of time until recovery from myelosuppression. That may take up to two months. My conception
is that the least toxic induction that achieves a high
percentage of complete clinical remissions should be used.
That's essentially what I have done. I'm using actinomycin-
D in combination with cisplatinum and vincristine during
the maintenance period, for a long time, and the results
are not different from the Einhorn regimen or the VAB
approach.

CHAIRMAN: Dr.Merrin, I don't think you mean a non-toxic
induction,but one that is less toxic than the PVB regimen
to use in combined modality. What is Dr.Skinner's
experience?

DR.SKINNER: I really want to support the Indiana PVB regimen. Since 1977, with the velban reduced to 0.3 milligrams per kilogram, we have really routinely utilized 4 courses of therapy, and then proceeded directly to our cytoreductive surgery, two weeks following completion of the last course of chemotherapy. And I simply have not seen this big problem of toxicity. It has been well tolerated. With some help of hyperalimentation these patients are doing very well. I do agree with Dr.Merrin that there is a magic time that you should go after these things surgically and not wait until the drugs are burned up and the patients are at the end of the road. You should have a very clear-cut protocol from the beginning in each individual patient. In my own experience, the Einhorn regimen modified with low dose velban has been extremely well tolerated.

CHAIRMAN: Dr.Young, do you have a comment?

DR.YOUNG:(Bethesda). Not a comment, just a question. It's always bothered me to use the term "maintenance therapy". I'm not sure it's valid in any disease. But this is certainly a situation in which one can seriously raise the question of what role maintenance chemotherapy plays in the impact of our curative approaches to the management of testicular tumors. Conversely it certainly makes an impact on late toxicities.
Is there data or is there a concept which would support the notion of maintenance therapy in this disorder?

DR.SKINNER: This is a big question. There is no data to say "Yes" or "No". Maintenance concepts relate back to the early actinomycin D experience when it took a long time to get a complete response. But, there is no data to support it.

DR.MERRIN: There is no data, but I had some patients who quit after induction. They all had recurrences.

DR.GOLBEY: Our basis for maintenance therapy was the way
we started. We didn't have an induction program, we just
had chronic, relatively low-dose therapy and we cured
a few people with it and we tended to stick to it. We
later superimposed a more aggressive initial treatment
which we called induction. It used to take us 3 to 6 months
to put a patient into complete remission, if we achieved
it. We now achieve complete remission in one to three
weeks, and sometimes faster than that. With our marker
data, it appears that we either cure or don't cure the
patient with the induction program. Now, with 3 -and in
some cases 4 induction courses- the patient is either
cured or not cured at that point. Our next protocol and
our current protocol are accumulating data on that
question. It is my belief that maintenance therapy, with
present-day induction therapy, plays no role at all. But
that's not to say that it didn't in the past.

DR.STOTER: Since nobody knows the answer, the E.O.R.T.C.
has also activated a protocol to answer this question,
following remission induction treatment with the PVB
regimen, patients are randomised to no treatment or one
year threeweekly velban and sixweekly platinum.

CHAIRMAN: Basically, the message is: we can be very
succesful in the treatment of testicular cancer.
We're still troubled with terminology problems and one
large question is: how to decrease morbidity.

PART THREE

OSTEOSARCOMA

23 CLASSIFICATION AND PROGNOSIS OF OSTEOSARCOMA

Th. G. van Rijssel

The classification of neoplasms of the skeleton is based on their histological structure, and the first distinguishing characteristic is the intercellular substance produced by the tumour cells.

When the tumour cells produce osteoid substance or bone, the classification is osteotumour, even when the tumour cells also produce cartilaginous substance or collagen fibres.

When the tumour cells produce cartilaginous substance but no osteoid, the tumour has to be classified as chondrotumour. Tumours with fibroblastic cells producing collagen fibres, but no osteoid nor chondroid substance, are fibrotumours. Moreover there are skeletal tumour types which do not produce any characteristic intercellular material (e.g. Ewing sarcoma, giant cell tumour etc.)

There are several types of osteotumours, some benign, others malignant, and also osteoplastic tumourlike lesions which are non-neoplastic.

Classification of osteotumours

malignant	benign	non-neoplastic bone forming lesions
osteosarcoma	osteoblastoma osteoid osteoma osteoma	fibrous dysplasia sclerosing osteomyelitis callus ossifying hematoma myositis ossificans

Malignancy means capability to metastazise; a bening tumour lacks this potential. Malignancy is a quality which occurs in very different degrees. Some tumours have a high degree of malignancy: they give rise to many metastases in nearly all cases and often early, i.e. when the primary tumour is still small. Other tumours have a low grade of malignancy;

in these cases treatment of the primary tumour cures most of
the patients. Osteosarcoma is the most frequently occuring
primary malignant bone tumour, forming circa 40% of all
skeletal sarcoma's in the files of the Netherlands Committee
on Bone Tumours. (see table 1).

Table 1

Netherlands Committee on Bone Tumours[*]
5000 skeletal lesions (1953-1978)

intraosseous osteosarcoma	642	
juxtacortical osteosarcoma	51	710
subperiostal chondro-sarcoma	17	
chrondrosarcoma	455	
fibrosarcoma (incl. M.F.H.)	156	
Ewing's sarcoma	279	
reticulosarcoma	54	
chordoma	38	
synoviosarcoma	37	
sarcomatous giant cell tumour	18	
Primary malignant skeletal tumours	1747	

[*] The work of the Netherlands Committee on Bone Tumours has
been supported since 1953 by the foundation "Koningin
Wilhelmina Fonds" (The Netherlands Cancer Society).

Osteosarcoma occurs:
   - inside the bone - intraosseous or central osteosarcoma
   - on the surface of the bone - subperiostal and juxtacortical or parosteal osteosarcoma
   - in the soft tissues - extraosseous osteosarcoma
The intraosseous site is far the most frequent:
nearly 90% of all osteosarcomas are localized within
the bones.

Intraosseous or central osteosarcoma
The usual localization of intraosseous osteosarcoma is the
metaphyseal region of the long bones. Circa 75% of these
tumours is localized in the lower extremities, 50% near the
knee.
The tumour fills the medullary cavity in the lesional area,
arrodes the inner surface of the shaft, invades the Haver-

sian cannals, destroys the cortical bone and spreads over
the surface of the shaft elevating the periosteum. This
can provoque an intense reactive periostal boneproduction
as lamellar deposits along the surface, as spicula protru-
ding from the surface of the shaft and as Codman's triangles
at the edges of the periostal elevation (fig 1).

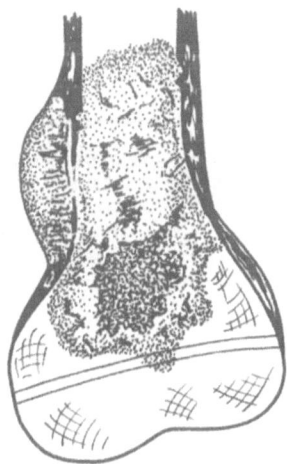

Fig 1. Intraosseous osteosarcoma. Sclerotic centre.
Arrosion and destruction of cortex.
Elevation of periosteum, with spicules and Codman's
triangles (upper and lower edge)
Lamellar deposits in periosteum on the other side.
Small perforation of epiphyseal plate.

The histological structure of osteosarcoma varies widely.
The tumour cells produce osteoid substance which may calcify
and become tumorbone, but usually an osteosarcoma contains
also areas where the cells produce cartilaginous substance
and other areas with fibroblastic tumour cells which produce collagen fibres.
The distrubution of these three patterns in osteocarcinoma
varies widely and according to the predominant intercellular material produced, osteoblastic, chondroblastic and
fibroblastic osteosarcoma types can be distinquished[3].
However, these types do not differ significantly in their
clinical behaviour and therefore this histological typing
is not of much use.

Even when a sarcomatous tumour shows great predominance of cartilaginous differentiation, and osteoid production by the tumour cells can be found only in a few areas, the tumour has to be classified as osteosarcoma and will behave as such, i.e. the course will be much more unfavourable than in the average chondrosarcoma.

In general intraosseous osteosarcoma is a highly malignant tumour: 5 years after adequate treatment of the primary tumour only 20-25% of the patients are surviving.

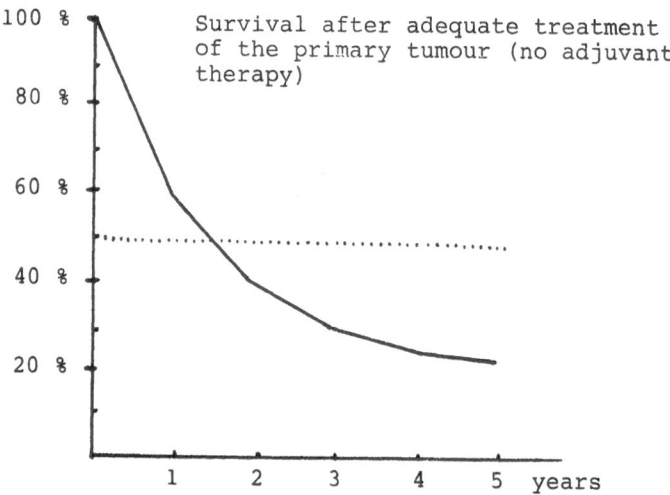

Fig 2. Intraosseous osteosarcoma (all types)

The other 75% died from metastases, usually in the lungs, sometimes in the skeleton. This means that in 75% of the patients with osteosarcoma who come for treatment, tumour cells have already been disseminated to the lungs, although metastases are not yet detectable then. This consideration is the base for the application of adjuvant therapy as complement to the treatment of the primary tumour.

Today the treatment of osteosarcoma consists of radical treatment of the primary tumour and adjuvant therapy to suppress and to eliminate disseminated tumour cells and to prevent the development of metastatic tumours.

This heavy treatment is justified for highly malignant neoplasms.

It is the task of oncological pathology to develop classifications of neoplasms which reflect as much as possible their clinical behaviour, i.e. the grade of their malignancy.

Certainly, not all intraosseous osteosarcomas are of the same grade of malignancy. Several attempts have been made to design grading systems for osteosarcomas.

As can be expected, the great majority of these tumours shows highly pleomorphic nuclei and anaplastic cells; in Broders grading system nearly 90% of the osteosarcomas are classified as high-grade malignant (grade 3 and 4). However, there are a few subtypes and some features which appear to be associated with a somewhat better prognosis than the average of the whole group.

On the other hand some intraosseous osteosarcomas show features which indicate an even worse prognosis than usual after adequate treatment of the primary tumour.

Some underlined unfavourable features are:

- Tumoursite inaccessible for radical treatment
- Osteosarcoma in Paget-bone

Histological:

- Teleangiectatic type of osteosarcoma
- Massive vaso-invasive growth
- Extreme mitotic activity

Radiological:

- Extensive extracortical tumour growth, of which only a small part is covered by reactive periosteal bone.

The teleangiectatic type of osteosarcoma, mentioned above, is characterized by the presence of wide blood-filled cystic spaces giving the tumour a sponge-like structure. The tumour usually grows rapidly and destructively. The neoplastic tissue is very cellular, containing many multinucleated giant cells, and forms septa between the cystic spaces. It is often not easy to distinguish this tissue from aneurysmal bone cysts, but the cellular atypia and the nuclear pleomorphism are indicative for sarcoma (8,9) The osteoid production by the tumour cells distinguishes it from angiosarcoma.

Teleangiectatic osteosarcoma may take a fulminant course, 5-year survival is between 10 and 20%.

Favourable features in intraosseous osteosarcoma are:

    Radiological:

- Well-defined cyst-like lesion
- Extensive periosteal bone production covers the tumour surface

    Histological:

- Low mitotic activity
- Pattern of interwoven bundles consisting of fibroblastic spindle cells and collagen fibres
- Well-differentiated osteosarcoma type, combining these favourable features

    Site:

        Localization in the yaw bones and in the peripheral parts of the extremities

Periosteal reaction

Cohen, radiologist of the Netherlands Cancer Institute, studied a series of 176 intraosseous osteosarcoma from the files of the Netherlands Committee on Bonetumours[2]. He found a correlation of the amount of ossifying periosteal reaction with the survival rate. The 25% of the patients who showed the most extensive periosteal bone formation as lamellae or spicula, had a significantly higher survival rate (fig. 3).

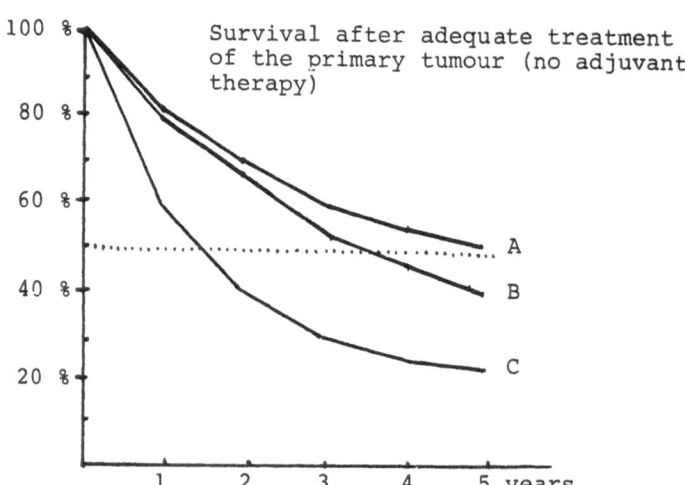

Survival after adequate treatment of the primary tumour (no adjuvant therapy)

Fig 3. A- intraosseous osteosarcoma with extensive reactive periosteal bone production
B- intraosseous osteosarcoma with low mitotic activity
C- intraosseous osteosarcoma (all cases)

Probably is the tumour growth in these cases slower, whereas rapidly growing tumours leave no opportunity for extensive periosteal bone production.

Mitotic activity

Van der Heul studied the mitotic activity in osteosarcomas in our Committee files[5]. He counted the number of mitoses, occurring among circa 3000 tumourcells in the cellular areas of peripheral parts of the tumours. He found a wide variation of mitotic activity among different tumours. The mitotic rate varied from 0,3 to 25 mitoses per 1000 tumour cells. He demonstrated that high mitotic activity was associated with low survival rate; in osteosarcomas with low mitotic rate, i.e. less than 8 mitoses per 1000 tumour cells, the course was slower, and the 5-year survival circa 40% (fig. 3).

Fibroblastic type of intraosseous osteosarcoma

Van der Heul noticed that some intraosseous osteosarcomas, apart from osteoblastic areas consisted completely of tissue with a fibrosarcomatous pattern of interwoven bundles of fibroblastic tumourcells with collagen fibres, resembling the pattern of juxtacortical osteosarcomas.
Often the mitotic rate in these tumours is low. The survival rate of patients suffering from this fibroblastic type of intraosseous osteosarcoma, was circa 60% (fig. 4).

Intraosseous well-differentiated osteosarcoma

This low-grade type was described by Unni et al[14]. It combines the two favourable histological features already mentioned; in the bundled fibroblastic tissue many heavy irregular woven bone trabeculae are present, whereas mitotic activity is not evident. The tumours grow slowly, but progression towards high-grade malignancy may develop. Metastasis is not frequent (15%) and without progression, metastasis probably does not occur. Long-term survival after adequate local treatment can be estimated at 80% or over (fig 4).

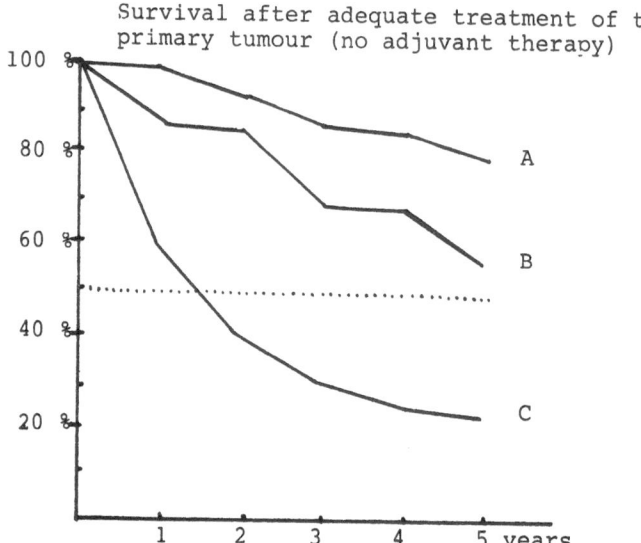

Fig 4. A- well differentiated intraosseous osteosarcoma
       B- fibroblastic type of intraosseous osteosarcoma
       C- intraosseous osteosarcoma (all cases)

The lesion can be mistaken for fibromatous growth and fibrous dysplasia, and in several cases the lesion was
initially diagnosed as benign. This low-grade tumour type
is rare: 1 or 2% of intraosseous osteosarcomas.

The occurence of osteosarcoma on the surface of the bone
is much less frequent than inside the bones.
It is remarkable that both types of surface osteosarcoma-
the juxtacortical and the subperiosteal type- have a
clinical behaviour which is completely different from
intraosseous osteosarcoma. In both surface-types metastasis
is rare, and a long term survival of over 80% can be
expected.

Juxtacortical osteosarcoma
This tumour type was recognized in the fifties and initially
described as parosteal osteoma. The tumour develops slowly
on the surface of the shaft, usually in the metaphyseal
region of a long bone (fig 5).

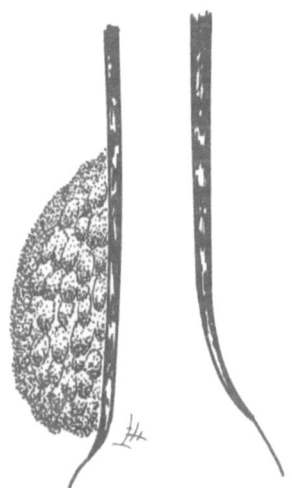

Fig 5. Juxtacortical osteosarcoma. Heavily ossified
       lobulated tumour mass is attached to the sur-
       face of the bone.
       Narrow free zone between lower part of the
       tumour and the cortex.

In the central area the tumour is attached to the bone, the
peripheral parts of the tumour may cover the bone as a
mushroom-like cap. Often a narrow free space between the
cortex and the tumour can be demonstrated on X-ray. The
tumour is a lobulated heavily ossified mass, consisting of
mature bone in well-differentiated fibrous tissue of
moderate cellularity especially in the central parts.
In a minority of cases the tumour tissue is more cellular
and pleomorphic with anaplasia.
In the peripheral zone the tumour bone is less mature and
merges in cellular tumour tissue consisting of spindle

cells and fine collagen fibres. This tissue is microscopically not well-defined from the surrounding soft tissues.
The tumour seems to have its origin in the periosteum, it
extends into the soft tissue, and may penetrate into the
cortical bone and after ultimately it may penetrate into
the marrow cavity. The tumour must be completely removed,
when the tumour is not too large, local surgery is usually
sufficient. Metastases do occur, but practically all cases
with metastasis were cases with a long course after
inadequate treatment, followed by repeated surgical inter-
ventions.

After adequate treatment the prognosis is good, the 5-year
survival rate is over 80% (fig. 6)

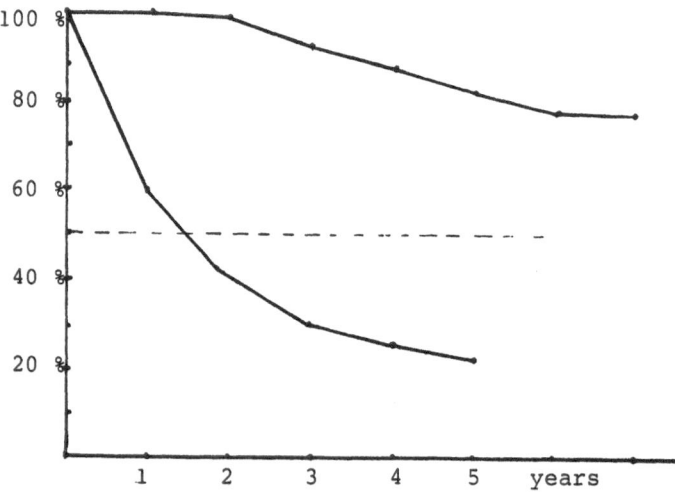

Survival after adequate treatment of the
primary tumour (no adjuvant therapy)

Fig 6. Juxtacortical osteosarcoma

Subperiosteal chondro-osteosarcoma

This tumour type is more rare than the juxtacortical osteo-
sarcoma. It has been described under different names:
Subperiosteal chondrosarcoma - Netherlands Radiological
Atlas of Bone tumours[4].
Juxtacortical chondrosarcoma - Histological typing of Bone
tumours, W.H.O. series no. 6 (1972), and Schajowicz
Periosteal osteogenic sarcoma- Unni, et al[13].
These tumours have a remarkable X-ray appearance.

The diaphyseal part of the shaft of a long bone is diabolo-
like thickened and is covered here by a thick brush of
long spikes (fig 7).

The tumour grows between cortex and periosteum and consists
of a mucoid gelatinous pale myxoid-chondroid tissue, which
surrounds partly, or totally the shaft, elevating the periosteum.

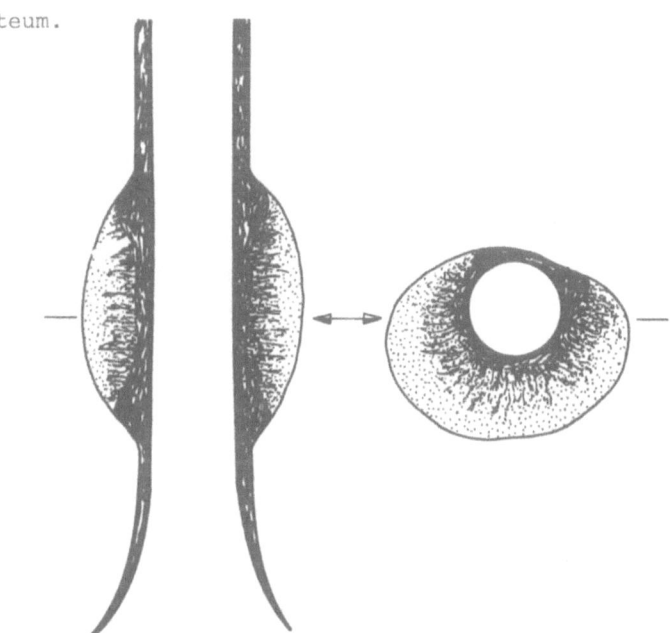

Fig 7. Subperiosteal chondro-osteosarcoma.
        Left: longitudinal section through a subperio-
        steal diaphyseal surface tumour.
        Right: transversal section through the shaft,
        which is for the greater part surrounded by the
        tumour. Intensive spicula formation, and trian-
        gular bony reaction at the edges (left).

The myxo-chondroid tissue is of low cellularity, with small
areas of more cellular tissue, which shows pleomorphism.
In the tissue a varying amount of atypical bony particles
has been formed. A great amount of bone spicula and a lot
of immature bone has been deposited on the surface of the
cortex. The tumour may invade the Haversian cannals,
extension in the medullary cavity is rare.

Nothwithstanding the alarming X-ray appearance, the tumour has a slow course and metastasis is infrequent. Of our 17 cases metastasis occurred in two patients.

Long-term survival after surgical removal of the tumour is of the same level as in juxtacortical osteosarcoma (over 80%).

Resuming, in osteosarcoma several types with marked differences of prognosis can be distinguished. In osteosarcomas on the surface of the bone the risk of metastasis is usually very low, whereas intraosseous and extraosseous osteosarcomas are highly malignant. In some cases of intraosseous sarcoma certain features occur which are associated with a more favourable course resulting in a higher survival rate (fig. 8).

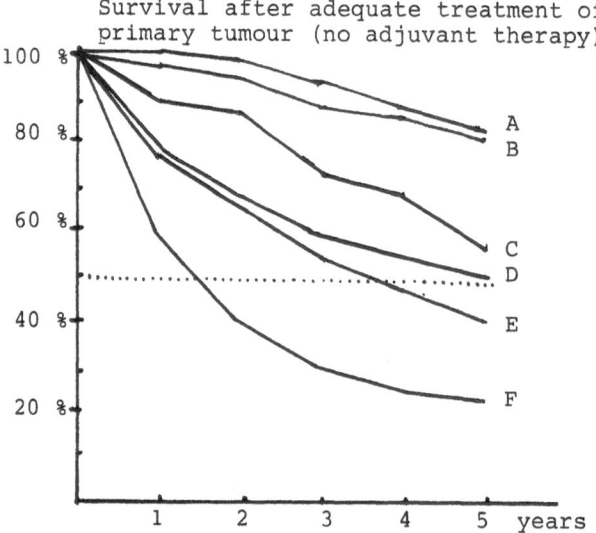

Survival after adequate treatment of the primary tumour (no adjuvant therapy)

Fig 8. A- surface osteosarcoma
       B- well-differentiated intraosseous osteosarcoma
       C- fibroblastic type of intraosseous osteosarcoma
       D- Extensive periosteal reaction intraosseous osteosarcoma
       E- low mitotic activity intraosseous osteosarcoma
       F- intraosseous osteosarcoma (all cases)

Unfortunately only a minority of all osteosarcomas belongs
to the low-grade types, or shows favourable features. Their
relative frequency is shown in table 2, together with the
5-years survival rates. These figures are,of course,
approximations.

Table 2   OSTEOSARCOMA VARIANTS

relative frequency		5-year-survival
	Intraosseous osteosarcoma	
100	all types	25%
2	teleangiectatic type	15%
15	with low mitotic activity	40%
25	with extensive periosteal reaction	50%
5	fibroblastic type	60%
1	well-differentiated low grade type	80%
2	subperiosteal osteosarcoma	80%
7	juxtacortical osteosarcoma	80%
2	extraosseous osteosarcoma	15%

Notwithstanding their rarity, these osteosarcoma variants
deserve attention, because otherwise there is a risk of
overtreatment, or, on the other side, of underrating the
nature of the lesion: low-grade osteosarcoma has been mis-
understood for fibrous dysplasia, and juxtacortical osteosarcoma for myositis ossificans.
The recognition of low-grade osteosarcoma types, and of the
histological and radiological features which can be informative concerning the degree of malignancy is a step towards
a more individual treatment. The necessary individualisation
of treatment will not only require adaptation of the treatment to the individuality of the patient, but also to the
biological individuality of his tumour.

298

REFERENCES

1) ALLAN, C.J., and E.H. SOULE.
   Osteogenic sarcoma of the somatic soft tissues.
   Cancer 27 (1971) 1121-1133.

2) COHEN, P.
   Osteosarcoma of the long bones, Clinical observations
   and experiences in the Netherlands.
   Europ. J. Cancer 14 (1978) 995-1004.

3) DAHLIN, D.C. and K.K. UNNI.
   Osteosarcoma of bone and its important recognizable
   varieties.
   Am. J. Surg. Pathology 1 (1977) 61-72.

4) HEUL, R.O. van der
   Netherlands Committee on Bone Tumours: Radiological
   Atlas of Bone Tumours. Vol. 1
   Baltimore, Williams & Wilkins, 1966, p. 20.

5) HEUL, R.O. van der, and J.R. von RONNEN.
   Juxtacortical osteosarcoma. Diagnosis, differential
   diagnosis, treatment and an analysis of eighty cases.
   J.B.J. Surg. 49-A (1967) 415-439.

6) MATSUNO, T., K.K. UNNI, R.M. MCLEOD, D.C. DAHLIN.
   Teleangiectatic osteogenic sarcoma.
   Cancer 38 (1976) 2538-2547.

7) RONNEN, J.R. von.
   Histological and radiographical classification of osteosarcoma in relation to therapy. A review of 245 cases
   located in the extremities.
   J. Belge Radiol. 51 (1968) 215-221.

8) RUITER, D.J. Th.G. van RIJSSEL and E.A. van der VELDE.
   Aneurysmal bone cysts. A clinicopatholigical study of
   105 cases.
   Cancer 39 (1977) 2231-2239.

9) RUITER, D.J., C.J. CORNELISSE, Th.G. van RIJSSEL and
   E.A. van der VELDE.
   Aneurysmal bone cysts and teleangiectatic osteosarcoma
   A histological and morphometric study.
   Virchows Arch. A. Path. Anat. and Histol. 373 (1977)
   311-325.

10) SCHAJOWICZ, F.
    Juxtacortical chondrosarcoma.
    J.B.J. Surg. 59-B (1977) 473-480.

11) TAYLOR, W.F. J.C. IVINS, D.C. DAHLIN, J.H. EDMONSON
    and D.J. PRITCHARD.
    Trends and variability in survival from osteosarcoma.
    Mayo Clinic Proceedings 53 (1978) 695-700.

12) UNNI, K.K., D.C. DAHLIN, J.W. BEABOUT and J.C. IVINS.
    Parosteal osteogenic sarcoma.
    Cancer 37 (1976) 2466-2475.

13) UNNI, K.K., D.C. DAHLIN and J.W. BEABOUT.
    Periosteal osteogenic sarcoma.
    Cancer 37 (1976) 2476-2485.

14) UNNI, K.K., D.C. DAHLIN, R.A. MCLEOD and D.J. PRITCHARD
    Intraosseous well-differentiated osteosarcoma.
    Cancer 40 (1977) 1337-1347.

24 SURGERY AND ADJUVANT CHEMO-IMMUNOTHERAPY IN OSTEOSARCOMA: REVIEW OF TREATMENT AT THE NATIONAL CANCER INSTITUTE

S. A. Rosenberg and W. F. Sindelar

ABSTRACT

A prospective, randomized study of adjuvant chemotherapy and chemoimmunotherapy following surgical resections of osteosarcoma was carried out on 39 patients at the National Cancer Institute. All patients, after evaluation to rule out disseminated disease, underwent definitive surgical resection of the primary tumor. After surgery, 21 patients were randomized to receive chemotherapy with high-dose methotrexate for 26 three-week cycles. Eighteen patients were randomized after surgical resection for treatment with 26 cycles high-dose methotrexate every three weeks and for immunotherapy with bacillus Calmette-Guerin (BCG) given by scarification between methotrexate doses. Disease-free interval and survival were similar in both chemotherapy and chemoimmunotherapy groups, suggesting no beneficial effect on osteosarcoma from adjuvant BCG immunotherapy. When the 39 protocol patients were considered as a group, combining chemotherapy and chemoimmunotherapy patients, and were compared to a historical control group of 23 patients treated by surgery alone, a significant prolongation of disease-free interval and survival was demonstrated in the protocol patients ($p < 0.05$). Improved disease control in the protocol patients was possibly due to the treatment with methotrexate. However the current protocol patients had a higher number of low grade lesions. When patients with high grade tumors were compared no difference in continuous disease-free survival was seen when comparing current protocol with historical patients. The three-year overall survival

A.T. van Oosterom et al. (eds.), Therapeutic Progress in Ovarian Cancer, Testicular Cancer and the Sarcomas, pp. 301-316. All rights reserved.
Copyright 1980 by Martinus Nijhoff Publishers, The Hague/Boston/London.

of protocol patients (67%) was significantly better than
that of controls (26%). It is believed that the aggressive
surgical resections of pulmonary metastases, which was performed for protocol patients but only sporadically for
controls, led to an increased absolute survival for patient
in the randomized osteosarcoma study.

INTRODUCTION

Osteosarcomas represent a class of malignant primary
bone tumors derived from osteoblasts. They tend to occur
in individuals below the age of 30, have a predominance in
males, and have a predilection for developing in the metaphyseal regions of the long bones. Osteosarcomas have a
tendency for hematogenous dissemination, particularly to
the lungs, and the prognosis has uniformly been grave.

The method of therapy for osteosarcoma has been excision of the involved bone and surrounding soft tissue.
Since most osteosarcomas occur in extremity long bones,
amputation has represented the standard treatment. However, despite radical surgical excisions, overall survival
has been poor due to frequent metastatic spread of the disease. From combined series (1,2), five-year survival
rates have averaged 20%, with median survivals of 16 months
following diagnosis and median time to detection of metastases ten months after treatment.

Attempting to improve survival in osteosarcoma following surgery, recent reports have suggested improvement in
survivals with treatment by chemotherapy (3,4,5). In addition, there has been interest in evaluating immunotherapy
as a possible adjunct to surgery in bone and soft tissue
sarcomas (6).

In an attempt to evaluate the efficacy of adjuvant
chemotherapy and immunotherapy following surgery for osteosarcoma, a prospective randomized protocol trial was carried out at the National Cancer Institute between 1975 and

1978. Specific questions of the study included: whether chemotherapy with methotrexate after surgery prolonged survival in osteosarcoma, and whether immunotherapy offered improvement in disease control of osteosarcoma when combined with chemotherapy after surgery. Early results of the protocol have been reported (7,8). The present paper represents an update of results to four years following institution of the study.

CLINICAL PROTOCOL

Protocol Schema

Patients with biopsy-proven osteosarcoma were entered into the protocol study. All patients received definitive surgery for their tumors, consisting of amputation for extremity lesions. Thirty-nine patients were entered into the study. Four patients received surgery prior to referral, while 35 patients had definitive surgery performed at the National Cancer Institute. Following surgery, patients were randomized to receive postoperative adjuvant chemotherapy or both adjuvant chemotherapy and immunotherapy. The randomizations in the treatment arms are illustrated in Figure 1.

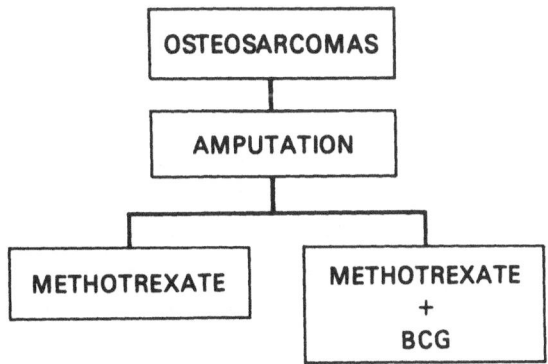

Fig. 1. Randomization in osteosarcoma protocol

Patient Population

All patients with histologically-documented localized osteosarcoma were admitted into the protocol. All had extensive evaluations to exclude metastatic disease, including blood count, serum chemistries, liver scan, bone

scan, and chest roentgenograpy including full lung tomography. All patients had significant renal disease excluded by urinalysis, serum urea and creatinine determinations,
and creatinine clearance. No patients had prior chemotherapy, radiation therapy, or immunotherapy. None had a history of malignant disease unrelated to osteosarcoma.
Patients were excluded from the protocol if they had a history of significant medical problems, such as cardiopul-
monary or renal disease, which would potentially complicate
surgery or postoperative adjuvant therapy. A total of 39
eligible patients were entered into the study.

Pathology

All patients had pathologic diagnosis of osteosarcoma
confirmed, classified, and graded by pathologists at the
National cancer Institute. Biopsy tissue was reviewed in
conjunction with roentgenography, and radiologic interpretation of the x-rays was provided by the diagnostic radiology staff of the National Institutes of Health. All tumors
were characterized by site of origin, (periosteal or medullary), histologic components (osteoblastic, chondroblastic,
fibroblastic, telangiectatic, anaplastic, or well differentiated), and grade (low grade or high grade).

Treatment Arms

Chemotherapy -- All patients in the protocol received
adjuvant chemotherapy with high-dose methotrexate following
surgical excision of the tumor. Chemotherapy was begun
as soon as the surgical incision was healed satisfactorily,
usually within two weeks of operation. All patients received high-dose methotrexate with leucovorin rescue in
21 day intervals for a planned total of 26 treatment cycles. In the initial 24 patients treated, methotrexate was
begun at a dose of 50 mg/kg, which was escalated at each
cycle by 50 mg/kg to a maximum of 250 mg/kg. The last 15
patients, in addition to methotrexate, received vincristine
2 mg infused 30 minutes prior to methotrexate at each cycle.
All methotrexate was given as a six hour intravenous infu-

sion, following 12 hours of vigorous intravenous hydration
which was maintained for 36 hours following completion of
infusion. Urine alkalinity was monitored and maintained by
bicarbonate administration with the hydration. All patients received citrovorum factor rescue following methotrexate. Leucovorin at a dose of 15 mg/m^2 was given two
hours after methotrexate and was repeated every six hours
for a total of eight doses. Additional leucovorin was
given to any patient who had an elevated serum methotrexate level at 48 hours after treatment. Chemotherapy schedule is illustrated in Figure 2.

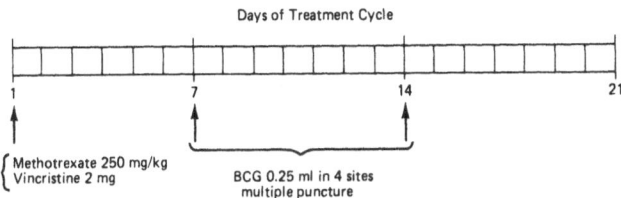

OSTEOSARCOMA

Fig. 2. Treatment cycle for chemotherapy and for immunotherapy. Citrovorum factor rescue not shown.

Immunotherapy -- Patients randomized to receive adjuvant postoperative immunotherapy received injections of
bacillus Calmette-Guerin (BCG) by scarification. The BCG
preparation (Connaught Laboratories, Ontario, Canada)
contained 40 mg of fresh-frozen organisms in 1 ml of ve-
hicle. Treatment consisted of one vial administered on
both the seventh and fourteenth days of each 21 day chemotherapy cycle. For each treatment, four separate areas
of the back were scarified by a multiple puncture technique. A 2x4 cm^2 area was cleansed, dried, and covered
with 0.25 ml of the BCG preparation. Each area was then
scarified in a standardized manner with 15 strokes of a
Heaf gun. Usually, BCG was administered to patients at
home by family members.

Followup during Treatment

        Prior to each treatment cycle, all patients had a com-
plete hematologic evaluation, serum chemical analysis,
urinalysis, creatinine clearance, and chest roentgenograph.

Full lung tomograpy was performed at intervals of three
months. Any findings on patient followup suspicious for
possible metastatic disease were vigorously pursued and
confirmed by biopsy.

Historical Control Group

Protocol patients were compared with a group of 23
historical control patients treated by surgery alone at the
National Cancer Institute between 1953 and 1974. Using
information extracted from hospital charts, all patients
used as historical controls fulfilled criteria for admission
to the study protocol.

Analysis

The 39 patients in the osteosarcoma study protocol
were randomized into two groups: adjuvant chemotherapy or adjuvant chemotherapy with immunotherapy. The two
protocol groups were compared directly as well as with
the 23 historical control patients. Groups were analyzed
for recurrence, disease free interval, and survival. A
generalized one-sided Kruskal-Wallis test was used for
statistical comparisons. The composition of the study
and control patients is summarized in Table 1.

RESULTS

The results and status of the study patients are presented in Tables 2 and 3. Protocol patients in the present analysis have been followed from 11 to 36 months, with
median interval of 27 months.

Twenty-one patients were randomized to receive post-
operative chemotherapy alone. There were 12 recurrences
(54.5%), with 11 patients showing initial recurrence in the
lungs. One patient had recurrence in the iliac crest, in
an area where bone chips were harvested to pack the area
of primary tumor in the tibia, following curettage for
what was thought to be a benign bony lesion. Eighteen
patients received both chemotherapy and immunotherapy postoperatively. Ten patients recurred (55.6%), with nine ini-

TABLE 1. COMPOSITION OF STUDY PATIENT POPULATION

Item	Number of Patients	
	Protocol	Historical Controls
HISTOLOGY		
Osteoblastic	32	20
Chondroblastic	2	0
Fibroblastic	0	1
Telangiectatic	1	0
Anaplastic	2	2
Well differentiated	2	0
GRADE		
Low grade	6	1
High grade	33	22
LOCATION OF TUMOR		
Upper extremity:		
Humerus	2	4
Radius-ulna	0	2
Lower extremity:		
Pelvis	1	0
Femur	23	15
Tibia-fibula	13	2
SEX		
Male	26	15
Female	13	8
RACE		
White	26	20
Black	13	3
AGE		
≤ 10	3	1
11-20	21	15
21-30	7	3
≥ 31	8	4
Median	18	16

308

TABLE 2. RESULTS OF TREATMENT PROTOCOL

Group	Patients	Recurrences	Difference (p value)	Median Time to Recurrence (Months)	Difference (p value)
PROTOCOL PATIENTS					
Chemotherapy	21	12 (54.5%)		8.9	
			>0.05		>0.05
Chemotherapy + immunotherapy	18	10 (55.6%)		11.6	
ALL PATIENTS STUDIES					
Protocol patients	39	22 (56.4%)		10.7	
			<0.05		<0.05
Historical controls	23	19 (82.6%)		6.0	

TABLE 3. SURVIVAL IN STUDY PATIENTS

Group	Patients	Deaths	Three-Year Survival (Actuarial)	Difference (p value)
PROTOCOL PATIENTS				
Chemotherapy	21	4	73%	
				>0.05
Chemotherapy + immunotherapy	18	5	61%	
ALL PATIENTS STUDIED				
Protocol patients	39	9	67%	
				<0.01
Historical controls	23	18	26%	

tially recurring in the lungs and one recurring locally
at the site of hemipelvectomy which was performed for a
pelvic osteosarcoma. No statistical difference in recurrence rate between chemotherapy and chemoimmunotherapy
groups was present. The median time to recurrence for the
chemotherapy alone was 8.9 months. Time to recurrence
for the chemoimmunotherapy group was 11.6 months, not
statistically different from the patients receiving chemotherapy alone.

Considering both the chemotherapy and the chemoimmunotherapy groups together, 22 treatment failures (56.4%)
were present out of the 39 protocol patients. Comparison
with the historical control group of 23 patients showed 19
recurrences (82.6%) among the controls. The median time
to recurrence in the protocol patients was 10.7 months,
as compared with 6.0 months for the control group. This
represented a statistically significant decrease in recurrence rate ($p<0.05$) for the protocol patients and a significant improvement in disease free interval ($p<0.05$)
for the protocol patients as compared with the historical
control group. Actuarial analysis of disease free interval for the protocol patients and controls is given in
Figure 3. If all protocol patients with only high grade
tumors are compared to historical controls with high grade

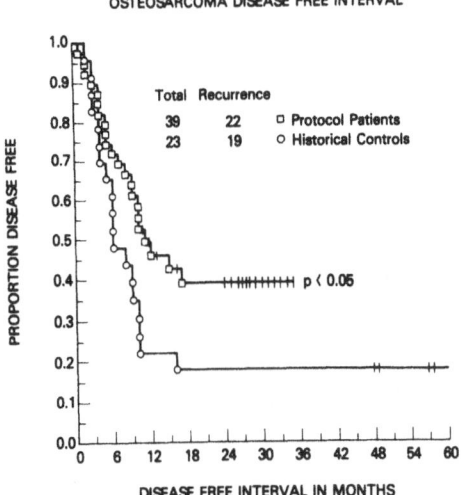

Fig. 3. Disease-free interval in osteosarcoma protocol

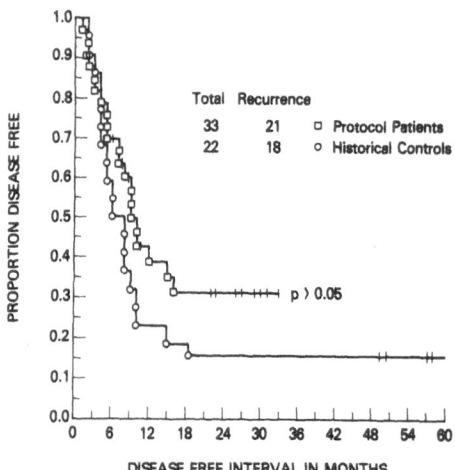

Fig. 4. Disease-free interval in osteosarcoma protocol for patients with high grade lesions.

lesions, the disease free interval of protocol patients is longer but not statistically different from the controls (Figure 4).

Actuarial survival in the 39 protocol patients, considering the chemotherapy and chemoimmunotherapy groups

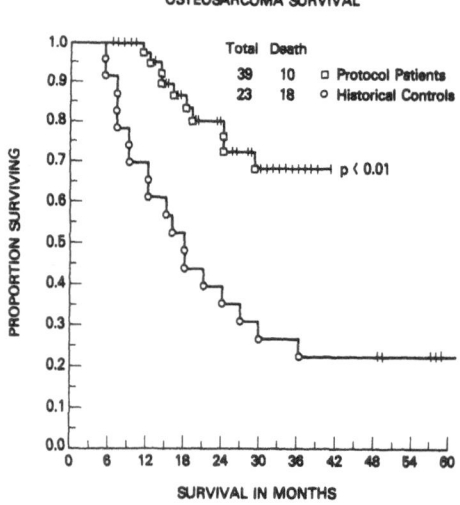

Fig. 5. Survival in osteosarcoma protocol

together, was considerably prolonged (p<0.01) as compared
to the 23 historical controls (Figure 5). Protocol patients who recurred frequently underwent surgical resections of metastatic deposits which prolonged survival.
Few historical control patients had resections of metastatic disease.

DISCUSSION

The treatment of osteosarcoma has involved radical
surgical excision of the involved bone and soft tissues
but has resulted in overall poor survival rates in the
range of 20% (1,2). There has been interest in attempting
to improve treatment results after surgery by utilizing
adjuvant chemotherapy (3,4,5) or immunotherapy (6).

The clinical trial performed at the National Cancer
Institute consisted of 39 patients with osteosarcoma randomized after definitive surgery to receive either adjuvant
chemotherapy with methotrexate or adjuvant chemoimmunotherapy with methotrexate and BCG. Control group consisted
of 23 patients treated at the National Cancer Institute
with surgery alone. Early results of the treatment protocols have been reported (7,8) and are updated in the present paper to a median followup of 27 months.

Comparison between the 21 patients randomized to chemotherapy and the 18 in the chemoimmunotherapy group showed no statistical differences in recurrence rate, disease
free interval, or survival (Tables 2 and 3). It was concluded that the addition of BCG immunotherapy to postoperative chemotherapy had no beneficial effects and that, at
present, BCG has no role in the treatment of osteosarcoma.

When a direct comparison is made between all protocol
patients (chemotherapy and chemoimmunotherapy patients
combined) with historical controls, a significant prolongation of disease free interval is demonstrated among the
protocol patients (Figure 3). It is tempting to conclude
that the improvement in disease control in the protocol
patients was due to the effects of high-dose methotrexate.
Such a demonstration of effective adjuvant chemotherapy

improving results after surgery would be of great importance in the overall management of all patients with osteosarcoma.

Because a historical control group was used in the present study, it is possible that the observed differences in treatment outcome between the protocol and control patients could be attributable to differences between the protocol and control group populations. The historical control group of 23 patients had a two-year disease free interval of 17% and a three-year actuarial survival of 26%, findings consistent with the clinical results of large series of osteosarcoma patients (1,2). There were no significant influences on disease free interval and survival and no significant differences between protocol and control groups with regard to histologic type of osteosarcoma, location of tumor, sex, race, or age. There were, however, small differences in histologic grade (Table 1). In the protocol group, six patients (15%) had low grade while 33 patients (85%) had high grade lesions. Among historical controls, one (4%) had low grade osteosarcoma and 22 (96%) had high grade tumors. The somewhat greater proportion of high grade lesions in the control group could have possibly influenced results by shortening survival or disease free interval in the control patients. This possibility is supported by comparison of disease free interval of protocol patients having high grade osteosarcoma with historical controls having high grade lesions (Figure 4). In such a comparison, the two-year disease free interval of protocol patients with high grade tumors was 31%, greater but not statistically different from the 15% disease free interval of control patients with high grade tumors.

Evaluation of metastatic disease status could also influence study results. If more sensitive screening measures for disseminated disease were used in the protocol patient group than in the control population, it is possible that the control group could contain patients with occult metastatic disease and thereby lower the overall

survival of the control group. Of 52 patients referred to
the National Cancer Institute for consideration of the
osteosarcoma study, 11 patients were discovered to have
pulmonary metastases and were excluded from the protocol.
In four of the 11 patients with metastases routine chest
x-rays were normal and pulmonary lesions were visible only
on full lung tomography. Among the historical control
group, initial screening for metastases by lung tomography was not consistent in all patients. It is conceivable
that the control population contained patients with un-
recognized early metastatic disease, and the control group
therefore might have diminished survival compared with
protocol patients.

Survival, with no regard for whether recurrences developed and were treated, in the protocol patients (67%
three-year survival) was significantly greater (p<0.01)
than among the historical controls (26% three-year survival); see Table 3 and Figure 5. The increase in absolute
survival in the protocol patients can be attributed to
aggressive surgical excision of metastatic lesions when
discovered. All protocol patients received chest roent-
genographs every three weeks and lung tomography every
three months. When pulmonary nodules were detected, patients were subjected to exploratory thoracotomy with
wedge resections of metastases. Out of the 39 protocol
patients, there were 22 total recurrences and 20 recurrences in the lungs. Of the 20 patients with pulmonary
metastases, two were thought to have unresectable disease
and did not have thoracotomy. Eighteen patients underwent
exploratory thoracotomy, and 11 had all detectable disease
resected. Seven of the 11 patients with resected metastases remained free of disease (minimum followup 12
months) and four patients subsequently recurred with further pulmonary metastases. The four patients with recurrences after thoracotomy underwent further resections,
were rendered free of detectable disease, and remained
free of metastases (followup minimum six months). Course
of the 39 protocol patients with respect to pulmonary re-

currence and resection of metastases is given in Figure
6. Among the 23 historical control patients there were
19 recurrences, one local recurrence and 18 patients with
pulmonary metastases. Out of the 18 control patients with
pulmonary metastases, only six were treated with thoracotomy and resection of metastatic lesions, as contrasted
to thoracotomies in 18 out of 20 protocol patients with
pulmonary recurrence. The prolongation of survival by
resection of pulmonary metastases in the protocol patients
led to the firm conclusion that aggressive resection of
metastatic disease, whenever possible, will prolong survival in osteosarcoma.

The National Cancer Institute osteosarcoma study indicated that following definitive surgery, adjuvant immunotherapy with BCG was of no benefit. Patients treated
postoperatively with adjuvant high-dose methotrexate did
have prolonged disease free survival. Since a historical
control group was used with the possibility of differences
in histological grade or presence of occult disseminated
disease between the control and protocol groups, no definite conclusion can be drawn at the present time that
methotrexate therapy is of benefit in the treatment of
osteosarcoma.

Currently, the National Cancer Institute is conducting a prospective protocol study of osteosarcoma where
patients, after definitive surgery, are randomized to receive chemotherapy with high-dose methotrexate given
weekly or to receive no adjuvant chemotherapy. Protocol
is diagrammed in Figure 7. All patients are followed, and
if pulmonary recurrences develop, patients are offered
thoracotomy and resection of metastases. Patients not receiving chemotherapy who develop recurrence are begun on
methotrexate after thoracotomy. Patients that have recurrence on methotrexate are randomized, following thoracotomy, to no further chemotherapy or to continued chemotherapy doxorubicin and cyclophosphamide. Any patient
randomized to no chemotherapy after methotrexate failure
is offered doxorubicin and cyclophosphamide therapy if

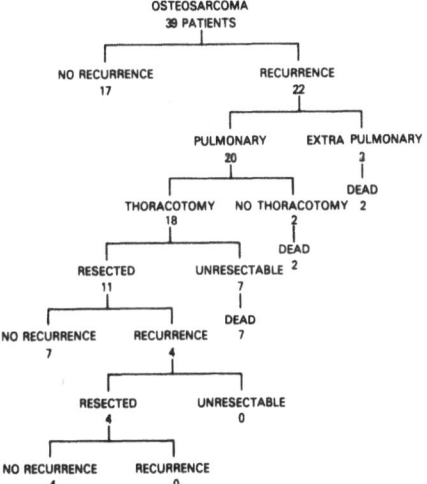

Fig. 6. Resection of pulmonary metastases in osteosarcoma
protocol

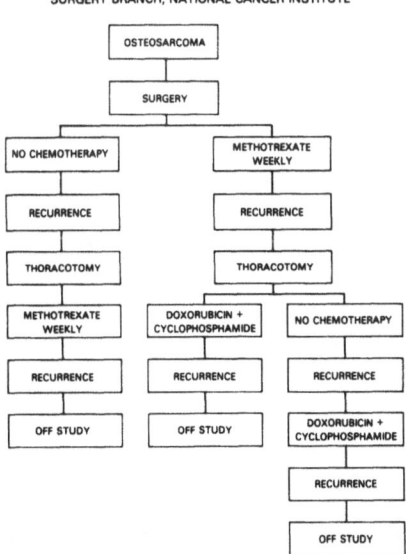

Fig. 7. Current osteosarcoma protocol at National Cancer
Institute

recurrences develop while not receiving chemotherapy. It
is expected the protocol will determine whether high-dose
methotrexate is of therapeutic benefit in osteosarcoma
and whether a combination of doxorubincin and cyclophosphamide has any efficacy in osteosarcoma following methotrexate failure.

316

REFERENCES

(1)   Marcove, R.C., Mike, V., Hajek, J.V., et al. Osteo-
      genic sarcoma under the age of twenty-one. A review
      of one hundred and forty-five operative cases. J.
      Bone Joint Surg. [Am.] 52-A:411-423, 1970.

(2)   McKenna, R.J., Schwinn, C.P., Soong, K.Y., et al.
      Sarcomata of the osteogenic series (osteosarcoma,
      fibrosarcoma, chondrosarcoma, parosteal osteogenic
      sarcoma, and sarcomata arising in abnormal bone).
      An analysis of 552 cases. J. Bone Joint Surg. [Am.]
      48-A:1-26, 1966.

(3)   Cortes, E.P., Holland, J.F., Wang, J.J., et al.
      Amputation and adriamycin in primary osteosarcoma.
      N. Engl. J. Med. 291:998-1000, 1974.

(4)   Jaffe, N., Frei, E., Traggis, D., et al. Adjuvant
      methotrexate and citrovorum-factor treatment of
      osteogenic sarcoma. N. Engl. J. Med. 291:994-997,
      1974.

(5)   Sutow, W.W., Gehan, E.A., Vietti, T.J., et al.
      Multidrug chemotherapy in primary treatment of
      osteosarcoma. J. Bone Joint Surg. [Am.] 58-A:629-
      633, 1976.

(6)   Morton, D.L., Joseph, W.L., Ketcham, A.S., et al.
      Surgical resection and adjunctive immunotherapy for
      selected patients wtih multiple pulmonary metastases.
      Ann. Surg. 178:360-366, 1973.

(7)   Rosenberg, S.A., Chabner, B.A., Young, R.C., et al.
      Treatment of osteogenic sarcoma. I. Effect of
      adjuvant high-dose methotrexate after amputation.
      Cancer Treat. Rep. 63:739-751, 1979.

(8)   Rosenberg, S.A., Flye, M.W., Conkle, D., et al.
      Treatment of osteogenic sarcoma. II. Aggressive
      resection of pulmonary metastases. Cancer Treat.
      Rep. 63:753-756, 1979

Acknowledgement

Results reported in the present study represent a coopera-
tive effort by many individuals in various branches and di-
visions of the National Cancer Institute. In particular,
efforts of the following were important in the completion
of the study: Surgery Branch -- A.R. Baker, M.F. Brennan,
P.B. Chretien, M.H. Cohen, E.V. deMoss, M.W. Flye, H.F.
Sears, C. Seipp, P.H. Sugarbaker; Medicine Branch -- R.C.
Young; Clinical Pharmacology Branch -- B.A. Chabner;
Pediatric Oncology Branch -- A.S. Levine; Laboratory of
Pathology -- J. Costa, T. A. Hanson; Biometric Research
Branch -- R.M. Simon.

25 THE ROLE OF RADIOTHERAPY IN THE TREATMENT OF THE PRIMARY AND IN ADJUVANT THERAPY

K. Breur

INTRODUCTION

Until about 10 years ago, the outlook for an improvement of the bad prognosis for patients with osteosarcoma seemed hopeless. As in the vast majority of cases the primary tumour originates from one of the bones of the limbs, ablative surgery can free the patient radically from this tumour. The bad prognosis is completely due to the appearance of metastases in about 3/4 of the cases. The lungs are almost always the first and main sites of these metastases, leading to the death of the patient. In about 40% of the cases the metastases become detectable on the chest X-rays within the first 6 months and in 60% within one year. Only in very few cases do they appear after more than two years. For a number of reasons, osteosarcoma establishes an excellent model in the human to study more quantitatively volume and time factors of growth, and the effects of cytotoxic agents. This in turn has lead to a more rational approach in the treatment of patients.

RADIATION TREATMENT OF THE PRIMARY TUMOUR

To circumvent the highly mutilating effect of ablative surgery, the possibilities of X-ray treatment have been explored for many years. Unfortunately it has been shown that this tumour type is rather radioresistant, meaning that local cures could only be obtained in a small percentage of the cases and that, for a better result, dosages were needed that would exceed the tolerance of surrounding normal tissues.

The advent of megavoltage radiation, which so markedly increased the potentials of radiotherapy, hardly improved results in osteosarcoma. However, some authors (1) have reported many local cures using doses of around 9000 rads in about 9 weeks. Due to late local complications and some recurrences, secondary amputation had to be performed in an appreciable number of cases. The overal 5-years survival was at least as good as reported for primary surgery.

Another attempt has been undertaken to prevent about 80% of all patients having to undergo a mutilating intervention, which within 2 years would prove to be of no importance for survival. The Dutch Bone Tumour Registry has advised, since the early fifties, the treatment of the primary tumour with radiation to a dose of around 6000 rads and that amputation should only be performed if after 6 months still no metastases are detectable. S. Cade (2) reported results of treatment based on a similar principle, in order to mutilate only that selected group of patients with a more favourable prognosis. Cohen (3) has published the results of the Dutch cases. The group selected for ablative surgery indeed proved to have a far better prognosis (39%), while the 5-years survival rate for the total group was no worse (22%) than that reported for cases treated by immediate amputation. However, the palliative effect in patients who were not amputated, proved to be unsatisfactory which, combined with improved prothesis techniques, lead to a renewed preference for ablative surgery as primary treatment. In most of the amputation specimens, the 6 months previously irradiated tumour was replaced by a necrotic mass in which clumps of viable looking tumour cells could still be found histologically.

To find a reason for this apparent low radio-

sensitivity of osteosarcomas we can consider the main
factors which influence radiation response of tumours
(Table I).

Table I: Factors influencing radiation response of tumours

1. Growth rate, growth fraction
2. Volume, number of viable tumour cells
3. Percentage of tumour cells in hypoxic condition,
   reoxygenation rate
4. Repopulation rate, repair of DNA damage, redistribution
   over cell cycle
5. "Intrinsic radiosensitivity"

According to the volume-doubling time of lung
metastases, osteosarcomas are usually rather fast-growing
tumours. In general such tumours, especially if a large
proportion of cells are in cell cycle, show a good radiosensitivity. This could indicate that other factors must
play a role in the relative resistance of osteosarcoma.

One of these factors could be the volume and number
of tumour cells present at the time of diagnosis. In a
series of cases from the Dutch Bone Registry, published by
Cohen (3), measurements on X-rays resulted in estimations
of volumes of primaries, ranging from 5 to 506 cc, with a
geometric mean of 108. This means that usually a large
number of tumour cells (in order of $10^{10}-10^{11}$) is present at
the onset of treatment. As for cure, an increase in dose is
needed with increasing number of tumour cells and tolerance
of normal tissues decreases with increased irradiated
volume, this results in a reduction of the therapeutic ratio.

Compared to well-oxygenated cells, those living under
hypoxic conditions are markedly more radioresistant. Many
tumours have an appreciable fraction of hypoxic cells,
which usually increases with tumour volume. In view of the
areas of necrosis in osteosarcomas, the tension in these
tumours in the limbs and the possibility of pressure on

afferent vessels, one can assume a large proportion of hypoxic radioresistant tumour cells. During fractionated radiotherapy a process called reoxygenation takes place. The first series of radiation doses will kill off mainly the well-oxygenated cells near the capillaries. Metabolic death and removal of these cells leading to tumour shrinkage, makes blood supplied oxygen available for the previously hypoxic cells, making these cells more sensitive to the following radiation fractions. The re-oxygenation rate has been shown to be different for different types of tumours. It is likely that the reoxy-genation rate is very low in osteosarcoma, in view of the slow tumour regression and the necrotic masses, which remain present for a long time. Also in experimental studies osteosarcomas were shown to have a small tendency for reoxygenation (6). Many French centres still prefer curative radiation therapy if the primary tumour, when detected, is still small. This could be based on favourable factors 2 and 3 for these cases.

For the other factors (4 and 5 in table I), there are no data to indicate that these could be responsible for the relatively low radiosensitivity of primary osteosarcomas.

Recent developments in radiotherapy hold promises for better results, especially in osteosarcoma. Most of them more or less eliminate the unfavourable influence of hypoxia. Fast heavy particle radiation, e.g. fast neutrons, affect hypoxic cells almost as efficiently as well-oxyge-nated cells. So called "hypoxic cell sensitizers" are drugs that selectively sensitize hypoxic cells almost to the same sensitivity as well-oxygenated cells. Other possibilities to be evaluated are radiation with a low dose rate or with multiple daily fractions. Finally combinations of chemo-therapy to reduce tumour volume and boosts of radiation should be explored as an attempt to avoid surgical mutilation.

RADIOTHERAPY FOR METASTASES

The form of treatment of the primary tumour hardly
influences prognosis, which is almost entirely determined
by the fact whether or not subclinical lung metastases are
present at the time of diagnosis. When already detectable
on the chest X-ray, radiation therapy can practically never
achieve cures, which is also due to the limited tolerance
of lung tissue to radiation. As improvement of prognosis
could only be achieved by suppressing the growth of
metastases, the Clinical Cooperative Group for Radiotherapy
of the E.O.R.T.C. decided in 1969 to investigate the
possibilities of whole-lung irradiation following radical
treatment of the primary in the absence of detectable lung
metastases. A rational justification was needed for a trial
that could be regarded as an experiment on humans.

From available clinical data 2000 rads on both lungs
in 10 sessions over 2 weeks was excepted as a safe
tolerance dose with regard to lung function (5). The D_{10},
being the dose needed to reduce the volume or number of
tumour cells to 10% of the original value could be assumed
to be in between 400 and 500 rads. A total dose of 2000
rads then could only cope with about 10^5 tumour cells. Such
a dose could thus only be effective in those cases in which
the number of disseminated tumour cells in the lungs is
still very small. The volume increase of the usually
globular lung metastases can be followed on subsequent
chest X-rays. It has been demonstrated before that, with
only very few exceptions, these metastases have a constant
growth rate, resulting in an exponental growth curve.
Extrapolation backwards in time can indicate the volume on
the date of treatment of the primary. In this way we found
that in 13 cases there were 3 in which the number of
tumour cells at the time of diagnosis could be estimated
to be 10^5 or less. If this were a representative probe, one
could expect the possibility of preventing manifestation of
lung metastases in 20-25% of the patients with subclinical

metastases.

In many cases the volume doubling time of lung
metastases has been determined. There is a log normal
spread of these values with a mean value of about 1 month.
From the percentage cumulative curve of the appearance of
lung metastases during follow-up after primary treatment
(Fig. 1), one can see that in about 20% of the cases, the
metastases appear after 12 months or more. In these cases
the metastases have at least to perform 12 volume doublings
to become visible on the chest X-ray with a diameter of
1 cm and about 10^8-10^9 tumour cells. This means for this
20% of the group also an estimated number of tumour cells
of 10^5 or less at the time of first treatment.

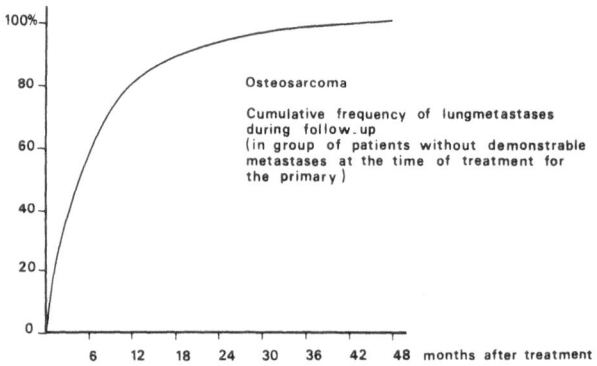

P. Cohen (1979)

Fig. 1.

When the time interval between first treatment and
the appearance of metastases becomes larger, the survival
time after detection of the metastases increases (11, 4).
This indicates a lower growth rate for the late appearing
metastases. Taking this factor into account together with
the time distribution of appearance of lung metastases, our
statistican, A.A.M. Hart could give an estimation of the

distribution of tumour cell numbers present in lungs for a
group of patients that later on had manifest metastases
(Fig. 2). A treatment that could kill 10^4-10^5 tumour cells
would be able to prevent growth of metastases in 20% of
these cases.

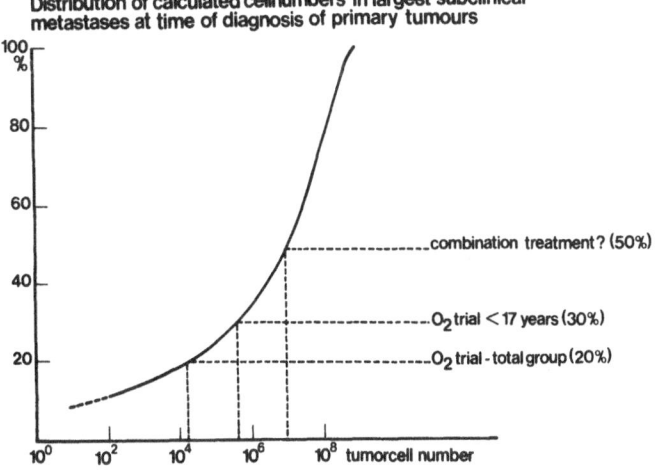

Distribution of calculated cellnumbers in largest subclinical metastases at time of diagnosis of primary tumours

A.A.M. Hart (1979)

Fig. 2.

On this basis a controlled clinical trial was started in
1970, in which 5 French and 2 Dutch centres participated.
Patients under 60 years of age with histologically
confirmed osteosarcoma in one of the limbs, with no
detectable metastases, were randomized in two groups after
radical treatment of the primary.

    A. no further treatment.

    B. adjuvant whole-lung irradiation

       (2000 rads in 2 weeks)

The main criterium for evaluation was the disease-free
survival time. In 4 years 86 patients were accepted in the
trial. The results were only evaluated more than two years
after the last patient entered the trial (8).

    It could be shown that the disease-free survival at

324

5 years in the lung-treated group was 45% compared to 28% in the untreated group. The results were more striking in the 64 patients under the age of 17. Here 48% remained disease-free compared to 28% of the controls (Fig. 3). The incidence of skeletal metastases was the same in both groups. Also the percentage 5-years survival was increased significantly. This means that this 2 weeks adjuvant therapy prevented clinical manifestation of metastases in respectively 20 and 30% of the cases. Newton and Barrett reported approximately the same result from a pilot study (10).

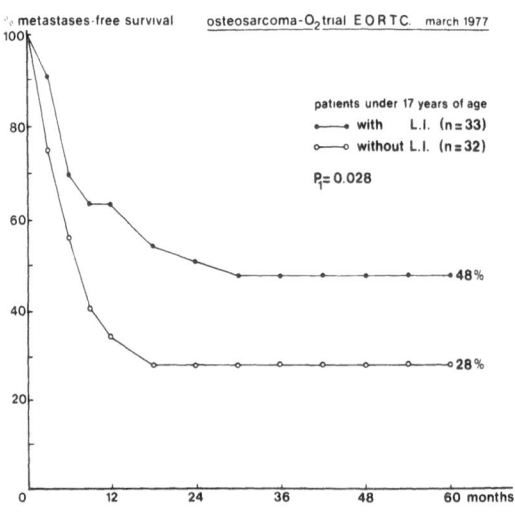

Fig. 3. Disease-free survival curves (Reference 8).

Although we would have preferred to collect a greater number of cases, the trial was terminated in 1974 because of the highly optimistic preliminary reports of adjuvant chemotherapy. This treatment was given in courses over a period of 12 or even 18 months. Oncologists already warned at that time that these publications were premature with regard to conclusions on final survival rate, as many of the patients were still under treatment. The initial suggestions were in the order of 60-80% two years disease-free survival, which was compared with rather bad results in historical series. The figures, after a longer follow-up period, have now dropped to around 40%, so the same level as reached with lung irradiation.

Despite a feeling of deception, it seems that intensive courses of chemotherapy can cope with about 4 decades of tumour cell numbers, although confirmation is still needed from randomized trials. It will therefore be very interesting to see what can be achieved by a combination of chemotherapy and lung irradiation. Looking at the estimated distribution of tumour cell numbers in the lungs in the group of patients which later would develop metastaes (Fig. 2), one can see that a few decades more than eliminated by irradiation alone could prevent development of metastases in half of these cases (9), which would have left the survival rate of the whole group at about 65%. Last year the E.O.R.T.C. [*] and S.I.O.P. [**] started a new trial. In this trial [***] patients are randomized after radical treatment of the primary into 3 groups (see Table II).

Table II: E.O.R.T.C. and S.I.O.P. trial on adjuvant treatment
in osteosarcoma of the limbs

    a. chemotherapy (HDMTX/CF, ADRIA, VRC, CFA)
    b. radiotherapy (lungirradiation, 2000 rad with air
          correction in 12 days)
    c. combination chemo- and radiotherapy (HDMTX/CF, ADRIA,
          VCR only induction therapy, followed by
          lung irradiation, 2000 rad)

[*] European Organization for Research on the Treatment of Cancer
[**] Société Internationale d'Oncologie Pediatrique
[***] The protocol for this trial can be requested from the secretary, Dr. E. van der Schueren, Department of radiotherapy, Wilhelmina Gasthuis, 1e Helmersstraat 104, Amsterdam

A group without adjuvant therapy, though desirable from a statistical point of view, was not included in the trial, as this was regarded as ethically not justifiable. As the selection criteria and the whole-lung irradiation scheme are identical, the untreated group from the first trial can serve as best historical control group. The main criterium for evaluation of results again will be the disease-free survival period during a follow-up of at least 2 years after the end of the adjuvant treatment. Up till December 1979 about a hundred patients were entered in the trial. The tolerance of the patient for the various treatment schedules will be compared. For this purpose lung function tests have to be performed at regular intervals. Up till now no untoward effects have been reported apart from one case of serious bone marrow depression after chemotherapy. In an annex study the possibilities of surgical removal of lungmetastases will be investigated. The suggestion that metastases still developing after adjuvant therapy will be strongly reduced in numbers, could make a higher proportion of these cases better managable for surgical intervention.

CONCLUSIONS

Treatment with megavoltage X-rays can achieve local cures of primary osteosarcomas when very high doses are applied. Unfortunately this is accompanied with a high complication rate. Chances for local cure are much better when the tumour is still small at the onset of treatment. Recent developments in radiotherapy, like the use of high LET radiation (e.g. fast neutrons), hypoxic cell sensitizers and unconventional time-dose schedules offer good perspectives and should be explored for osteosarcomas. Whole-lung irradiation has already shown to be effective as adjuvant treatment.

Both for the primary and the suppression of

metastases combinations of radio- and chemotherapy could
further improve the fate of patients struck with this type
of malignant tumour. Rather than expressing effects in
partial and complete response rates, a more quantitative
analysis of the efficacy of chemotherapeutic agents should
be employed.

REFERENCES

1   J. Papillon and L. Duton:
    Traitement par Cobalt 60 des Sarcomes Osteogeniques.
    In: Symposium Ossium (Eds. A.M. Jelliffe and B. Strick-
    land), p. 133-134. E. & S. Livingstone, Edinburgh and
    London, 1970.
2. S. Cade:
    Bone Sarcoma.
    J. Roy. Coll. Surg. Edinb. 12, 83, 1967.
3. P. Cohen:
    Het osteosarcoom van de lange pijpbeenderen.
    Thesis, Amsterdam, 1974.
4. P. Cohen:
    Osteosarcoma of the long bones.
    Europ. J. Cancer, 14, 995-1004, 1979.
5. J.S. Abbatucci, A. Boulier, J. Fabre and J.C. Lozier:
    Functional evaluation of pulmonary irradiation effects.
    Europ. J. Cancer, 14, 781-785, 1979.
6. L.M. van Putten, P. Lelieveld and J.J. Broerse:
    Response of a poorly reoxygenating mouse osteosarcoma
    to x-rays and fast neutrons.
    Europ. J. Cancer, 7, 153-160, 1971.
7. K. Breur:
    Growth rate and radiosensitivity of human tumours.
    Europ. J. Cancer, 2, 157, 1966.
8. K. Breur, P. Cohen, O. Schweisguth and A.M.M. Hart:
    Irradiation of the lungs as an adjuvant therapy of
    osteosarcoma of the limbs.
    Europ. J. Cancer, 14, 461-471, 1978.
9. K. Breur and E. van der Schueren:
    Adjuvant therapy in the management of osteosarcoma:
    need for critocal reassessment.
    In: Recent Results in Cancer Research, vol. 68.
    (Eds. G. Bonadonna, G. Mathé and S.E. Salmon).
    Springer Verlag Berlin Heidelberg 1979.
10. K.A. Newton and A. Barrett:
    Prophylactic lung irradiation in the treatment of
    osteogenic sarcoma.
    Clin. Radiol., 29, 493, 1978.
11. G.M. Jeffree, D.H.G. Price and H.A. Sissons:
    The metastatic patterns of osteosarcoma.
    Brit. J. Cancer, 32, 87-107, 1975.

26 CHEMOTHERAPY OF OSTEOSARCOMA - AN OVERVIEW

C. B. Pratt

Oncologists, both medical and pediatric, expressed little interest in or concern for treatment of patients with osteosarcoma prior to 1972. The reasons for this apathy were the dismal results of the past and the natural history of osteosarcoma to metastasize to the lungs within months of diagnosis, followed by the early death of the patients from pulmonary insufficiency (1,2).

Few studies before 1972 demonstrated any benefits of chemotherapy for metastatic osteosarcoma (1). It was a custom of the past to amputate if possible the affected part and to follow the patient expectantly for the development of metastases. In many instances, chest radiographs were not obtained routinely, and thus determination of the time to development of pulmonary metastases was not recorded with certainty (2).

Within this communication there will be attempts to outline the influences of chemotherapy on the treatment of osteosarcoma - in the treatment of metastatic disease, in the treatment of primary tumor, as well as in the adjuvant situation.

Single Agent Effects On Metastatic Osteosarcoma

Table 1 indicates the responses obtained with the use of single agents cyclophosphamide (3-6), phenylalanine mustard (5), mitomycin C (1), high-dose methotrexate (7-11), adriamycin (12-19) and cis-platinum (20-28). Responses were rare with cyclophosphamide, phenylalanine mustard and mitomycin C, but occurred with predictable frequency in 20 to 30% of the patients treated with high-dose methotrexate, adriamycin and cis-Platinum.

Table 1. Single Activity Against Advanced Osteosarcoma

Agent	Number Complete + Partial Responses/Number Treated	References
Cyclophosphamide	4/28	3-6
Phenylalanine Mustard	5/32	5
Mitomycin C	11/76	1
High-Dose Methotrexate	13/31	7-11
Adriamycin	39/183	12-19
Cis-diammine-dichloroplatinum	12/48	20-28

Effects Of Combination Chemotherapy On Metastatic Osteosarcoma

Against osteosarcoma with either pulmonary, bony or soft tissue metastases, with combinations using 2 to 4 agents including mitomycin C, phenylalanine mustard, vincristine, adriamycin, DTIC, cyclophosphamide, high-dose methotrexate, bleomycin and dactinomycin, responses (Table 2) occurred with predictable frequency in from 30 to 90% of the patients, indicating the effectiveness of these agents given in combination for affecting complete or partial responses following treatment (10,13,29-33). Of particular note was the response of almost one-third of the patients receiving combinations including adriamycin. Additionally, the frequency of response following the treatment of patients with weekly high-dose methotrexate in combination with vincristine, as reported by Jaffe (23), provided impetus for continuation of efforts for

Table 2. Combination Chemotherapy Activity in Patients with

　　　　　Advanced Osteosarcoma

Agents	Number Complete + Partial Responses/Number Treated	References
Mito C-PAM-VCR	0/10	29
Mito C-PAM-VCR	6/18	30
Adria-DTIC-VCR	16/46	13
Cyclo-VCR-Adria-DTIC	7/29	13
HDMTX-Adria	7/13	31
HDMTX-VCR	4/10	32
HDMTX-VCR-weekly	7/8	7
HDMTX-Adria-Cyclo	4/16	10
Bleo-Cyclo-Dact	8/13	33

Mito C = Mitomycin C
PAM = Phenylalanine Mustard
VCR = Vincristine
Adria = Adriamycin
DTIC = Imidazole Carboxamide
Cyclo = Cyclophosphamide
HDMTX = High-Dose Methotrexate
Bleo = Bleomycin
Dact = Dactinomycin

treatment of patients with metastatic disease. The frequency of responses in patients receiving a combination of
bleomycin, cyclophosphamide and dactinomycin (33) led to
the inclusion of this 3-agent combination into the multidrug treatments for patients receiving adjuvant treatment
at Memorial Hospital in New York (34). Most of the agents
as listed in Table 2 have found their way into adjuvant
chemotherapy schemes, with the exception of mitomycin C.

Sutow included phenylalanine mustard into the CONPADRI I and COMPADRI II and III protocols of the Southwest Oncology Group (35); from these protocols results, the contribution of phenylalanine mustard was not certain, in that another alkylating agent, cyclophosphamide, was used additionally.

Adjuvant Chemotherapy for Osteosarcoma

Without the availability of agents which were effective, or partially effective, against pulmonary metastases, there were only a few early efforts at treatment using adjuvant chemotherapy. Treatments given by Sutow and his associates (Table 3) at the M.D. Anderson Hospital (36) and Hustu and his associates at St. Jude Children's Research Hospital (37) with a combination of vincristine plus cyclophosphamide with or without dactinomycin yielded inconclusive results which were approximately the same as expected without the addition of chemotherapy. Another early study, as performed by Necheles and his associates at the Tufts New England Medical Center (42), has used high dose cyclophosphamide at 3 month intervals for a period of 18 months; three of the 6 patients have been long-term survivors.

By 1971, data suggested that the effectiveness of methotrexate might be increased in experimental animal tumors by the delivery of this agent in higher dosages, the toxicity of which could be avoided by the administration of citrovorum factor (38). Djerassi (39) applied this rationale to the treatment of patients with lung cancer, and later Jaffe utilized these methods in the treatment of patients with metastatic osteosarcoma (32). The use of high dose methotrexate with citrovorum factor rescue produced measurable complete or partial responses in patients with metastatic osteosarcoma (7,32). With the indication that the cellular efflux of methotrexate could be enhanced by pretreatment of animal tumors with vincristine, Jaffe added this agent to the regimen of high dose methotrexate.

Also by 1972 the effectiveness of adriamycin was demonstrated against many tumors, including osteosarcoma (12-19). Adriamycin was introduced into adjuvant chemotherapy trials at the Roswell Park Memorial Institute, and by investigators of the Cancer and Leukemia Group B (40,41). These adjuvant studies as reported by Holland and Cortes have indicated a 61% 2-year disease-free survival for the patients who have received treatment with adriamycin 30 mg/m^2 daily for 3 days every 4 weeks, for a total cumulative dose of 540 mg/m^2. For the individuals who were considered to have had chemotherapy or surgical violations, the 2-year disease-free survival was 39%, which is somewhat improved over that which would be expected from an untreated control group who had had no chemotherapy following amputation.

Of particular interest are those protocol studies which included high dose methotrexate and adriamycin, alone or in combination. The ongoing comparative study of adriamycin vs. high-dose methotrexate with adriamycin, as reported by Cortes and associates (46) earlier this year, has indicated no superiority of either treatment regimen with the median disease-free survival of 50% at 12 months. Of additional interest is the low-dose methotrexate, adriamycin, vincristine study as reported by Campanacci in which more than 50% of the patients were surviving disease-free at 2 years (47).

Studies of Jaffe (43) and Rosenberg (44,45) with methotrexate in combination with vincristine with and without BCG led to 42% and 38% 2-year disease-free survival. The study as reported by Rosenberg has an improvement in overall survival because of the aggressive resection of pulmonary metastases which developed in 22 of 39 patients.

Table 3. Adjuvant Chemotherapy of Osteosarcoma

Agents	Number Patients	Percentage 2-year Survival		Reference
		Overall	Disease-Free	
VCR-Cyclo-Dact	11		27	36
VCR-Cyclo	14		21	37
Cyclo	6		50	42
HDMTX-VCR	12		42	43
HDMTX-VCR ± BCG	39	76	38	44,45
HDMTX-VCR-Adria	22		73	8
Intensive HDMTX-VCR-Adria	30		80[1]	8
HDMTX-VCR-Adria-Cyclo Amputation (T-4)	23	72		34
En bloc resection (T-5)	31	85		34
En bloc resection + Bleo-Dact (T-7)	61		88[2]	34
HDMTX-VCR-Adria- Cyclo-PAM				
COMPADRI II	60		51	35
COMPADRI III	44		42	35
HDMTX-VCR-Adria ± BCG	18	35	26	48
HDMTX-VCR-Adria-Cyclo	29	70	50	48
HDMTX-Adria-Cyclo	26	65	55	37

HDMTX-Adria	31		50[3]	46
Adria	88		61	40,41
Adria	31		50	46
Adria	13	72	42	51
Adria-Cyclo-VCR-PAM (CONPADRI I)	44		55	35
Adria-VCR-MTX (low dose MTX)	37		62	47
Adria-VCR-Cyclo-DTIC	25		60	50
Adria-CDDP	11		91[4]	53

[1] at 19 months
[2] at 22 months
[3] at 12 months
[4] at 21 months

Adria = Adriamycin
PAM = Phenylalanine Mustard
DTIC = Imidazole Carboxamide
CDDP = Cis-diamminedichloroplatinum

VCR = Vincristine
Cyclo = Cyclophosphamide
Dact = Dactinomycin
HDMTX = High-Dose Methotrexate
BCG = Bacillus Calmette Guerin

The 2 studies utilizing high dose methotrexate, vincristine and adriamycin as reported by Jaffe (8) from the Sidney Farber Cancer Center have predicted 73 and 80% 2-year disease-free survival rates.

The combination adjuvant chemotherapy studies of Rosen and his associates at the Memorial Sloan Kettering Cancer Center, following amputation or following pretreatment with chemotherapy prior to amputation have led to impressive over-all survival as well as the impressive predicted disease-free survival of 88% of the patients admitted to the T7 protocol (34).

The results of the CONPADRI I protocol have been minimally better than the results of the COMPADRI II and III protocols, the latter of which included the addition of high-dose methotrexate (35).

The reported experiences from Stanford (48), St. Jude (37), UCLA (49), M.D. Anderson (50), and Milan (51) have shown about 50% 2-year disease-free survival, whereas the Mayo Clinic adjuvant studies with HDMTX-VCR-Adria yielded less favorable results (52).

As reported by Ettinger and associates (52), an ongoing Roswell Park Memorial Institute study using adriamycin and cis-Platinum has resulted in the disease-free survival of 10 of 11 patients treated for a median of 21 months. The only relapse among the group of 11 patients thus far reported has been that of a patient with a radiation-associated osteosarcoma of the temporal bone.

Effects of Chemotherapy on Primary Osteosarcoma

Table 4 indicates the responses obtained by several investigators using high dose methotrexate. Among 4 patients treated by Jaffe, 3 patients obtained complete response and 1 patient developed a partial response after treatment with high-dose methotrexate delivered in a weekly dosage of 7500 mg/m^2 (8). Rosen has recently reported 9 complete and 11 partial responses among 30 patients with primary and metastatic osteosarcoma treated at Memorial Hospital (9). In our institution none of 6

Table 4. Effect of HDMTX on Primary Osteosarcoma

Dosage Schedule	Number Complete + Partial Responses/Total	Reference
7500 mg/m^2/wk	4/4	8
8000-12000 mg/m^2/wk	20/30*	9
1250-15000 mg/m^2/wk	0/6	10
	24/40	

*Primary and metastatic

patients with primary osteosarcoma developed responses following treatment with increasing dosages of methotrexate delivered at weekly intervals (10).

In ongoing studies at the M.D. Anderson Hospital, Mavligit, Jaffe and associates have recently observed the effect of intraarterial cis-Platinum on primary osteosarcoma; 7 of 10 patients developed partial responses (54). Responses were estimated by imaging techniques including bone scans, and by histologic evidences of proportions of viable tumor cells following several treatments using cis-Platinum in a dosage of 120 mg/m^2 delivered as a 3-4 hour infusion every 2 weeks.

Rosen has examined the histologic effects on primary extremity osteosarcoma treated with preoperative high-dose methotrexate, vincristine, adriamycin with or without bleomycin, cyclophosphamide and dactinomycin (34). The survival of patients was found to be directly related to the quality of response obtained with presurgical chemotherapy. By the T5 protocol 31 patients were treated, of which 16 patients developed partial responses and 9 patients survive, of which 6 were reported to be free of evidence of active disease. For the 15 patients who developed complete or almost complete response, all survive without evidence of disease. For the 20 patients treated by the T7 protocol, 16 patients developed complete or almost complete responses; the effect of this treatment on survival of these latter patients was not reported.

DISCUSSION

Friedman and Carter (1), in a review of 17 reported series of osteosarcoma patients, found that the 5-year survival rate of patients with this tumor ranged from 5% to 23% after amputation, radiotherapy, or a combination of the two. Few studies before 1972 demonstrated any benefit derived from chemotherapy for the treatment of patients with osteosarcoma. Since 1972 many studies have been reported indicating the benefits of chemotherapy for metastatic and non-metastatic osteosarcoma. Yet definitive answers for the treatment of this aggressive tumor are not yet available.

Is adjuvant chemotherapy necessary? Most of the reported results of adjuvant chemotherapy have indicated a 2-year disease-free survival rate of about 50%. The Mayo Clinic experience for the treatment of osteosarcoma has indicated an increasing survival rate among patients treated at that institution up to 1974, and continuing to the present time (55). Most of the institutional reports other than from the Mayo Clinic have indicated a comparison of the adjuvant chemotherapy results with historical controls obtained from patients data recorded prior to 1972. Only the Mayo Clinic recorded improved results during recent years prior to the institution of aggressive adjuvant chemotherapy (56). The ongoing Mayo Clinic trials compare the use of high dose methotrexate with vincristine given in the adjuvant setting to the results obtained following amputation alone. At this time no data is available from these studies. Results of adjuvant chemotherapy studies elsewhere have indicated disease free survival rates ranging from 26 to 91%. The success of adjuvant chemotherapy must be measured in terms of disease-free survival percentages rather than in overall survival (57) because of survival of increased numbers of patients following resection of pulmonary metastases, as noted particularly by the studies of Rosenberg and his associates (44,45).

Following the indication of favorable responses of the pulmonary metastases of osteosarcoma after treatment with high dose methotrexate (32), there was prompt acceptance of this method of treatment for this tumor. There were indications that patients who failed to respond at dosages of 2500 mg/m^2 often developed responses when the dosages were increased to 7500 mg/m^2 (7). Methotrexate was included in many adjuvant chemotherapy protocols without the evidence of dose response relationships or classical Phase III trials determining the merits of this agent in concurrent trials using various dosages.

What is the optimum duration of adjuvant chemotherapy administration for osteosarcoma? Most metastases which develop within patients who receive adjuvant chemotherapy are detected within 1 year from diagnosis. Late metastases have developed in our patients as late as 32 months (58), in Rosen's patients as late as 33 months (34), in Sutow's patients as late as 36 months (35) and in Jaffe's patients as late as 48 months (8). Patients who develop pulmonary metastases while receiving chemotherapy may have a greater number of metastases than those patients who develop late metastatic disease, and multiple thoracotomies may be unsuccessful for the patients with "early" metastases. Two-thirds of our patients who developed metastases following amputation had these metastases detected within the year during which they received chemotherapy; one-third developed metastases after completion of chemotherapy.

Is drug toxicity necessary for the effective adjuvant treatment of osteosarcoma? Djerassi has observed that the antitumor effect of high dose methotrexate is not dependent upon the development of methotrexate-related toxicity (59). The same is probably true for other agents such as adriamycin, cyclophosphamide and cis-platinum. The late morbid effects of these latter 3 agents are fully appreciated at this time in relation to cardiac, reproductive and renal dysfunction. To date, no similar problems have been associated with high dose methotrexate administration. Leukoencephalopathy has been reported in some younger patients receiving weekly high dose methotrexate at Memorial Hospital (60); this complication has not been reported from other institutions. At the time that long-term survivors are examined for evidences of late metastatic disease, evaluation should be performed for evidences of subtle changes that might be considered late effects of chemotherapy.

In recent years great emphasis has been placed upon specifically designed treatment plans for individuals with of leukemia or tumors with special features which might place the individual at high risk for lack of response or for early recurrence of disease. Approximately one-third of osteosarcoma patients admitted to treatment centers do not qualify for admission to adjuvant chemotherapy schemes because of evidences of metastatic tumor or other complicating situations. It is from these patients that the results of primary treatment should be carefully evaluated for application into future adjuvant chemotherapy schemes.

The major options for chemotherapy for osteosarcoma today include the use of high dose methotrexate and adriamycin alone or in combination with vincristine, bleomycin, cyclophosphamide, dactinomycin and cis-diamminedichloroplatinum. As yet there is no evidence that vincristine or bleomycin contributes significantly to the responses obtained with other agents. It has been suggested that dosages of vincristine necessary to affect cellular influx of methotrexate cannot be administered to human subjects (61). The nephrotoxic effects of cis-Platinum have been shown to delay the excretion of methotrexate in patients who received treatment with cis-Platinum prior to high dose methotrexate (62). There have been no studies reported of the combined use of platinum and high-dose methotrexate. Although promising results have been reported with the combination of cis-Platinum and adriamycin in an adjuvant situation (53), the effects of these agents in patients with measurable indicators of disease activity have yet to be reported.

In conclusion, there have been few reports regarding the results of treatment for patients with primary or metastatic osteosarcoma with single agents or combinations of agents. It is from these experiences and reports that the future therapy for osteosarcoma will be determined. Additionally, it may be mandatory in the future that all patients with osteosarcoma be screened in uniform and consistent manners in order to examine the prognostic factors which have been derived from the treatment of patients of the past. Such examinations of necessity may include bone scans, computed tomographic scans of the lungs, with considerations regarding the site, size and histology of the primary tumor.

ACKNOWLEDGEMENT

Supported in part by U.S. Public Health Service Childhood Cancer Center Grant CA 23099 and Cancer Center Support (CORE) Grant CA 21765 from the National Cancer Institute, and by ALSAC.

REFERENCES

1. Friedman, M.A., and Carter, S.K. The therapy of osteogenic sarcoma: current status and thoughts for the future. J. Surg. Oncol. 4:482-510, 1972.

2. Marcove, R.C., Mike, V., Hajek, J.V., et al. Osteogenic sarcoma under the age of twenty-one. A review of 145 operative cases. J. Bone Joint Surg. 52A: 411-423, 1970.

3. Pinkel, D. Cyclophosphamide in children with cancer. Cancer 15:42-49, 1962.

4. Haggard, M. Cyclophosphamide in the treatment of children with malignant neoplasms. Cancer Chemother. Rep. 51:403-405, 1967.

5. Sutow, W.W., Vietti, T.J., Fernbach, D.J., et al. Evaluation of chemotherapy in children with metastatic Ewing's sarcoma and osteogenic sarcoma. Cancer Chemother. Rep. 55:67-81, 1971.

6. Finklestein, J.Z., Hittle, R.E., and Hammond, G.D. Evaluation of a high dose cyclophosphamide regimen on childhood tumors. Cancer 23:1239-1242, 1969.

7. Jaffe, N., Frei, E., III, Traggis, D., and Watts H. Weekly high-dose methotrexate-citrovorum factor in osteogenic sarcoma. Cancer 39:45-50, 1977.

8. Jaffe, N. High dose methotrexate: A review of adjuvant treatment and limb salvage in osteosarcoma. Cancer Treat. Rep. (In press).

9. Rosen, G., Juergens, H., Nirenberg, A., et al. Response of primary osteogenic sarcoma to high dose methotrexate-single agent chemotherapy. Proc. 11th Int. Congress of Chemotherapy and 19th Interscience Conf. on Antimicrobial Agents and Chemotherapy. Oct. 1-5, 1979, Boston, Massachusetts (Abstract 535).

10. Pratt, C.B., Howarth, C., Ransom, J.L., et al. High-dose methotrexate alone and in combination therapy for measurable primary or metastatic osteosarcoma. Cancer Treat. Rep. (In press).

11. Ambinder, E.P., Perloff, M., Ohnuma, T., et al. High dose methotrexate followed by citrovorum factor reversal in patients with advanced cancer. Cancer 43:1177-1182, 1979.

12. Cortes, E.P., Holland, J.F., Wang, J.J., and Glidewell, O.: Adriamycin (NSC-123127) in 87 patients with osteosarcoma. Cancer Chemother. Rep. (Part 3) 6:305-313, 1975.

13. Gottlieb, J.A., Baker, L.H., O'Bryan, R.M., et al. Adriamycin (NSC-123127) used alone and in combination for soft tissue and bony sarcomas. Cancer Chemother. Rep. (Part 3) 6:271-282, 1975.

14. Wang, J.J., Holland, J.F., and Sinks, L.F. Phase II study of adriamycin (NSC-123127) in childhood solid tumors. Cancer Chemother. Rep. (Part 3) 6:267-270, 1975.

15. Bonadonna, G., Monfardini, S., DeLena, M., et al. Clinical trials with adriamycin. Results of three-years' study. In International Symposium on Adriamycin (Carter, S.K., Di Marco, A., Ghione, M., et al., Eds.) New York, Springer-Verlag, 1972, pp. 139-152.

16. Tan, C., Rosen, G., Ghavini, F., et al. Adriamycin (NSC-123127) in pediatric malignancies. Cancer Chemother. Rep. (Part 3) 6:259-266, 1975.

17. Pratt, C.B., and Shanks, E.C. Doxorubicin in treatment of malignant solid tumors in children. Am. J. Dis. Child. 127:534-536, 1974.

18. Evans, A.E., Baehner, R.L., Chard, R.L., et al. Comparison of daunorubicin (NSC-83142) with adriamycin (NSC-123127) in the treatment of late-stage childhood solid tumors. Cancer Chemother. Rep. 58:671-676, 1974.

19. Ragab, A.H., Sutow, W.W., Komp, D.M., et al. Adriamycin in the treatment of childhood solid tumors: a Southwest Oncology Group Study. Cancer 36:1567-1576, 1975.

20. Kamalakar, P., Freeman, A.I., Higby, D.J., et al. Clinical response and toxicity with cis-dichloro-diammineplatinum (II) in children. Cancer Treat. Rep. 61(5):835-839, 1977.

21. Catane, R., Douglass, H.O., Jr., and Mittelman, A. A Phase II study of high dose cis-diammine-dichloro-platinum II (DDP) in non-testicular tumors. Proc. Amer. Assoc. Cancer Res. 18:115, 1977.

22. Ochs, J.J., Freeman, A.I., Douglass, H.O., Jr., et al. cis-Dichlorodiammineplatinum (II) in advanced osteogenic sarcoma. Cancer Treat. Rep. 62:239-245, 1978.

23. Leventhal, B.G., and Freeman, A. Cis diamminedi-chloroplatinum. A Phase II study in pediatric malignancies. Proc. Amer. Assoc. Cancer Res. 20:197, 1979.

24. Nitschke, R., Starling, K.A., Vats, T., and Bryan, H. Cis-diamminedichloroplatinum (NSC-119875) in childhood malignancies: a Southwest Oncology Group Study. Med. Pediatr. Oncol. 4:127-132, 1978.

25. Rosen, G., Nirenberg, A., Juergens, H., and Tan, C. Phase II trial of cis-platinum in osteogenic sarcoma. Proc. Am. Assoc. Cancer Res. 20:363, 1979.

26. Baum, E., Greenberg, L., Gaymon, P., et al. Use of cis-diamminedichloroplatinum in osteogenic sarcoma in children. Proc. Amer. Assoc. Cancer Res. 19:385, 1978.

27. Gaymon, P., Baum, E., Greenberg, L., et al. A Phase II trial of cis-platinum diammine dichloride (DDP) (NSC 119825) in refractory childhood tumors: A CCSG trial. Proc. Amer. Assoc. Cancer Res. 20:394, 1979.

28. Pratt, C.B., Hayes, F.A., Green, A.A., et al. Phase II-pharmacokinetic study of cis platinum diamminedichloride (CDDP) in children with solid tumors. Proc. Amer. Assoc. Cancer Res. 20:361, 1979.

29. Jaffe, N., Traggis, D., and Enriquez, C. Evaluation of a combination of mitomycin C (NSC 26980), phenylalanine mustard (NSC 1420), and vincristine (NSC 67574) in the treatment of osteogenic sarcoma. Cancer Chemother. Rep. 55:189-193, 1971.

30. Nathanson, L., Hall, T.C., Dederick, M.M., et al, S. Initial pharmacologic studies of three types of combination chemotherapy. Cancer Chemother. Rep. 50:259-264, 1966.

31. Rosen, G., Suvanisirikul, S., Kwon, C., et al. High-dose methotrexate with citrovorum factor rescue and adriamycin in childhood osteogenic sarcoma. Cancer 33:1151-1163, 1974.

32. Jaffe, N. Recent advances in the chemotherapy of metastatic osteogenic sarcoma. Cancer 30:1627-1631, 1972.

33. Mosende, C., Guitterez, M., Caparros, B., and Rosen, G. Combination chemotherapy with bleomycin, cyclophosphamide and dactinomycin for the treatment of osteogenic sarcoma. Cancer 40:2779-2786, 1977.

34. Rosen, G., Marcove, R.C., Caparros, B., et al. Primary osteogenic sarcoma. The rationale for preoperative chemotherapy and delayed surgery. Cancer 43:2163-2177, 1979.

35. Sutow, W.W., Gehan, E.A., Dyment, P.A., et al. Multidrug adjuvant chemotherapy for osteosarcoma; interim report of the Southwest Oncology Group Studies. Cancer Treat. Rep. 62:265-270, 1978.

36. Sutow, W.W., Sullivan, M.P., Wilbur, J.R., and Cangir, A. Study of adjuvant chemotherapy in osteogenic sarcoma. J. Clin. Pharmacol. 7:530-533, 1975.

37. Pratt, C.B., Shanks, E.C., Hustu, H.O., et al. Adjuvant multiple drug chemotherapy for osteosarcoma of the extremity. Cancer 39:51-57, 1977.

38. Goldin, A., Mantel, N., Greenhouse, S.W., et al. Effect of delayed administration of citrovorum factor on the antileukemic effectiveness of aminopterin in mice. Cancer Res. 14:43-48, 1954.

39. Djerassi, I., Rominger, C.J., Kim, J.S., et al, Phase I study of high doses of methotrexate with citrovorum factor in patients with lung cancer. Cancer 30: 22-30, 1972.

40. Cortes, E.P., Holland, J.F., Wang, J.J., et al. Amputation and adriamycin in primary osteosarcoma. N. Engl. J. Med. 291:998-1000, 1974.

41. Holland, J.F., and Cortes, E.P. The role of adriamycin in the treatment of osteogenic sarcoma and future directions for its use. J. Natl. Cancer Inst. (In press).

42. Shepp, M., Necheles, T.F., Banks, H.H., et al. Adjuvant of osteogenic sarcoma with high-dose cyclophosphamides. Cancer Treat. Rep. 62:295-296, 1978.

43. Jaffe, N., Frei, E., III, Watts, H., et al. High-dose methotrexate in osteogenic sarcoma: A 5-year experience. Cancer Treat. Rep. 62:259-264, 1978.

44. Rosenberg, S.A., Chabner, B.A., Young, R.C., et al. Treatment of osteogenic sarcoma. I. Effect of adjuvant high-dose methotrexate after amputation. Cancer Treat. Rep. 63:739-751, 1979.

45. Rosenberg, S.A., Flye, M.W., Conkle, D., et al. Treatment of osteogenic sarcoma. II. Aggressive resection of pulmonary metastases. Cancer Treat. Rep. 63:753-756, 1979.

46. Cortes, E.P., Necheles, T.F., Holland, J.F., Glidewell, O. Adriamycin (ADM) alone versus ADM and high dose methotrexate citrovorum factor rescue (HDMTX-CF) as adjuvant to operable primary osteosarcoma: A randomized study by cancer and leukemic group B (CALGB). Proc. Am. Assoc. Cancer Res. 20:412, 1979.

47. Campanacci, M., Pagani, P.-A., and Guinti, A. La chimiotherapie systematioue post-operative des osteo-sarcomes localises aux extremites. Nouv. Presse. Med. 7:3462, 1978.

48. Etcubanas, E., and Wilbur, Jr. Adjuvant chemotherapy for osteogenic sarcoma. Cancer Treat. Rep. 62: 283-287, 1978.

49. Eilber, F.R., Grant, T., and Morton, D.L. Adjuvant therapy for osteosarcoma: Preoperative and post-operative treatment. Cancer Treat. Rep. 62:213-216, 1978.

50. Murphy, W.K., Benjamin, R.S., Eyre, H.J., et al. Adjuvant chemotherapy in osteosarcoma of adults. In, Salmon, S.E., Jones, S.E. (Eds.). Adjuvant Chemo-therapy of Cancer, Amsterdam, Elsevier/North Holland Biomedical Press, 1977, p. 399.

51. Fossati-Bellani, F., Gasparini, N., Gennari, L. Adjuvant treatment with adriamycin in primary oper-able osteosarcoma. Cancer Treat. Rep. 62:279-281, 1978.

52. Gilchrist, G.G., Ivins, J.C., Ritts, R.E., Jr., et al. Adjuvant therapy for non-metastatic osteogenic sarcoma: an evaluation of transfer factor versus adjuvant chemotherapy. Cancer Treat. Rep. 62: 289-294, 1978.

53. Ettinger, L.J., Douglass, H.O., Jr., Higby, D.J., et al. Adriamycin in (Adr) and cis-diamminedichloro-platinum (CDDP) as adjuvant therapy in primary osteo-sarcoma (OS). Proc. Amer. Assn. Cancer Res. 20:438, 1979.

54. Mavligit, G., and Jaffe, N. Personal communications.

55. Taylor, W.F., Ivins, J.C., Dahlin, D.C., et al. Trends and variability in survival from osteosarcoma. Mayo Clinic Proc. 53:695-700, 1978.

56. Frei, E., and Polli, E. Discussion pp 229-232. In, Periti, P. (Ed) Proceedings of the High Dose Metho-trexate International Workshop, June 13-14, 1978, Firenze, Italy. Firenze:Editrice Guintina, 1978.

57. Muggia, F., Catane, R., Lee, Y.J., and Rozencweig, M. Factors responsible for therapeutic success in osteo-sarcoma: A critical analysis of adjuvant trial results. pp. 383-390, 1979. In Adjuvant Chemo-therapy of Cancer II, S. Salmon and S. Jones (eds).

58. Pratt, C.B. Selected applications of methotrexate alone and in combination in osteosarcoma. Cancer Treat. Rep. (In press).

59. Djerassi, I. Discussion pp. 173-174. In: Periti, P. (ed) Proceedings of the High Dose Methotrexate International Workshop, June 13-14, 1978. Firenze, Italy. Firenze:Editrice Guintina, 1978.

60. Allen, J.C., and Rosen, G. Transient cerebral dysfunction following chemotherapy for osteogenic sarcoma. Ann. Neurology 3:441-444, 1978.

61. Bender, R.A. The membrane transport of methotrexate pp. 23-35 In: Periti, P. (ed) Proceedings of the High Dose Methotrexate International Workshop, June 13-14, 1978. Firenze, Italy. Firenze:Editrice Guintina, 1978.

62. Pitman, S.W., Minor, D.R., Papac, R., et al, Sequential methotrexate-leucovorin (MTX-LCV) and cisplatinum (CDDP) in head and neck cancer. Proc. ASCO 20:419, 1979.

27 THE SUCCESSFUL MANAGEMENT OF METASTACTIC OSTEOGENIC SARCOMA: A MODEL FOR THE TREATMENT OF PRIMARY OSTEOGENIC SARCOMA

G. Rosen, B. Caparros, A. Nirenberg, H. Juergens and A. G. Huvos

Summary

From September 1976 through August 1979, 79 consecutive patients with fully malignant (grade 2 or 3) osteogenic sarcoma of an extremity (69 with primary tumor and 10 with primary tumor and pulmonary metastases) and no prior surgery other than a biopsy were treated with preoperative chemotherapy prior to surgery. On histologic examination of the resected primary tumor, 40 of the 69 patients with primary tumor only (58%) showed complete or near complete necrosis of the primary tumor attributable to chemotherapy. All 40 of these patients (100%) have remained free of recurrent or metastatic disease demonstrating that the effect of preoperative chemotherapy on the primary tumor is a strong prognostic indicator of the effect of that chemotherapy as adjuvant chemotherapy on disease-free survival. Sixty-one of the entire group of 69 patients (88%) have not developed recurrent or metastatic disease from 3+ to 37+ months (median 16+ months). All 8 patients who relapsed did not show a favorable effect of preoperative chemotherapy on the primary tumor. These 8 patients relapsed at a median time of 13 months. Three of the 10 patients presenting with primary tumor and pulmonary metastases did not show a favorable effect of preoperative chemotherapy on the primary tumor and all 3 are currently alive with disease on other treatment. Seven patients are currently free of disease from 2+ to 24+ months (median 13+ months). All 7 of these patients, in addition to having a good clinical response of their primary tumor and pulmonary metastases to preoperative chemotherapy, showed evidence of complete or near complete tumor necrosis on histologic examination of the resected residual primary tumor and pulmonary metastases. The favorable disease-free survival rate reported here for osteogenic sarcoma is attributed to the aggressive use of preoperative chemotherapy, including the proper dosage of high dose methotrexate ($12gm/M^2$ in children and $8gm/M^2$ in older adolescents), and to the careful timing of surgery following preoperative chemotherapy after all evidence of gross disease (primary tumor and metastases) has shown evidence of either stabilization or regression for at least 3 months. This approach was learned through our experience in treating patients with overt pulmonary metastases, and has proven to be equally as successful with patients with primary tumor only (and presumably microscopic metastases).

(Supported by Clinical Cancer Research grant CA05826-18)

INTRODUCTION

Since 1972 we have treated more than 225 patients with osteogenic sarcoma at the Memorial Sloan-Kettering Cancer Center. More than 75 of these patients presented to us with advanced metastatic disease. The majority of the remaining patients with primary tumor only were treated with drug therapy prior to surgery. This experience has allowed us to evaluate the effects of drugs on osteogenic sarcoma, and to arrive at what we believe is the optimal timing of systemic drug therapy and local surgery for the treatment of this disease.

In 1978 we reported the results of treatment of 45 patients with metastatic osteogenic sarcoma (1). Thirty-one of those patients had diffuse inoperable pulmonary metastases. Many of these patients had multiple thoracotomies at varying times before and during systemic chemotherapy. At that time we reported a median survival of more than 30 months in those patients. Indeed, 7 of those patients are still surviving at a median of 5½ years from the time of

presenting for treatment with inoperable pulmonary metastases. One of those patients still has residual disease in
the heart and mediastinum. His metastatic osteogenic sarcoma has remained exquisitely sensitive to high dose methotrexate with citrovorum factor rescue, and this patient has
been maintained on that treatment given every three weeks
for the past six years (Figure 1). All 7 of the prolonged
survivors from that initial group owe their survival to initial dramatic responses to high dose methotrexate with citrovorum factor rescue and its continued use in their management (Figure 2).

Analysis of the favorable responses of very poor risk
patients led us to conclude that the optimal timing of
therapy for the patient with disseminated disease was the
use of systemic chemotherapy for a period of at least 3
months. If at that time all manifestations of disease are
well controlled with drug therapy, surgery should be done
to remove residual disease, both primary tumor and metastatic nodules. Past experience had shown that without surgical resection disease usually recurred following
the cessation of chemotherapy.

The timing of the modalities of treatment for the patient with disseminated disease can be extended to the patient with only primary osteogenic sarcoma, since the majority of these patients do harbor disseminated metastatic
disease, albeit only microscopic. This approach to the
patient with primary tumor was proven to be of value in a
study completed in 1978 (2). We had shown that the delay
in surgery to give preoperative chemotherapy to the patient
was not detrimental, and actually resulted in a higher
disease-free survival rate. This approach allowed us to
determine the proper dose of high dose methotrexate in
many patients who would not have received adequate dosage
of that drug had they been treated on an adjuvant protocol
following amputation. It was shown that children who had
not yet achieved their adolescent growth spurt required the
threshold dose of $12gm/M^2$ of methotrexate in order to a-
chieve regression of their primary tumor. This study also
showed that the effect of chemotherapy, particularly high

352

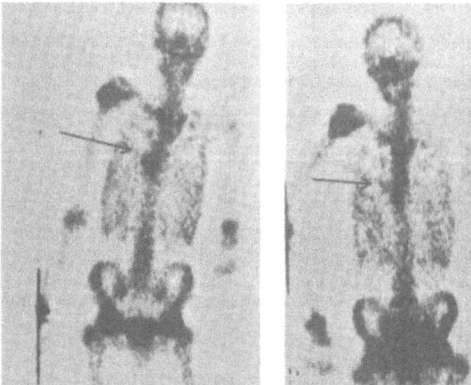

Figure 1. Serial bone scans document the response of inoperable osteogenic sarcoma to high dose methotrexate in a patient who presented with bilateral pulmonary metastases in December 1973. Mediastinal metastases occurred in July 1977 after an interruption in his chemotherapy. He has been maintained on high dose methotrexate with citrovorum factor rescue every 2-3 weeks for the past 6 years.

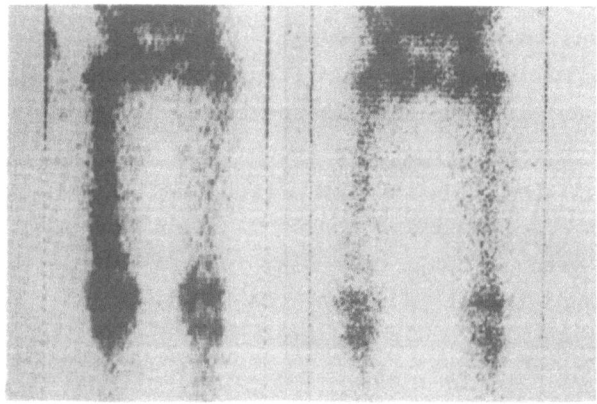

Figure 2. This 15-year old boy presented with osteogenic sarcoma of the right femur and bilateral pulmonary metastases. Following initial response to chemotherapy he underwent bilateral thoracotomies, and subsequently amputation. He was then continued on high dose methotrexate with citrovorum factor rescue, adriamycin and BCD for one more year. This patient has now remained free of all evidence of metastatic or recurrent disease for almost six years.

dose methotrexate with citrovorum factor rescue, on the
primary tumor directly correlated with the prolonged
disease-free survival in that patient when continued on the
same chemotherapy following surgery (3).

In addition to high dose methotrexate with citrovorum
factor rescue and adriamycin, the combination of bleomycin,
cyclophosphamide and dactinomycin (BCD) has been shown to
be effective in the treatment of both metastatic and primary
osteogenic sarcoma (4). This combination can cause regression of metastatic disease (Figure 3) and it has also been
shown to be effective in the initial treatment of primary
tumor in 18/22 patients with evaluable primary tumors undergoing preoperative chemotherapy where the combination of
bleomycin, cyclophosphamide and dactinomycin was used as the
initial chemotherapy (5).

Sixty-one patients were treated with our T-7 chemotherapy protocol which included high dose methotrexate with
citrovorum factor rescue given at the dose of $8gm/M^2$ to
adolescents and adults, and $12gm/M^2$ to prepubescent children. Surgery for both primary tumor and metastatic disease was delayed until approximately 3 to 4 months after the
start of therapy. Only 38 of those 61 patients received
preoperative chemotherapy with the T-7 protocol; the remain-
der of the patients were referred following amputation (Figure 4). Of that entire group of 61 patients 52 have remained free of metastatic disease (85%) at a median follow-up
time of 27+ months.

In July 1978 the T-7 chemotherapy protocol was modified to include only high dose methotrexate with citrovorum
factor rescue given as a single agent prior to surgery in
an effort to further evaluate the effectiveness of that
treatment as a single agent in osteogenic sarcoma. The
initial results of this study showed that there was a 75%
objective response rate in patients with evaluable primary
tumor, and primary tumor with pulmonary metastases, to
treatment with single agent high dose methotrexate with
citrovorum factor rescue (6). Following surgery and evaluation of the response to high dose methotrexate, patients are
continued on adjuvant chemotherapy which includes, in ad-

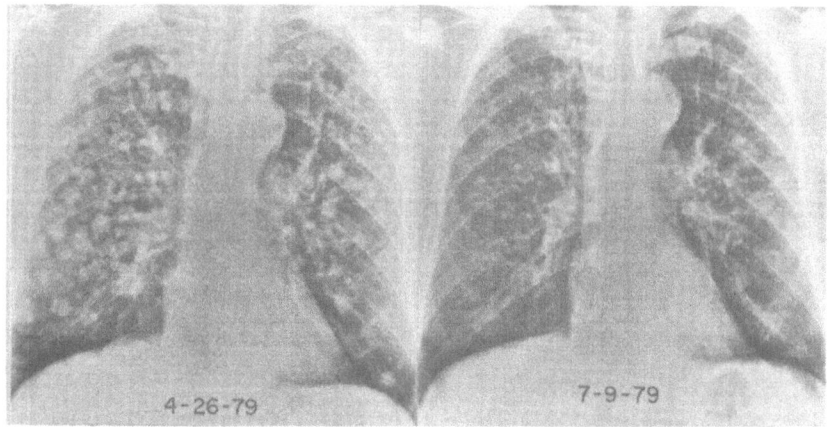

Figure 3. Serial chest x-rays of a 64-year old man with metastatic osteogenic sarcoma arising in Paget's disease. The response shown above was obtained following treatment with both BCD and adriamycin chemotherapy. He was unable to receive high dose methotrexate with citrovorum factor rescue due to poor renal function.

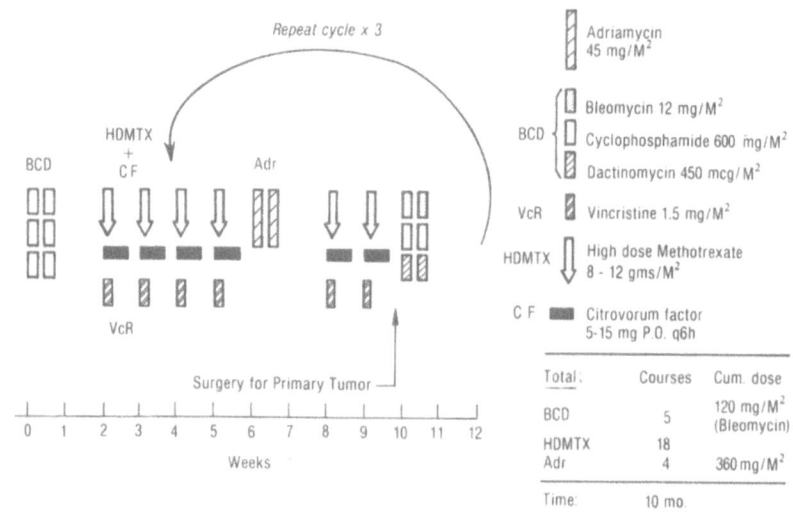

Figure 4. T-7 chemotherapy for osteogenic sarcoma.

dition to high dose methotrexate with citrovorum factor
rescue, adriamycin and the combination of bleomycin, cyclophosphamide and dactinomycin. In the patient with pulmonary metastases, in addition to surgery for the primary tumor, bilateral thoracotomies are performed to remove residual pulmonary nodules.

Histologic examination of the resected residual tumor
tissue allowed us to further evaluate the efficacy of chemotherapy (Figure 5) and to correlate the histologic response
to the patients' disease-free survival (Figure 6) (2, 3).

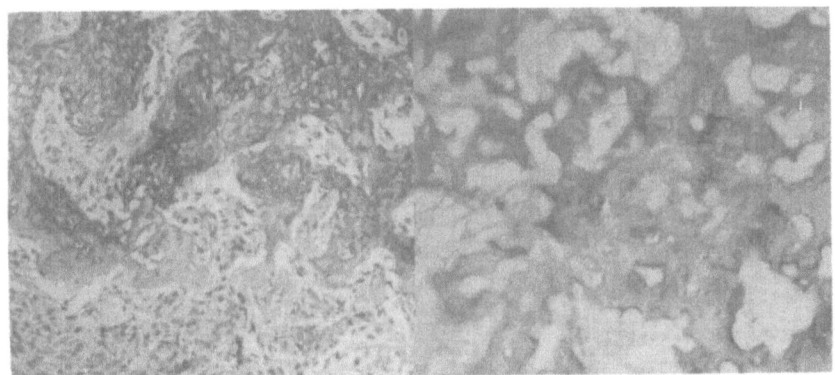

Figure 5. Histologic response of osteogenic sarcoma to high dose
methotrexate with citrovorum factor rescue treatment. Prior to therapy
an abundant tumor cell stroma producing tumor osteoid is seen (A). In
responding patients, following treatment, only the tumor osteoid remains
with no tumor cells in the supporting stroma (B). This latter finding
in all sections examined from the resected specimen is defined as a
favorable histologic response to preoperative chemotherapy.

From September 1976 through August 1979, 79 consecutive
patients with osteogenic sarcoma (69 primary tumor only, 10
primary tumor and pulmonary metastases) were started on preoperative chemotherapy for the treatment of their disease.
Review of these 79 patients demonstrates that the patient's
response to preoperative chemotherapy is an important factor
determining that patient's subsequent survival, even for patients presenting with metastatic disease to the lungs. The

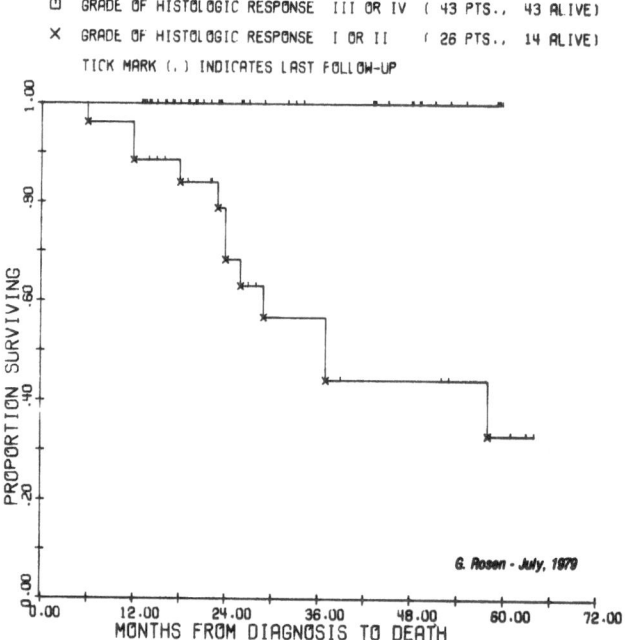

□ GRADE OF HISTOLOGIC RESPONSE III OR IV (43 PTS., 43 ALIVE)
× GRADE OF HISTOLOGIC RESPONSE I OR II (26 PTS., 14 ALIVE)
TICK MARK (.) INDICATES LAST FOLLOW-UP

PROPORTION SURVIVING

MONTHS FROM DIAGNOSIS TO DEATH

G. Rosen - July, 1979

Figure 6. The correlation of the histologic response to preoperative chemotherapy and survival in 69 patients with primary osteogenic sarcoma. Thirty-eight were treated with T-7 preoperative chemotherapy and 31 were treated on an earlier protocol (T-5) with preoperative chemotherapy. Forty-three of the patients demonstrated either a complete lack of viable tumor (grade IV), or only a few foci of viable tumor cells (grade III) on histologic examination of more than 30 sections taken from the primary tumor. 100% of these patients are disease-free survivors. The minority of patients not having a good histologic response to preoperative chemotherapy are at a high risk for relapsing. In these latter patients other therapy may be indicated postoperatively.

timing of surgery and the subsequent removal of all residual disease, both primary and metastatic, is also an important factor in the patient's ultimate chance for survival.

METHODS

From September 1976 through August 1979, 79 previously un-treated patients with primary osteogenic sarcoma (10 with

primary tumor and pulmonary metastases) who received preoperative chemotherapy were studied.

Pretreatment evaluation included review of the biopsy
slides. Only patients with fully malignant (grade 3 or 4)
osteogenic sarcoma were included in this study. Of the 69
patients with primary tumor only, 39 patients had lesions
in the femur, 16 patients had lesions in the humerus, 14 in
the tibia, 1 in the fibula, and 1 in the pelvis. Of the 10
patients presenting with pulmonary metastases, 8 patients
had femur primaries, and 2 patients had primary lesions in
the tibia. Of the entire group of 79 patients, 9 patients
were above the age of 21. Seven of the latter were in their
third decade of life, and 2 patients were 32 years of age.
These latter 9 patients all had classic osteogenic sarcoma
of an extremity which was fully malignant on histologic examination of the biopsy. Two of the older patients had
humerus lesions, two tibia lesions, and five femur lesions
(one with pulmonary metastases).

None of the 79 patients had metastatic bone disease on
examination of the bone scan; however, increased uptake in
the limb, either proximal or distal to the primary tumor,
was noted in 12 of the patients, and assumed to be hyper-
emia secondary to the tumor in that limb. Full chest tomography was performed on all patients whose PA and lateral
chest x-ray failed to reveal metastatic disease. In the 10
patients presenting with metastatic disease, 7 of them had
pulmonary nodules evident on the plain, PA or lateral chest
x-ray. Computerized transaxial tomography of the chest was
not performed to rule out pulmonary metastases.

Bone scans were repeated at monthly intervals, and
chest x-rays were repeated at monthly intervals. Determination of the serum alkaline phosphatase was done twice
weekly and proved to be valuable in following the course of
patients whose initial serum alkaline phosphatase was ab-
normally elevated.

Chemotherapy was given to the first 38 patients according to the T-7 protocol (Figure 4). The next 41 patients were started on weekly high dose methotrexate with
citrovorum factor rescue given for 4 to 6 weeks prior to

surgery. In patients with evaluable pulmonary metastases, and in some patients who were awaiting endoprostheses for the total femur and knee, chemotherapy was continued pre-operatively with the inclusion of BCD and adriamycin after the initial evaluation of the first four weekly high dose methotrexate treatments. BCD and adriamycin as well as high dose methotrexate was given postoperatively as is in the T-7 protocol.

High dose methotrexate was given to prepubescent children at the dose of $12gm/M^2$, and to older adolescents and adults at the dose of $8gm/M^2$. All patients received doses of methotrexate of between 10 and 20gm. Citrovorum factor rescue was given orally at a dose of 10-15mg every 6 hours for 10 doses beginning 24 hours from the start of the high dose methotrexate infusion. The methods of following the patient after high dose methotrexate to insure that severe toxicity does not ensue have been previously reported (2, 7, 8).

Following surgery representative areas from all parts of the resected primary tumor-bearing bone as well as all pulmonary metastases removed were decalcified and carefully examined by the same pathologist who determined the effect of preoperative chemotherapy on tumor tissue. A good effect of chemotherapy (grade III or IV, Figure 5) was considered no evidence of viable tumor or only a few foci of tumor cells noted after reviewing all of the representative sections from the primary tumor and pulmonary metastases. A poor effect of chemotherapy (grade I or II) was defined as uniform sheets or clusters of tumor cells apparent in any one of the sections examined. A grade II effect may show greater than 50% necrosis or total necrosis and lack of viable tumor in some of the sections, but confluent areas of tumor cells may be seen in other sections examined. This was also considered a poor effect of chemotherapy. The effect of chemotherapy on the resected tumor was considered to be over and above the necrosis that can normally occur spontaneously in primary or metastatic osteogenic sarcoma (2).

After preoperative chemotherapy surgery was performed for the primary tumor (and for the removal of residual pulmonary nodules in patients with pulmonary metastases). Twenty-seven of the 79 patients underwent amputation of the primary tumor. Fourteen of the 16 patients with proximal humerus lesions underwent resections of the shoulder joint and proximal humerus. Twenty-two of the 37 patients with femur lesions had resection of the femur and endoprosthetic replacement of the bone and knee joint (9).

Two weeks following resection of the primary tumor bilateral thoracotomies were performed in 6 of the 10 patients presenting with pulmonary metastases. Unilateral thoracotomy was performed in 4 patients for the removal of residual metastatic disease. Patients were continued on adjuvant chemotherapy within two weeks of surgery.

RESULTS

Toxicity

As previously reported there was one toxic death due to high dose methotrexate in a patient started on therapy in July 1976 (2). Since that time there have been no toxic deaths or severe toxicity noted from the high dose methotrexate with citrovorum factor rescue. Some patients required reduction in their dose of adriamycin from $90mg/M^2$ per course to $75mg/M^2$ per course due to severe leukopenia and thrombocytopenia following $90mg/M^2$. The total cumulative dose of adriamycin received by all patients was $360mg/M^2$ or less. No clinical evidence of cardiomyopathy was observed at the above dosage of adriamycin. The toxicity of BCD chemotherapy has been previously reported (4, 5) and no patient had deterioration in pulmonary function after completing chemotherapy.

There were 2 surgical deaths in this group of patients; one patient expired with "shocked lung" syndrome which manifested itself as respiratory failure following surgery for the primary tumor. Surgery was performed at another institution and the cause of acute respiratory failure was not

determined. Another patient expired of a pulmonary infection while being treated for an infected endoprosthesis.
This latter patient was not leukopenic, having been off
chemotherapy for approximately two months at the time of her
demise. Autopsy performed on both patients failed to reveal
any evidence of residual or metastatic disease.

Response to therapy

Of the 69 patients with primary tumor only, 40 (58%) had a
good response of the primary tumor to preoperative chemotherapy as determined by histologic examination of the resected tumor (grade III-IV). Twenty-three patients (33%)
demonstrated 50% or greater necrosis of their primary tumor
following preoperative chemotherapy (grade II effect), and
6 patients (9%) showed no effect of preoperative chemotherapy on the primary tumor on histologic examination of the
resected specimens. Thirty-six of the 47 patients with ab-
normally elevated serum alkaline phosphatase showed a return
to normal of this tumor marker while on preoperative chemotherapy.

Sixty-one of the 69 patients with primary tumor only
(88%) have remained continuously free of all evidence of
metastatic disease from 3+ to 39+ months (median 16+
months). All 8 of the patients who relapsed demonstrated
a poor effect of preoperative chemotherapy on the primary
tumor on histologic examination of the resected specimen
(grade I-II). Seven of the relapsing patients developed
pulmonary metastases and one patient developed a solitary
bone metastasis. The median time for the development of
metastases in these patients was 13 months.

Of the 10 patients presenting with pulmonary metastases
7 showed clinical evidence of regression of primary tumor.
These 7 patients also had greater than 75% regression of all
measurable pulmonary metastases while on preoperative chemotherapy. All 7 patients having a favorable response of preoperative chemotherapy on the primary tumor and pulmonary
metastases are all surviving free of disease 2+ to 24+
months (median 13+ months) from the start of therapy. None

of the 3 patients who relapsed had a favorable effect of preoperative chemotherapy on the primary tumor. One patient was found to have subclinical multicentric bone disease at the time of above-the-knee amputation. He also had a residual osteogenic sarcoma in the pulmonary nodules following their removal at thoracotomy. Another patient had residual osteogenic sarcoma in one of two pulmonary nodules removed at the time of thoracotomy. The third patient had no residual tumor found in two pulmonary nodules removed at the time of thoracotomy, but he relapsed with a solitary bone metastasis 14 months from the start of therapy. In this latter patient, although the pulmonary metastases responded favorably to preoperative chemotherapy, the lack of a favorable histologic response of the primary tumor to preoperative chemotherapy could have been predictive of his increased risk for developing metastases which he eventually did.

DISCUSSION

The results of treatment in this group of 79 patients continues to demonstrate the value of preoperative chemotherapy. The 88% disease-free survival rate in 69 patients with primary tumor only is certainly as good as, if not better than, any disease-free survival rate reported for patients being treated with amputation followed by adjuvant chemotherapy. Forty, or approximately 60%, of those patients had a favorable histologic effect of preoperative chemotherapy on their resected primary tumor, and past experience has shown us that at least that portion of patients can be expected to be disease-free survivors with a prediction of 100% based on our prior studies and published work (Figure 6) (2, 3). In addition, approximately 50% of the remaining 29 patients can be expected to be cured on the same adjuvant chemotherapy, again based on our prior experience (2, 3).

However, we now have the distinct advantage of having defined a poor risk group (those patients who did not have a favorable histologic response of preoperative chemotherapy

on examination of the primary tumor). It may be preferable
in this latter group of patients, at an appropriate time in
their therapy, to discontinue high dose methotrexate with
citrovorum factor rescue and institute other effective
therapy for the treatment of osteogenic sarcoma such as
cis-platinum or combination cis-platinum and adriamycin (11)
(Figure 7).

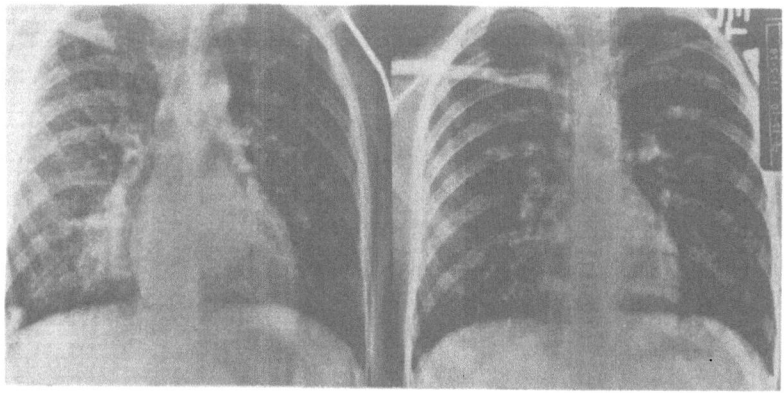

Figure 7. *Serial chest x-rays demonstrating the effect of cis-platinum
(120mg/M^2 with mannitol diuresis) in combination with adriamycin
(60mg/M^2) in a patient who developed pulmonary metastases unresponsive
to high dose methotrexate.*

The high proportion of favorable responses to high dose
methotrexate with citrovorum factor rescue is attributable
to the use of high dose methotrexate in its proper dosage
form. This includes the dose of 12gm/M^2 for prepubescent
children who have not achieved their full adult stature
(2). It is only at this dose level that we have seen the
response of evaluable osteogenic sarcoma to high dose methotrexate. The use of lower dosage forms is just as potentially toxic but will rarely be of value to the patient. We
have had experience in obtaining complete responses in
patients with metastatic osteogenic sarcoma who had been
treated at other institutions with doses of 4, 8 and 10gm
of high dose methotrexate. Upon presentation to our insti-

tution the higher dose, which has been in the range of 12 to
16gm has produced complete regression of evaluable metastatic osteogenic sarcoma.

In the majority of patients who demonstrate a good effect of high dose methotrexate with citrovorum factor rescue on their primary tumor, this treatment is most valuable,
and if continued in that group of patients in combination
with other effective agents it can be expected to produce
a 100% disease-free survival (Figure 6.

We have demonstrated that approximately 75% of patients with osteogenic sarcoma respond to high dose methotrexate with citrovorum factor rescue when used as a single
agent in the treatment of this disease (6). Investigations
are underway to try to define what factors play a role in
making methotrexate effective in patients with osteogenic
sarcoma (10). Continued investigations into its use and
the pharmacokinetics of both methotrexate and reduced fo-
lates in patients receiving this treatment must be carefully studied to not only determine that the treatment will be
safe, but to determine how one can make it effective in all
patients (8).

The use of systemic chemotherapy prior to surgery has
been shown at the very least not to decrease the cure rate
for this disease, but indeed it has been shown to increase
it through the application of knowledge that we have gained
observing favorable responses to therapy. Every patient is
his own clinical investigation, and stands to benefit by a
therapeutic trial of optimal chemotherapy for his disease
prior to surgical ablation of the primary tumor. Those few
patients who do not demonstrate a favorable response can
then be identified and offered other therapy that may be of
greater value to them. In addition, a further dividend of
preoperative chemotherapy has been the successful application of resectional therapy as an alternative to amputation
in the majority of patients with osteogenic sarcoma who are
now expected to survive their disease.

REFERENCES

1. Rosen, G., Huvos, A.G., Mosende, C., Beattie, E.J.,
   Jr., Exelby. P.R., and Marcove, R.C.
   Chemotherapy and thoracotomy for metastatic osteogenic
   sarcoma: A model for adjuvant chemotherapy and the ra-
   tionale for the timing of thoracic surgery.
   Cancer 41, 841-849, 1978.

2. Rosen, G., Marcove, R.C., Caparros, B., Nirenberg, A.,
   Kosloff, C., and Huvos, A.G.
   Primary osteogenic sarcoma: The rationale for preopera-
   tive chemotherapy and delayed surgery.
   Cancer 43, 2163-2177, 1979.

3. Rosen, G., Nirenberg, A., Juergens, C., Kosloff, C.,
   Metha, B., Marcove, R.C., and Huvos, A.G.
   Osteogenic sarcoma: Three year disease-free survival
   in excess of 80% with combination chemotherapy including
   effective high-dose Methotrexate with citrovorum factor
   rescue.
   J. Natl. Cancer Inst. (in press).

4. Mosende, C., Gutierrez, M., Caparros, B., and Rosen, G.
   Combination chemotherapy with Bleomycin, Cyclophosphamide and Dactinomycin for the treatment of osteogenic
   sarcoma.
   Cancer 40, 2779-2786, 1977.

5. Juergens, H., Nirenberg, A., Caparros, B., and Rosen, G.
   Response of primary osteogenic sarcoma to combination
   chemotherapy with Bleomycin, Cyclophosphamide and Dactinomycin.
   Cancer Treat. Rep. (in press).

6. Rosen, G., Nirenberg, A., Juergens, H., Caparros, B.,
   and Huvos, A.G.
   Response of primary osteogenic sarcoma to high-dose
   Methotrexate with citrovorum factor rescue single-agent
   chemotherapy.

(Abst) Proceedings of 11th International Conference
of Chemotherapy and 19th Interscience Conference on
Anti-microbial Agents and Chemotherapy, October 1979.

7. Nirenberg, A., Mosende, C., Mehta, B.M., Gisolfi, A.L.,
and Rosen, G.
High-dose Methotrexate with citrovorum factor rescue:
Predictive value of serum Methotrexate concentrations,
and corrective measures to avert toxicity.
Cancer Treat. Rep. 61, 779-783, 1977.

8. Mehta, B.M., Juergens, H., Allen, J.G., Rosen, G., and
Hutchinson, D.J.
Distribution of Methotrexate, citrovorum factor and
5-methyltetrahydrofolate following high-dose Methotre-
xate-leucovorin rescue in osteogenic sarcoma.
(Abst) Proceedings of 11th International Conference
of Chemotherapy and 19th Interscience Conference on
Anti-microbial Agents and Chemotherapy, October 1979.

9. Marcove, R.C., Lewis, M.M., Rosen, G., and Huvos, A.G.
Total femur replacement.
Comprehensive Therapy 3, 13-19, 1977.

10. Juergens, H., Kosloff, C., Nirenberg, A., Mehta, B.M.,
Huvos, A.G., and Rosen, G.
Clinical and pharmacokinetic prognostic factors in the
response of primary osteogenic sarcoma to pre-operative
chemotherapy (high-dose Methotrexate with citrovorum
factor rescue).
J. Natl. Cancer Inst. (in press).

11. Rosen, G., Nirenberg, A., Caparros, B., Juergens, H.,
Tan, C., and Gutierrez, M.
Cis-diamminedichloro-platinum (II) in metastatic osteo-
genic sarcoma in Current Status and New Developments
with Cisplatin.
Ed. Crooke, S.T., and Carter, S.
Academic Press, 1980.

28 CURRENT AND FUTURE MANAGEMENT OF OSTEOSARCOMA
Panel Discussion, held on December 8th, 1979

Chairman: J. F. Holland (New York)
Panel members: K. Breur (Amsterdam), Ch. B. Pratt (Memphis),
G. Rosen (New York), G. van Rijssel (Leiden) and
W. Sindelar (Bethesda)

CHAIRMAN :

I will show you an important general item to begin with.
The figure is from the National Cancer Institute:

CANCER MORTALITY AND U.S. POPULATION TRENDS
1954 - 1976*

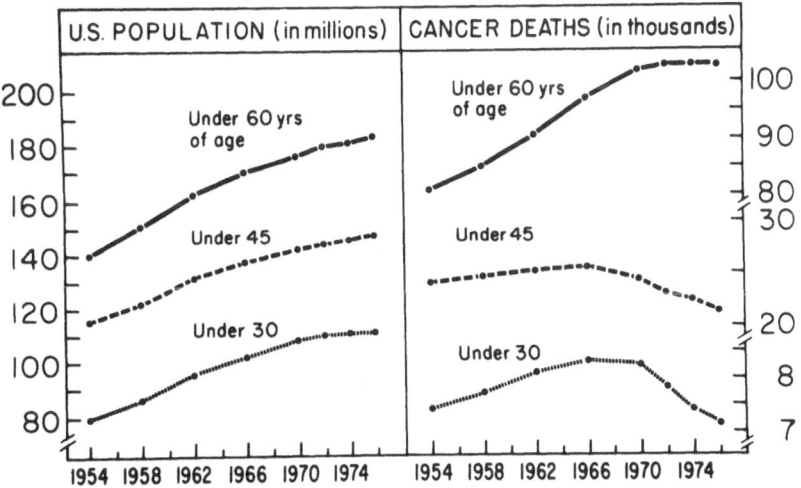

* Source of data U S Public Health Service Statistics

On the left hand side is the population of the United
States and on the right hand side are plotted cancer
deaths. There has been a sharp decrease in the number of

cancer deaths in individuals under the age of 30, in the
lower line, despite the population increase. Under the age
of 45, there is a decrease. There is a plateau in cancer
deaths, in all individuals under the age of 60, despite the
fact that there has been, if anything, a sharp increase in
the number of total Americans under the age of 60. So the
continuing increase in cancer deaths in the United States
is related to the increasing incidence of cancer in the
elderly population. Diseases which in part can be cured by
chemotherapy such as osteosarcoma, acute lymphoblastic
leukemia, ovarian cancer, Hodgkin's disease, Wilms tumor,
and some other sarcomas are the ones making an impact in
the changing statistics of the younger age groups. Although
there are improvements in surgery and radiotherapy as well,
beginning in 1970, the increased funding of the National Cancer Program, effected a major transfer of the information concerning chemotherapy from the research centers to the practice of medicine, which has lead to better overall results.

We will deal with 1) the operation, 2) the sequence and
type of treatment, 3) the proper drugs to use, 4) new concepts,
5) pulmonary metastases at the time of diagnosis, 6) pulmonary
metastases, later, 7) follow-up.

1. The operation

We discuss now the proper operation.
We have already heard of limb-salvage and the need for
orthopedic oncologists. Perhaps we should start with the
biopsy and ask Dr. Rosen whether there are any circumstances
where you undertake treatment before biopsy of the primary
lesion.

DR. ROSEN : Never.

CHAIRMAN : We should now discuss the possibility of frozen
section and whether or not frozen section is a useful
technique. Dr. van Rijssel, could you help us with that ?

DR. VAN RIJSSEL : It is possible to make a definite
diagnosis on frozen sections. But, it's a requirement that
the pathologist has a vast experience in bone-tumor
pathology. Bone tumors are rare and there are only very few

pathologists who have the opportunity to see more than a
few cases a year.

CHAIRMAN : Do you think there is anything lost by waiting ?
Is it preferable to have a frozen tissue diagnosis ?

DR. VAN RIJSSEL : I do not think that much is lost by
waiting.

CHAIRMAN : What do you think of radical amputation which
involves hip disarticulation as distinct from trans-
medullary amputation of the femur.

DR. SINDELAR : In the past total bone removal in osteosarcoma was the rule. And since most tumors occur in the
distal femur, this has resulted in a lot of hip
disarticulations which give functionally poor results.

Our own experience, at the National Cancer Institute, has
been, in the distal lesions - to perform trans-medullary
amputations. In approximately 37 of such amputations, there
has been only one local recurrence. Trans-medullary
amputation can be performed in the majority of the patients
It is a safe procedure. Exceptions to that would be very
large bulky tumors, with possibility of trans-medullary or
soft-tissue extension. This extension should be assessed by
tomography, and CT-scans.

CHAIRMAN : Dr. Rosen, have you any differential results in
your patients who've had less than amputation ?

DR. ROSEN : No, except in one or two anecdotal patients.
I've personally gone over with Dr. Huvos over 100 femurs
that were disarticulated. Only two had skip areas. In one
the tumor was right up practically to the skip. The second
one, had other bone metastasis. The proper use of bone scan
is to facilitate planning for a trans-medullary amputation
without incurring in additional risk.

DR. PRATT : There are some familial cancer syndromes that
are associated with osteo-sarcoma and rhabdomyosarcoma.
A hip disarticulation for disease of the femur may be

necessary in these patients because they often have multi-focal osteo-sarcoma.

CHAIRMAN : One kind of limb-salvage procedure has been undertaken by Morton and his colleagues (UCLA), which involves local treatment to the lesion with chemotherapy and radiation, followed by curettage of the bone. Bone chips of either autologous or cadaver origin are implanted. What do you think of this technique, Dr. Rosen ?

DR. ROSEN : They're not curettaging the tumor, but they're trying to resect it following local perfusion with adriamycin. They've had healing problems with perfusion and radiation, and they've eliminated the radiation. The Stanford Group had similar experience.

CHAIRMAN : As of two weeks ago, he was carrying out such a program. Maybe we don't have enough information to make any authoritative statements.

DR. ROSEN : The concept of curettage seems to me extremely dangerous for recurrence, no matter what preceding treatment.

CHAIRMAN : Dr. Breur, would you like to speak of the role of radiation after having seen some of the data presented by other colleagues who spoke after you ?

DR. BREUR : First of all, I feel a little bit lost among all these great American dreams that are represented here. One of the problems we are faced with is that we don't define very well the end points. Chemotherapy, may have a great influence on the tumor, and on prolongation of life. In Dr. Pratt's paper he didn't give us figures about the length of treatments. We should be careful not to present too early too great successes. It could be a disappointment later, as it was with Jaffe before.

Another remark : If we present data, we should show what the survival is after all patients have finished treatment.

I already pointed out that treating cancer is multidisciplinary, and radiotherapy of the primary tumor combined with chemotherapy should be explored. This could also achieve a functioning limb. Possibilities in the near future include types of radiation and drugs that sensitize hypoxic cells.This combined effort should always be performed in controlled clinical trials.

CHAIRMAN : I think that Dr. Rosen and I and Dr. Pratt did present data of all our patients. None dropped out. There were long periods of follow-up. The charts go back 7 years.

DR. BREUR : For part of the patients.

CHAIRMAN : Yes. Dr. Pratt, did you take all the patients treated with chemotherapy and plot their survival in the same way as has been done for radiotherapy ?

DR. PRATT : No. None of the patients were treated for more than 2 years. These disease-free survival percentages that were presented were all done, except in 4 instances, longer than 2 years after the initiation of the treatment protocols, and with at least a 2-year survival for those patients to be presented.

DR. WELVAART (Leiden): Does frozen section play a role in deciding whether you should perform a trans-medullary resection or a disarticulation ? Why should we rely on the bone scan ? What is the role of frozen section in surgery with regard to the level of resection.

DR. VAN RIJSSEL : When the surgeon has some suspicion about the possible presence of tumor near the level where he wants to perform his amputation, he will take a frozen section. It may be very difficult to make a diagnosis and one may have to wait for the paraffin sections.

CHAIRMAN : I thought your answer, Dr. van Rijssel, was going to be that there are very few bone pathologists who are qualified to look at frozen sections. Therefore Dr. Rosen's use of bone scanning may be helpful, and new techniques such as with N-13 glutamate add further interest.

DR. SINDELAR : What is our practice at the Cancer Institute? When a trans-medullary amputation is planned, we try to get all the data beforehand together, and we have found that CT scans probably provide the most useful determinant of the extent of tumor. Bone scans are also quite useful. However, we routinely, at the site of transsection, do send tissue for frozen section.

DR. CARDOZO (Leiden): I haven't heard the word "cytology" pronounced here, except in connection with peritoneal washings. But there is the hard fact that on 50 tumor cells I can make a diagnosis. I think there is a place for cytology, also for early relapse.

CHAIRMAN : Thank you. Do you imply that there is a place for needle biopsy of the primary tumor ?

DR. CARDOZO : Yes, I had several cases myself.

DR. ROSEN : We've had experience with needle biopsy. You can make the diagnosis based on X-ray, and an elevated alkaline phosphatase. However, you need accurate data on the type of tumor, the variant of osteogenic sarcoma and the histologic grade in order to reach a decision about chemotherapy. A good, adequate biopsy should be done before anyone is treated for future reference.

DR. MUGGIA : I would like to comment further on a topic that Dr. Breur raised : the combination of radiation and chemotherapy on the primary. I have heard data from a recent study, from the Institute Curie in Paris, where they have treated 14 patients with this combination. The radiotherapy having been given over a period of 7 weeks at a total dose of 7200 rads. Seven patients are without any recurrence, median follow-up being 14 months, the shortest one being 10 months and the longest 30 months. Four patients had a local problem, of which 3 had recurrent tumor, one had a fracture, but no tumor at amputation. The 3 with local recurrences and two others have had pulmonary metastases. These results are better than radiation alone in the past.

2. *The sequence and type of treatment*

CHAIRMAN: I think we've handled those areas well and ought to move on then to chemotherapy. Dr. Rosen, we've seen you change drugs in the last cycle, taking different things and putting them first. Dr. Pratt made a number of observations of response activities in different sequences. Do you think that the optimal chemotherapy or the optimal sequence of drugs is known, or is it still a topic of research?

DR. ROSEN: It's still a topic of research. The most information can be gained by treating the patients pre-operatively. It's also important for the continued investigation and search of effective treatments for this disease.

DR. PRATT: It has been mentioned that high-dose methotrexate has been available to a number of institutions for a few years. It is very important to recognize the E.O.R.T.C. and their S.I.O.P. collaborators, as well as the Children's Cancer Study Group and the Medical Research Council have not reported their results using more moderate doses of methotrexate. There are also additional studies that were not cited, for which no long-term follow-up results are available from Spain and Austria, except as cited by Dr. Rosen.

We certainly dit not intend to omit the reference to these people, but I think until we have other long-term follow-ups, we can't make some recommendations about what the optimal schedules for ostea-sarcoma are.

CHAIRMAN: This implies that the ad hoc treatment of specific individual patients with osteo-sarcoma is ill-advised and they should be entered in the protocol studies, so that this rare tumor where enormous progress is being made can be better cured.

I doubt that there are many people who feel as Dr. Sindelar does that there is a question as to whether adjuvant chemotherapy is active. We've seen doubling or even tripling or even quadrupling of the background history of

relapse in disease-free individuals in a number of studies.
Do you have any information from your review, Dr. Pratt,
that would relate to the duration of treatment?

DR. PRATT : Most of the recurrences in patients treated
with adjuvant therapy for a period of about a year have
occurred during treatment. Therefore, this period of one
year should not be exceeded as the optimal duration of
treatment. A 6-month treatment period as in the CALGB study
is perhaps also very acceptable. I'm afraid that we're not
in the ideal situation as was discussed by the
urologic surgeons, that we can afford the luxury of not
giving adjuvant chemotherapy, or of cutting down the length
of time of chemotherapy. We do not know whether short-term
effective chemotherapy exists today and, therefore, we take
the more cautious attitude of treating the patients for
longer periods of time.

3. Proper drugs to use

CHAIRMAN : Dr. Rosen, I'd like to hear your opinion on the
differences in the impact of high-dose methotrexate, in
different people's hands. Is there a relation with infusion
time and serum levels?

DR. ROSEN : We have looked at the serum levels after a
four-hour infusion. A four-hour infusion was convenient,
and it turned out to be succesful. It may be the initial
high concentration that enters into the tumor cell and is
responsible for the effect. We've seen no responses in
patients who failed the four-hour infusion, when given a
six- or twenty-four-hour infusion. We have changed the
dose schedule of citrovorum factor in non-responding
patients and found that we can delay rescue to 48 hours,
without a difference in the response rate. We have also
escalated the dose above 20 grams. Contrary to Dr. Djerassi
we do not find significant responses above that dose range.
We have given unsuccessfuly high-dose methotrexate for two
days in a row in some patients refractory to 14 or 16 grams.
Total duration of our current adjuvant protocol is 45 weeks.
But, remember any patient that has achieved complete
remission following pre-operative chemotherapy has a

prolonged disease-free survival. In the earlier protocols, we gave only 6 high-dose methotrexate infusions and 6 courses of adriamycin. The patients that responded were cured. Prolonging treatment by giving high-dose metho- trexate intermittently with the other drugs, gives a higher percentage of complete remissions.

DR. MUGGIA : There is an essential paradox in some of the high-dose methotrexate results. There are at least two studies, one from the CALGB, the other from Sutow and the COMPADRI regimens where high-dose methotrexate does not add to their previous experience, or to a simultaneous comparison with regimens without methotrexate. In the COMPADRI regimens, Sutow did switch to the weekly metho- trexate regimens. But they still did not obtain better results in their latest COMPADRI,than in their first combination that did not have high-dose methotrexate It's this particular paradox, and the experience at the N.C.I. that is the key to the new N.C.I. trial. They believe that other regimens may be associated with significant morbidity, whereas the high-dose methotrexate is attractive because it has little acute toxicity and is devoid of serious long-range effects.

DR. SINDELAR : I just wanted to comment to Dr. Holland after he casually cast me in the role of the devil's advocate as to questioning whether or not adjuvant therapy could be given. I personally feel that it is still an open question the data of Dr. Rosen notwithstanding. There is ample data at the present time to indicate that a proportion of patients - possibly as high as 50 percent - treated with surgery, may never recur after this treatment alone. We will never know the answer to the efficacy of adjuvant chemotherapy, unless that particular question is asked and answered in a randomized control fashion. Let me add one thing. A more important question is; can failures be salvaged by chemotherapy ? If they can, then I think the whole question of adjuvant therapy is open for discussion.

DR. MUGGIA : The surgical resection is a very important problem. It is related to the biology of osteogenic sarcoma. There is a contrast between Dr. Rosen's patients with pulmonary metastases, and those identifed to have metastases on a prospective survey. There may be a difference between those two groups of patients not only related to the number of metastases or the operability. The patients in Dr. Martini's series, treated with surgical resection alone have as good long-term survival as the ones you treated agressively with chemotherapy. Now this was a very selected series of unilateral single lesions. However, if you pick them up prospectively, it is open to question if metastases of a certain critical size, may stimulate the appearance of more metastases. This is a possibility which the N.C.I. prospective trial will actually address itself to.

DR. SINDELAR : The question that hasn't been answered - what is the remission rate in patients who had adjuvant chemotherapy and failed ? Do they respond?

DR. ROSEN : Usually not very well. When patients relapse it's very rare to have a solitary operable pulmonary metastasis. The reason why we were able to salvage 5 of 10 of the younger patients is because they were still responsive to high-dose methotrexate. You can produce a remission in these patients again with chemotherapy, but you never cure them unless you can remove the residual disease surgically. Without adjuvant chemotherapy the majority of your patients will have inoperable disease that is going to kill them. Therefore we should put everyone on adjuvant chemotherapy resulting in at least a 50 % cure rate and in our institution and at M.D. Anderson up to 80 % and 90 %. There is absolutely no question in my mind about the usefulness of adjuvant chemotherapy.

4. New concepts

CHAIRMAN : Now, we shall discuss interferon and newer aspects of treatment. Interferon is a natural substance of human origin that has been reported by Strander and his colleagues from Sweden to have produced a response rate, given adjuvantly for osteo-sarcoma, equivalent to the response rate of adriamycin in CALGB study.

Dr. Rosen, I can't believe that you haven't dallied in interferon somewhere along the line.

DR. ROSEN : If we could get it, we would treat half of our patients with interferon in a study. We want to use it in a therapeutic dose up front, as part of the pre-operative treatment, to see if we can affect evaluable disease. We haven't used it yet because it's been unavailable to us. The doses suggested for treating established disease have been in the order of 10 million units a day. Dr. Strander, in his adjuvant studies has been using 2 to 3 million units a day.

DR. PRATT : We have not used interferon.

DR. SINDELAR : We have no experience but the pediatric oncology branch of het N.C.I. has done some preliminary work with interferon. There are 5 patients with advanced metastatic disease so treated, none have responded at all.

CHAIRMAN : This is, of course, a greater challenge for any drug than the adjuvant circumstance. This compound is a natural product and therefore of great interest.

5. Pulmonary metastases at the time of diagnosis
A lot was said about the possibility that we have changed things by better diagnostic staging The proposition is that you are selecting patients better for surgery because of recognition of pulmonary metastasis at the time of entry. What is the frequency of finding people with metastatic disease, when they come to you ? Dr. Rosen, Pratt, Sindelar.

DR. ROSEN : (passes).

DR. PRATT : Since 1973, we've admitted 86 patients with osteo-sarcoma, of which 29 did not fit the criteria for admission to adjuvant chemotherapy protocols, either because of pulmonary metastases, pelvic disease that crossed the mid line, diseases of flat bones rather than the extremity lesions (we've admitted only patients with extremity lesions to adjuvant treatment protocols), and radiation-associated osteo-sarcomas. There are certainly innumerable types other than the pure classical osteo-sarcoma of the extremities that should not be admitted to adjuvant chemotherapy protocols. About one-third of our patients do not fit adjuvant-therapy schemes because of these special situations. Nearly half of the 29 patients had pulmonary metastases at the time of diagnosis.

CHAIRMAN : So, that's about 15 out of 86, or nearly 20 %. I'm trying to develop the proposition that those who say that the surgery today is better surgery are excluding an only small segment of patients presenting with metastases who would have been included in Marcove's or Sindelar's historical data.

DR. SINDELAR : In our series, 11 out of 52 patients were discovered to have metastatic disease at the time of referral. That percentage of patients referred to our Institution, with supposedly localized disease in which we uncover metastases continues to hold up at 15 to 20 %.

CHAIRMAN : How many are diagnosed by chest X-ray as distinct from tomography or other techniques that might not have been used in the past ?

DR. SINDELAR : I would say about one-third.

DR. BREUR : In the material of the Dutch Bone Tumor Registry, published by Cohen, there were about 5 % of patients coming with metastases. These were patients from all over the country. It is certain that, in a center where you look closer, you will find by better examination a higher percentage at diagnosis. I'm sure that all the new methods, tomography, CT scan, will raise that figure. And that's one of the reasons why you can't use historical controls.

CHAIRMAN : In the three institutions that are using exquisitely sensitive techniques of diagnosis, a maximum of 25 % might have been subtracted from adjuvant studies. Thus the change in survival from the 20 % historical base

could be to 40 or 50 % at the very most. We already see
substantial survivals over and above that due to the
treatments administered.

DR. ROSEN : Most of Marcove's patients did have chest tomography particularly in those in updated reports after his
1970 publication of 121 patients. Now he includes 210
patients and there is still a 17 % cure rate for those
additional 89 patients and I can guarantee you that all
those 89 patients did have initial tomography.

6. Pulmonary metastases, later

CHAIRMAN: The last topic concerns the pulmonary metastatic lesion and should we always resect it after it regresses on
chemotherapy. You have pointed in that direction, Dr. Rosen.
Are there those who think one need not undergo thoracotomy
or even bilateral thoracotomy ? Should this be done through
a mid-line sternal incision, doing both lungs simultaneously?
Or separate thoracotomies ? Should it be done per primam,
with chemotherapy afterwards or chemotherapy first ?

DR. SINDELAR : If there is suspicion or radiologic evidence
of a lesion - even though it has regressed - one still
feels obliged to explore the chest. I recommend thoracotomy
in all cases where metastatic disease is suspected.
Generally, osteosarcomas occur in young people who
tolerate thoracotomies extremely well. They're up and out
of the hospital usually within a week to ten days.
We advocate a median sternotomy and bilateral exploration
of both chests through a single incision, at a single
operation. This is not always possible, particularly when
lesions occur in the posterior portion of the left upper
lobe. I would say the vast majority of patients can have
their disease resected very adequately through a median
sternotomy.

DR. BREUR : It is possible that adjuvant therapy, either
radio- or chemotherapy decreases the number of metastases
and renders them more amenable to surgical extirpation.

CHAIRMAN : This has been described by the Sidney Farber
Cancer Group (Jaffe, ASCO, 1978). Dr. Rosen would have us

believe that he reduces them to zero, in a high proportion patients.

DR. ROSEN : But I still think they should come out, because they recur when you stop chemotherapy.

DR. PRATT : In addition to the effect on the pulmonary metastases, there may have been some change in the natural history of osteo-sarcoma in patients who develop metastatic disease. I think that Dr. Jaffe and Dr. Rosen have both mentioned at other meetings the influence of pulmonary metastases and their probable ability to create metastases in other areas of the body, specifically the long bones and the spine.

CHAIRMAN : A number of patients in the failing period have developed trans-section of the cord.

DR. ROSEN : When you keep a patient who has pulmonary metastasis alive with systemic therapy ; you keep them alive with multiple thoracotomies. In those patients brain metastases and visceral metastases occur.

DR. HOSSFELD (Essen): Does anybody have experience in treatment of metastatic disease with adriamycin and cisplatinum ?

DR. ROSEN : We showed a response of a very large retro-cardiac mass to adriamycin and cisplatinum. Dr. Ettinger (Roswell Park) has also treated some metastatic patients with the sequential combination of adriamycin and cisplatinum at doses of 90 mg per m^2 and 100 mg per m^2 respectively. We use 60 milligrams per m^2 of adriamycin because our patients have had trouble with the higher dose in combination.

DR. HOSSFELD : Were these patients previously untreated ?

DR. ROSEN : No, all three patients had received up to 360 milligrams per m^2 of adriamycin. We've seen objective responses in all 3 and it's very encouraging.

CHAIRMAN : It's a very active combination in a whole spectrum of tumors. Other comments ?

DR. CLETON : I would like to ask something on pulmonary tumorectomy. Is there a certain time when you do not expect new metastases to occur anymore ? If they start within half a year and you take them out and you get new ones and you take them out again for up to two years, do you expect them no to occur anymore ? Or will they continue to occur because they arise from previous metastases ?

DR. ROSEN : In the patients in which we have seen a complete response to chemotherapy and no viable tumor in the metastasis, they have not come back following thoracotomy. However, in patients where there is still viable tumor, we have seen them relapse up to three years after thoracotomy. That's why we follow them very carefully, and put them back on chemotherapy. Sometimes it makes no difference and they'll relapse usually, within the first year but exceptionally up to five years.

7. Follow-up

CHAIRMAN : What is the proper follow-up ?
What should be the frequency of films or scans ?
Dr. Pratt, do you still wait 6 months between tomograms ?

DR. PRATT : No, we wait 4 months, but use CT scans and not tomograms any longer. We do routine chest radiographs at 5 weekly intervals, because that happens to fit into the present cycle of the chemotherapy. We also do bone scans at 6 monthly intervals, during the first two years after the diagnosis.

CHAIRMAN : Could I ask Dr. Sindelar : with what frequency do you find metastases on the chest X-rays, distinct from the CT scan ?

DR. SINDELAR : I would estimate that about half of the patients have them determined by CT scans as opposed to the regular radiographs. In some instances (3 out of 24) the findings at thoracotomy were other than metastases.

DR. ROSEN : I recently had an infant referred to me who was seen at the Mayo Clinic, where they said the CT scans showed diffuse pulmonary metastases from a fibrosarcoma. We reviewed the histologic material and sent the patient home. These presumed lesions have not changed in three years. I think certain places may be over-reading the CT scans.

CHAIRMAN : The quality of the radiologic studies and their interpretation is crucial. All films made in follow-up require review at an experienced center.

DR. BREUR : In the protocol of our last trial, we include 3 or 4 weeks' waiting after detection of metastases, to study growth rate and also to see if new metastases appear during that period. Do you agree with this procedure ? In early publications, it was always said that growth rate of less than 40 days doubling time had a worse prognosis than those with slower growth. A slower time of appearance (i.e. after 6 months) is also more amenable to surgery. Such a period of observation would also exclude the possibility of benign lesions.

DR. ROSEN : We wait at least three months. We try to observe a stopping of the growth rate of the tumors and at least a stabilization in growth before we take them out.

CHAIRMAN : Do you wait a month before you initiate chemotherapy ?

DR. ROSEN : No. We start chemotherapy right away. We don't observe the growth rate but we observe it regressing - hopefully.

DR. BREUR : A correlation between the regression rate from chemotherapy and growth rate would be an interesting study.

DR. PRATT : Our surgeon would prefer to resect the metastases as soon as they are found. We prefer the unilateral thoracotomy approach rather than sternum-splitting incisions.

CHAIRMAN : Dr. Rosen, do you use the sternum split ?

DR. ROSEN : No, our surgeons do not. When I'm asked what to do with the appearance of pulmonary metastases during chemotherapy I recommend higher doses of methotrexate or trial of cisplatinum and subsequent resection.Histologic examination can then be very informative regarding the effect of chemotherapy.

DR. SINDELAR : I can't let you get away totally with that statement. There are situations where we frequently see pulmonary metastases excised on no therapy, that show considerable necrosis. Interpretation of histologic changes in metastatic deposits must be done with great caution. Conclusions drawn from that must be appropriately tempered.

DR. WAGENER (Nijmegen): Has chemotherapy an influence on the bone scan ?

DR. ROSEN : Yes it does. You can have reactive bone increasing uptake although initially lesions were not detected.

DR. HOSSFELD : Could we hear about the application of adriamycin intra-arterially ?

DR. SINDELAR : I have no such experience.

DR. ROSEN : No experience.

CHAIRMAN : We have done it for 100 hours with 1 milligram per m^2 per hour. The outcome has been dubious,relative to the total tumor necrosis expected from Dr. Rosen's regimens. Morton and his colleagues have used a similar approach but combine it with radiation in the immediate post-infusion period, so one cannot assess the effect of adriamycin alone. More rapid infusion leads to endarteritis.
The Sidney Farber Group has abandoned the treatment.

PART FOUR

SOFT TISSUE SARCOMA

29 SOFT TISSUE SARCOMA - CLASSIFICATION AND PROGNOSIS

J. A. M. van Unnik and Ch. E. Albus Lutter

The relationship between the histologic type of a soft tissue tumour and prognosis is well established. However, in nearly each type a subdivision is made in several grades of differentiation or - perhaps better - grades of malignancy. It is even stated that grades of malignancy are more important in this field of oncology than the histogenetic diagnosis. To examine the value of different parameters patients with soft tissue sarcomas, who were treated in the Netherlands Cancer Institute in Amsterdam, and who had a follow-up of at least 10 years were studied. Data were collected of 126 patients.

Liposarcomas form the largest group (fig. 1) closely followed by fibrosarcomas, malignant fibrous histiocytomas (M.F.H.) and the relatively benign groups of agressive fibromatosis and dermatofibrosarcoma. Smaller groups are the myosarcomas (mostly rhabdomyosarcomas), angiosarcomas and groups which were not classifiable because of the undifferentiated character of these tumours. Other less frequently encountered diagnoses e.g. malignant synovioma, epithelioid cell sarcoma, alveolar soft part sarcoma etc. were represented in this material by only 1 or 2 patients each. They were not suitable for further analysis. Together they accounted for only 7% of the total number of patients. Accordingly the groups given in fig. 1 comprise 93% of the total number of patients studied.

Setting the group of fibromatosis in which only 1 out of 19 patients died during the follow-up period apart, liposarcoma has the best prognosis during the first 10 years (fig. 2).
The difference in prognosis with fibrosarcoma and M.F.H. is statistically significant. The group of myo- and angiosarcoma has the worst prognosis, comparable with undifferentiated sarcoma (not shown in this figure). The prognostic results of all cases taken together are poor compared to most figures given in the literature.

A.T. van Oosterom et al. (eds.), Therapeutic Progress in Ovarian Cancer, Testicular Cancer and the Sarcomas, pp. 387-396. All rights reserved.
Copyright 1980 by Martinus Nijhoff Publishers, The Hague/Boston/London.

388

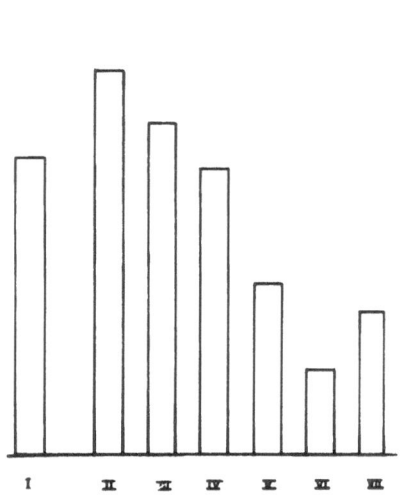

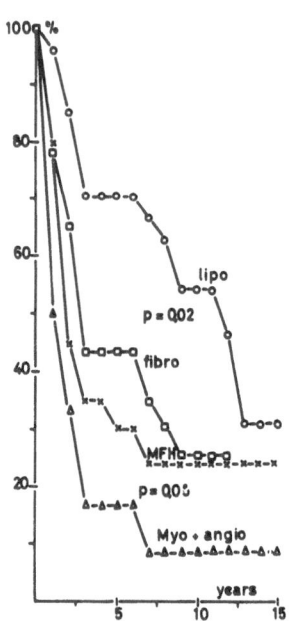

Fig.1. *Distribution of soft tissue tumours according to the diagnosis made in 1979. I. Fibromatosis, II. liposarcoma, III.fibrosarcoma, IV. M.F.H., V. Myosarcoma, VI. Angiosarcoma, VII. unclassifiable.*

Fig.2. *Survival curve of patients with liposarcoma, fibrosarcoma, M.F.H., myosarcoma and angiosarcoma.*

In all probability this is due to a selection of patients with a bad prognosis; most of them were treated primarily in another hospital and often after recurrence referred to the Cancer Institute.

In figure 3 the distribution is given according to the original diagnoses. They were made at least 10 years ago but often they date back from 15 to 20 years. The diagnosis of M.F.H. was non-existent at that time and the group of fibromatosis was not yet as clearly defined as it has become in more recent times. Accordingly fibrosarcoma is the most frequent diagnosis and it has a fair prognosis comparable with liposarcoma (fig. 4). Myosarcoma and angiosarcoma have a bad prognosis again.

Comparing these figures with the diagnoses of 1979 it may be concluded that the separation of fibromatosis certainly is an improvement. It was known, of course, in former times that "highly differentiated fibrosarcoma"did rather well, but now the diagnosis of this non-metastasizing variety is made with more certainty. In our material the separation of M.F.H. from fibrosarcoma did not have much bearing on prognosis. Most cases of M.F.H. in fact are derived from the former

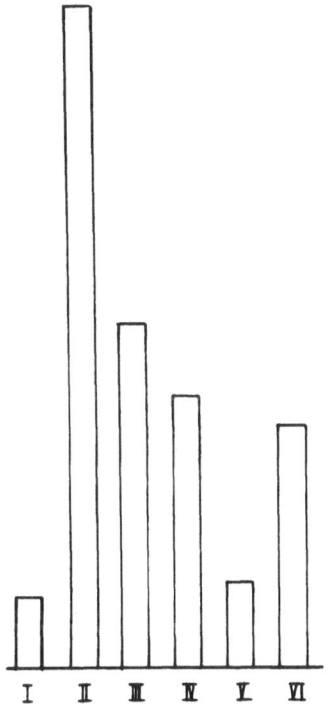

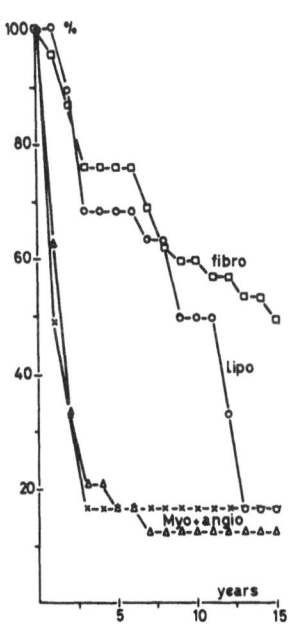

Fig. 3. Distribution of soft tissue tumours according to the original diagnosis made at least 10 years ago. I. fibromatosis, II. fibrosarcoma, III. liposarcoma, IV. myosarcoma, V. angiosarcoma, VI. unclassifiable.

Fig.4. Survival curve according to the original diagnoses (fibrosarcoma, liposarcoma, myosarcoma and angiosarcoma).

fibrosarcomas, some cases from the rhabdomyosarcomas and others from the group of pleomorphic liposarcomas. In the cases on which a firm diagnosis is not possible on account of the undifferentiated character of the constituents a useful designation for practical purposes is still possible, as these tumours have a bad prognosis.

Aside from the histogenetic diagnosis numerous parameters are mentioned in the literature as prognostic indication in soft tissue tumours e.g. in myxoid chondrosarcoma the degree of cellularity and mitotic activity, but not the size of the tumour (Enzinger a.o. 1972); in tendosynovial sarcoma the anatomic site and size of the tumour, the histologic type (biphasic versus monophasic pattern) and the presence of lymph node metastases (Hadju a.o. 1977); in haemangiopericytoma mitotic activity, the presence of necrosis, haemorrhage and the degree of cellularity, the size of the tumour having no influence (Enzinger 1974); in myxoid M.F.H. the degree of cellularity, the size of the tumour and the presence of myxoid intercellular material in more than 50% of the tumour, the mitotic index, however, being rather unimportant

(Weiss and Enzinger 1977); in M.F.H. superficial versus deep localization of the tumour, the presence of an inflammatory infiltrate and the presence of myxoid intercellular material (Enzinger and Weiss 1978) again in M.F.H. a low mitotic index as indicator of a rather good prognosis (Enzinger 1977); in fibrosarcoma mitotic index, size and anatomic site of the lesion (v.d. Werf and v. Unnik 1965).

In the patients of this study a statistical significant (P=0.05) correlation was found between size and prognosis, when all cases were divided into 2 groups, 5 cm accepted as a borderline. Restricting this parameter to the group of liposarcomas, fibrosarcomas and M.F.H. the correlation was no longer significant, probably due to the rather small number of patients. In only 67% of the cases it was possible to trace the size of the primary tumour.

Lymph node metastases were found in 8% of these patients (in 9.3% of all cases minus fibromatosis), which is in accordance with figures from literature. When lymph node metastases were present the patient nearly always died within a few years. Lymph node metastases in sarcomas are less frequent than in carcinomas but when found they are a very ominous sign.

The amount of collagen fibres is positively related to prognosis (fig. 5). The group with much fibre formation certainly includes a large number of the fibromatosis group but a significant difference in prognosis was even found between the cases with a moderate degree of fibre formation and the groups with only a few or no collagen fibres In any case it seems a prognostic favourable point when a soft tissue tumour makes collagen fibres and the more it does the better.

The presence of myxomatous parts in these tumours in our material did not correlate with the prognosis. This feature was studied particularly in lipo- and fibrohistiocytic sarcomas. Only the liposarcomas with more than 50% mucous parts did somewhat better than other liposarcomas, i.e. 50% 10 years survival against 30% of the other liposarcomas. A difficulty encountered was that in the original descriptions the amount of myxomatous tissue was often scarcely mentioned, so we had to rely only on histologic sections.

Regarding the liposarcomas it was found that the cases which were well differentiated according to the WHO classification behaved better than the other types, i.e.60% 10 years survival of the well differentiated against 20% of the other groups. On the other hand

liposarcomas with much polymorphy had a very bad prognosis, i.e. only
14% 10 years survival. The results were very relevant when these
patients with liposarcoma were divided according to the mitotic index.
In this way it was possible to separate a group in which no mitoses
were found and which had a very good prognosis (fig. 6).

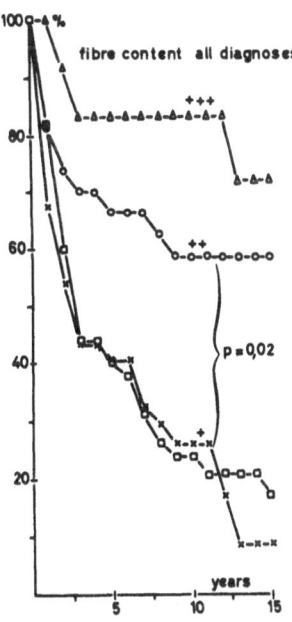

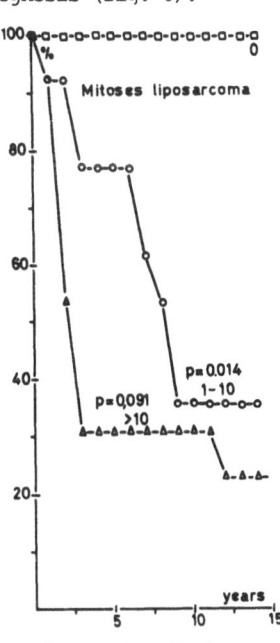

*Fig. 5. Survival curve of patients
with soft tissue tumours (all
diagnoses) according to: much collagen fibre formation (+++), moderate
fibre formation (++), little fibre
formation (+) and no fibre formation.
The difference between the group
with moderate fibre formation and
little or no fibre formation is
statistically significant (P= 0.02).*

*Fig. 6. Survival curves of
patients with liposarcoma.
Respectively 0 mitoses found
in 10 high power field (HPF),
1-10 mitoses in 10 HPF and
>10 mitoses in 10 HPF. The
difference between the first
two groups is significant
(P=0.014).*

A high degree of polymorphy and a very low mitotic rate seem to be
the most relevant prognostic indicators in liposarcomas respectively
for a very bad and a very good prognosis. In M.F.H. no relation
between mucous formation and prognosis was found. A significant
relation, however, was seen between mitotic activity and prognosis
(fig. 7).

The same relation was seen in fibrosarcoma (fig. 8). The
question arises whether the tumours with no mitoses will have to be
included in the group of fibromatosis at second examination.

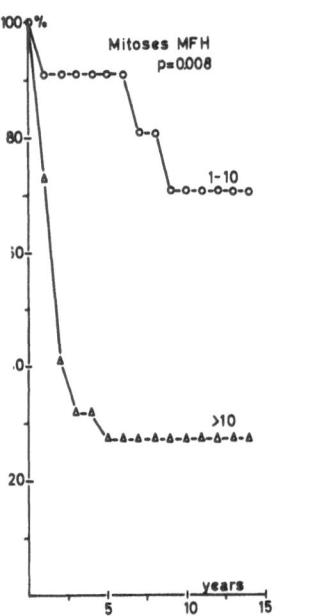

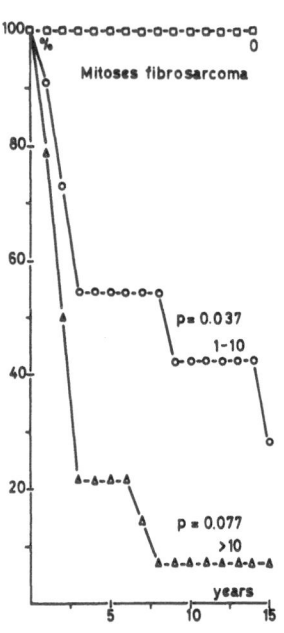

Fig. 7. Survival curves of patients with M.F.H. The group with 1-10 mitoses in 10 HPF has a significant better prognosis than the group with 10 mitoses in 10 HPF (P=0.008).

Fig. 8. Survival curves of patients with fibrosarcoma. Th group with 0 mitoses in 10 HPF has a significant better prognosis than the group with 1-10 mitoses in 10 HPF.

A very interesting feature is the relation between the presence of inflammatory infiltrate and prognosis. From the study of Weiss and Enzinger (1978) it is known that an inflammatory infiltrate in M.F.H. may be regarded as a good prognostic sign. The infiltrates within and around the tumours were studied separately. It appears that an infiltrate inside the tumour has no relation to prognosis (fig. 9).
An infiltrate outside the tumour, however, is related to a better prognosis (fig. 10). This is the case when all types of soft tissue tumours are taken together. It was felt that the better prognosis in these cases could be explained by assuming the more frequent presence of an inflammatory infiltrate in the neighbourhood of fibromatosis. However, after excluding the cases of fibromatosis the difference

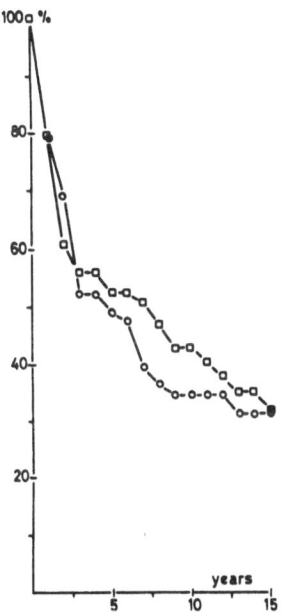

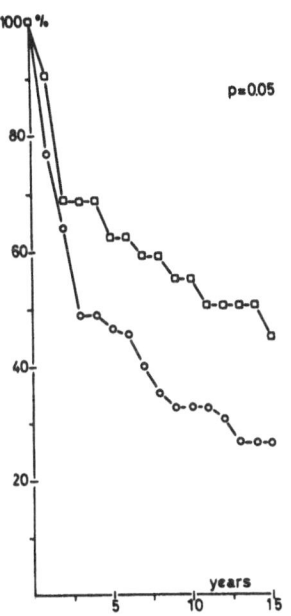

Fig. 9. *Survival curves of all cases of soft tissue tumours divided according to the presence of inflammatory infiltrate inside the tumour (□) or absence of such an infiltrate (0). No difference was found.*

Fig. 10. *Survival curves of all cases of soft tissue tumours divided according to the presence of inflammatory infiltrate outside the tumour (□) or absence of such an infiltrate (0). The difference is significant (P=0.05).*

became all the more clear (fig. 11).

This relationship has to be analysed in more detail.

Summarizing the conclusion seems warranted that besides histogenetic classification other parameters may have a strong relation to prognosis. The results of this study show that the mitotic index in lipo-,fibro- and-fibrohistio sarcomas together with other parameters like fibre formation and pleomorphism can give valuable information in addition to the histogenetic diagnosis of these tumours. These three groups of soft tissue tumours together represent $\pm$ 60% of the total number of cases of this study,

The significance of the inflammatory infiltrate around the tumour merits further study.

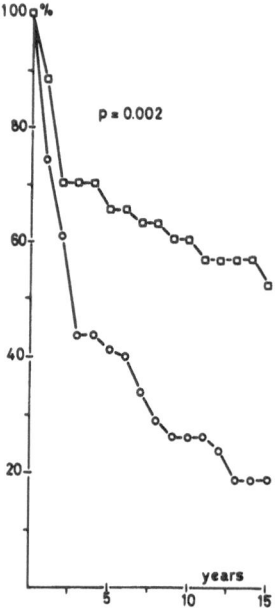

Fig. 11. Survival curves of all cases of soft tissue tumours minus fibromatosis divided according to the presence of inflammatory infiltrate outside the tumour (▭) or absence of such an infiltrate (0). The difference is significant (P=0.002).

REFERENCES

Enzinger, F.M. & Shiraki, M.   Extraskeletal myxoid chondrosarcoma. Human Pathology 3 - 421 (1972).

Enzinger, F.M. & Smith, B.H.   Haemangiopericytoma. Human Pathology 7 - 61 (1976)

Enzinger, F.M.   Recent developments in the classification of soft tissue sarcomas in Management of primary bone & soft tissue tumours. Year book Medical Publishers inc. Chicago - London, p. 219 (1977).

Hadju, S.I., Shiu, M.H.   Tendosynovial sarcoma.
& Fortner, J.G.   Cancer 39-1201 (1977).
Weiss, S.W. & Enzinger,   Myxoid variant of malignant fibrous
F.M.   histiocytoma.
                           Cancer 39-1672 (1977).
Weiss, S.W. & Enzinger,   Malignant Fibrous Histiocytoma.
F.M.   Cancer 41-2250 (1978)
V.d. Werf-Messing, B.   Fibrosarcoma of the soft tissues.
& V. Unnik, J.A.M.   Cancer 18-1113 (1965).

Acknowledgement.

The statistical work was done by Dr. J.A.J. Faber
and mr. A.J. de Meijer of the Institute for Mathematical
Statistics, State University of Utrecht.

Authors addresses:

J.A.M. van Unnik
    Department of Pathology
    State University, Utrecht, The Netherlands

Ch.E. Albus Lutter
    Department of Pathology
    Netherlands Cancer Institute, Amsterdam, The Netherlands

30 SURGERY AND ADJUVANT RADIATION-CHEMO-IMMUNOTHERAPY IN SOFT TISSUE SARCOMAS: RESULT OF TREATMENT AT THE NATIONAL CANCER INSTITUTE

S. A. Rosenberg and W. F. Sindelar

ABSTRACT

A prospective randomized evaluation of limited surgical excision with adjuvant radiotherapy, chemotherapy and immunotherapy was carried out at the National Cancer Institute on 49 patients with soft tissue sarcomas. Twenty-six patients with sarcomas of the extremities were randomized to receive amputation with adjuvant chemotherapy (doxorubicin and cyclophosphamide, followed by methotrexate); limb-sparing conservative surgery with radiotherapy and chemotherapy; or conservative surgery with radiotherapy, chemotherapy, and immunotherapy (Corynebacterium parvum). No differences in disease free interval or survival were present among the groups. Patients with sarcomas of the head-neck and trunk were randomized to receive surgery, radiation therapy, and chemotherapy or to receive surgery, radiotherapy, chemotherapy, and immunotherapy. The groups showed similar therapeutic results. The sarcoma protocol patients, when compared to a similar historical control patient group, showed significant improvement in disease free interval and in survival. The study suggested that limited surgery with radiotherapy may be efficacious for local control of sarcomas. Immunotherapy was not demonstrated to be beneficial. Adjuvant chemotherapy appeared to be considerable benefit in preventing or delaying distant recurrences.

A.T. van Oosterom et al. (eds.), Therapeutic Progress in Ovarian Cancer, Testicular Cancer and the Sarcomas, pp. 397-412. All rights reserved.
Copyright 1980 by Martinus Nijhoff Publishers, The Hague/Boston/London.

INTRODUCTION

Sarcomas of the soft tissues represent a disease group of malignant neoplasms arising in tissues of mesenchymal origin. Soft tissue sarcomas are relatively uncommon, accounting for under 1% of all adult malignancies. However, they have a predilection for younger age groups, and sarcomas of soft tissues comprise approximately 7% of malignancies occurring under the age of 25. Soft tissue sarcomas carry a poor prognosis, with five-year survival rates under 50% in most collected series (1,2).

Soft tissue sarcomas tend to locally invade surrounding tissue extensively. Because of local tumor extension, it has been repeatedly demonstrated in surgical series that limited local tumor resections frequently result in recurrence. Recurrence rates for local excisions have been reported up to 80% (2,3). Wide, radical excisions have proven more successful in locally controlling soft tissue sarcomas, but such operations can carry significant morbidity. Radical excisions of extremity sarcomas generally require amputation. Even with amputation, local recurrences can be expected in about 20% of patients (1,2,3). Besides local invasion, soft tissue sarcomas may metastasize widely, generally by the hematogenous route. Distant metastases may occur in over half of patients treated for sarcomas (1,3). Successful efforts to control soft tissue sarcomas, therefore require methods to provide local eradication of tumor as well as prevention or elimination of metastatic deposits.

Because of limitations in survival rates from surgery alone, interest was generated in the use of additional modalities in treating soft tissue sarcomas, particularly the use of radiotherapy (4) and chemotherapy (5,6). Immunotherapy (7) also showed evidence of efficacy in the treatment of certain sarcomas. Interest has been given to treatment and survival of various classifications of sarcomas (8). In order to determine the efficacy of limited, function-preserving surgery and the role of adjuvant radiotherapy, chemotherapy, and immunotherapy in the treatment of soft tissue sarcomas, a prospective randomized trial was carried out at the National Cancer Institute between 1975 and 1977. Specific questions toward which the study was directed included: whether local tumor control achieved by limited excision with postoperative adjuvant radiotherapy was comparable to radical surgical excision often involving amputation of an extremity, whether adjuvant postoperative combination chemotherapy improved survival by diminishing the incidence of metastatic disease, and whether adjuvant immunotherapy was of any benefit in disease control in the soft tissue sarcomas. Early results of the protocol studies have been reported (1). The present paper represents an update of the data to four years following initiation of the studies.

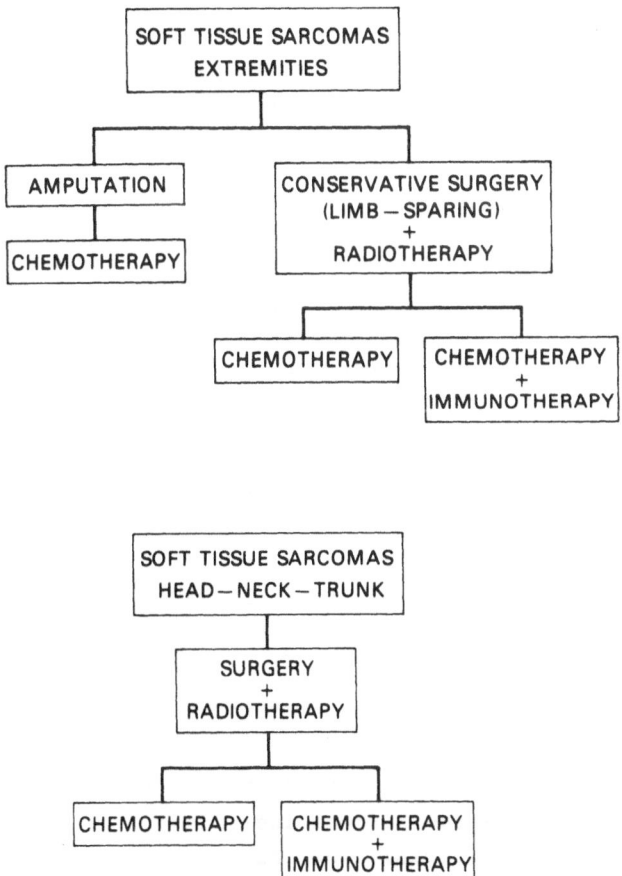

Fig. 1. Randomizations in soft tissue sarcoma protocols

CLINICAL PROTOCOL

Schema

Patients with soft tissue sarcomas were studied in one
of two protocols, depending on site of primary: extremity
lesions, or tumors of the head-neck and trunk. All patients were investigated in a prospective, randomized fashion. Patients with extremity lesions were randomized to
receive: amputation as the "standard surgical therapy"
followed by postoperative adjuvant chemotherapy; to receive
limited "limb-sparing" surgery which removed gross tumor
but preserved a functional extremity, followed by post-
operative radiotherapy to the tumor bed and adjuvant chemotherapy; or to receive limited surgery, radiation therapy, chemotherapy, and immunotherapy. Patients with sarcomas of the head-neck or trunk all received surgery to
excise all gross tumor followed by postoperative radiotherapy. Patients were then prospectively randomized to receive chemotherapy, or both chemotherapy and immunotherapy.
The randomizations in the treatment arms are illustrated in
Figure 1.

Patient Population

Patients up to the age of 65 with sarcomas diagnosed
within six months were included in the protocol study. All
had extensive evaluations showing no evidence of metastatic
disease. No patient had received prior radiation or chemotherapy, and none had a history of previous unrelated malignant disease. Patients were excluded from the study if
they had any history of significant medical problems, such
as cardiovascular disease or renal dysfunction, which
would increase the risk of either surgery or adjuvant therapy.

Tumor Histology

Patients were eligible for study with a biopsy-proven
diagnosis of soft tissue sarcoma including: liposarcoma,
fibrosarcoma, angiosarcoma, synovial sarcoma, undifferentiated sarcoma, malignant fibrous histiocytoma, or malignant mesenchymoma. All lesions were classified and graded

by pathologists at the National Cancer Institute. Patients were stratified by grade (low and intermediate against high grade lesions) and type of tumor (undifferentiated sarcoma, synovial sarcoma, and angiosarcoma against liposarcoma, fibrosarcoma, rhabdomyosarcoma, leiomyosarcoma, mesenchymoma, and fibrous histiocytoma). Patients were also stratified by time of diagnosis (referral within two months of diagnosis against referral after two months), by recurrence status (no local recurrence against local recurrence after excision), and by location in extremity (lesions with proximal location against distal location).

Treatment Arms

Surgery-- Patients with sarcomas of an extremity randomized to the radical surgery treatment arm received amputation through or above the joint proximal to the tumor. Extremity sarcoma patients randomized to receive limited limb-sparing surgery had operations designed to remove all gross tumor while preserving a functional extremity. Such operations included wide resections and muscle group excisions. No amputations were performed in the limited surgery group. Microscopically positive margins were accepted if tumor was located adjacent to bone, vessels, nerves, or other structures vital to preserving the integrity of the extremity. All patients with head-neck or trunk sarcomas underwent wide excisions of the primary tumor. Vital structures were preserved even at the expense of microscopically positive surgical margins.

Radiation Therapy -Patients with extremity sarcomas randomized to receive limb-sparing surgery all received postoperative radiotherapy in fields designed to cover all soft tissues at risk for potential local recurrences. Generally, wide fields covering the area between joints proximal and distal to the tumor were used to a dose of 4000-5000 rads. Shrinking fields were then used to deliver 6000-7000 rads to the tumor bed. Head-neck and trunk sarcoma patients also received postoperative radiotherapy to the area of resection. Total dose varied depending on area

and local normal tissue toxicity but generally range between 4000 and 5000 rads. Typically, radiotherapy was
given daily at a fractionation of 200 rads/day. Treatment
was begun as soon as wounds were healed, usually two to
three weeks postoperatively. Tangential ports, rotating
fields, compensators, and other radiotherapeutic techniques
were employed to minimize toxicity to normal structures.

SOFT TISSUE SARCOMA

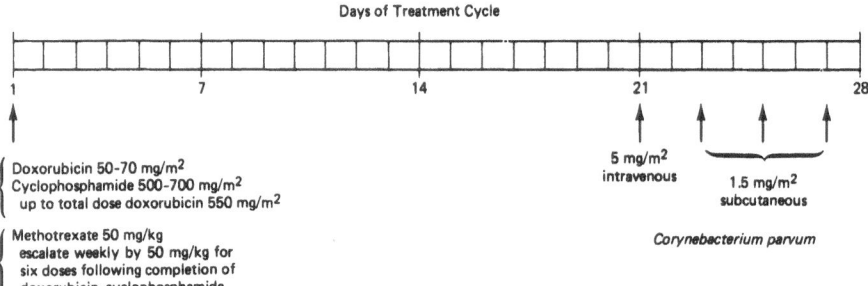

Days of Treatment Cycle

Doxorubicin 50-70 mg/m^2
Cyclophosphamide 500-700 mg/m^2
up to total dose doxorubicin 550 mg/m^2

Methotrexate 50 mg/kg
escalate weekly by 50 mg/kg for
six doses following completion of
doxorubicin-cyclophosphamide

5 mg/m^2
intravenous

1.5 mg/m^2
subcutaneous

Corynebacterium parvum

Fig. 2. Treatment cycle for chemotherapy with doxorubicin,
cyclophosphamide, and methotrexate with citrovorum
factor rescue (see text), and for immunotherapy
with Corynebacterium parvum.

Chemotherapy —All patients received adjuvant postoperative chemotherapy, begun after recovery from surgery and
initiated typically three days prior to radiation therapy,
for those patients randomized to receive both chemotherapy
and radiotherapy. Treatment schedule is given in Figure 2.
Chemotherapy was administered every 28 days. Initial
therapy consisted of a combination of intravenous doxorubicin (Adriamycin^{TM}) and cyclophosphamide (Cytoxan^R)
given on the first day of the 28 day cycle. Doxorubicin
was begun in doses of 50 mg/m^2 and escalated as tolerated
to 70 mg/m^2. Cyclophosphamide was initiated at 500 mg/m^2
and escalated to 700 mg/m^2. Treatment was continued to
maximum doxorubicin dose, 550 mg/m^2. Patients were then
given six cycles of intravenous methotrexate with leucovorin rescue. Initial methotrexate dose was 50 mg/kg, and
dosage was escalated in increments of 50 mg/kg up to a
maximum of 250 mg/kg. Chemotherapy with doxorubicin-cyclo-

phosphamide was given on an outpatient basis, and methotrexate infusions were administered only to inpatients. Serum levels of methotrexate were monitored, as was patient hydration and status of urine alkalinization.

Immunotherapy -Patients randomized to immunotherapy treatment groups received intravenous infusion of Corynebacterium parvum at dose of 5 mg/m² on day 21 of the treatment cycle, followed by subcutaneous injections at 1.5 mg/m² on days 23, 25, and 27 of each 28 day cycle (see Figure 2).

Historical Control Group

Study patients were compared with a group of 66 historical control patients with soft tissue sarcomas treated at the National Cancer Institute by radical surgery alone between 1953 and 1974. All patients used as historical controls fulfilled criteria for admission to the study protocol.

Study Patients

Forty-nine patients were enrolled into the randomized protocol study. An additional six patients with extremity sarcomas who were unsuitable for randomization between limb-sparing and amputative surgery were treated with chemotherapy after surgery; some patients received radiotherapy as well. Patients in the various treatment groups were compared directly as well as with the 66 historical controls. Compositions of the study and control patient groups are summarized in Table 1. Numbers of patients in the treatment arms are given in Table 2.

RESULTS

Status of patients allocated to the protocol treatment groups is presented in Tables 2 and 3. Protocol patients in the present analysis have been followed from 27 to 52 months, with median followup of 38 months.

Twenty-six patients with extremity sarcomas were randomized into three treatment arms. Ten patients received

TABLE 1. COMPOSITION OF STUDY PATIENT POPULATION

Item	Number of Patients	
	Protocol	Historical Controls
HISTOLOGY		
Liposarcoma	13	13
Fibrosarcoma	1	1
Neurofibrosarcoma	4	3
Rhabdomyosarcoma	5	6
Leiomyosarcoma	7	6
Angiosarcoma	1	1
Synovial sarcoma	7	6
Undifferentiated sarcoma	6	14
Malignant fibrous histiocytoma	5	15
Malignant mesenchymoma	0	1
GRADE OF HISTOLOGY		
Low grade	12	24
High grade	37	42
LOCATION OF TUMOR		
Extremity	26	46
Head-neck and trunk	23	20
SEX		
Male	34	36
Female	15	30

radical surgery (amputation) with postoperative adjuvant chemotherapy. There were two treatment failures (recurrent disease) and no deaths during the followup interval. Nine patients received conservative limb-sparing surgery with postoperative radiotherapy and chemotherapy. Three patients failed treatment and one patient died. Seven patients received conservative surgery with radiotherapy, chemotherapy, and immunotherapy. Three treatment failures and one patient death occurred. No statistical differences

TABLE 2. RESULTS OF SOFT TISSUE SARCOMA TREATMENT PROTOCOLS
OF EXTREMITY LESIONS AND HEAD-NECK-TRUNK LESIONS

		Number of Patients			
	Total	Recurrence (Treatment Failure)			Death
		Total	Local	Distant	
EXTREMITY LESIONS					
Protocol patients	26	8	1	7	2
Amputation + chemotherapy	10	2	0	2	0
Conservative surgery + radiation + chemotherapy	9	3	1	2	0
Conservative surgery + radiation + chemotherapy + immunotherapy	7	3	1	2	0
Historical controls	46	26	3	23	23
HEAD-NECK-TRUNK LESIONS					
Protocol Patients	23	6	2	4	5*
Surgery + radiation + chemotherapy	11	3	1	2	1
Surgery + radiation + chemotherapy + immunotherapy	12	3	1	2	4*
Historical controls	20	10	4	6	6

* Includes three patients dead with no malignant disease as a result
of treatment complications.

in disease free interval and survival were observed among
the three treatment arms as determined by actuarial analysis using a one-sided generalized Wilcoxon test. In all
treatment arms, the group of 26 protocol patients had eight
failures and two deaths. A group of 46 comparable historical patients treated by surgery alone had 26 treatment
failures and 23 deaths.

TABLE 3. COMBINED RESULTS OF SOFT TISSUE SARCOMAS
         TREATMENT PROTOCOLS

		Number of Patients	
	Total	Recurrence (Treatment Failure)	Death
Protocol patients	49	14	7*
Historical controls	66	36	29
p value		<0.01	<0.01

* Includes three patients dead with no malignant disease as a result
  of treatment complications.

Twenty-three patients with sarcomas of the head-neck
and trunk were randomized into two treatment groups. Eleven patients received surgery, postoperative radiation therapy, and chemotherapy. There were three recurrences and
one death. Twelve patients were randomized to receive surgery, radiotherapy, chemotherapy, and immunotherapy. Three
patients failed treatment. Four patients died, but only
one patient had malignant disease at autopsy. Three patients died without tumor as a result of treatment: one
patient from doxorubicin-related congestive heart failure,
one from complications of cyclophosphamide cystitis, and
one following surgery for radiation-induced enteritis. The
group of 20 historical control patients had ten treatment
failures and six deaths. Considering all 49 protocol patients together, the 14 treatment failures represented a
significant improvement in disease-free interval (p<0.01)
as compared to the 36 failures in the group of 66 historical control patients (see Figure 3). In addition, the seven deaths among protocol patients represented a significantly greater survival rate (p<0.01) than the 29 deaths in
the control group (see Figure 4).

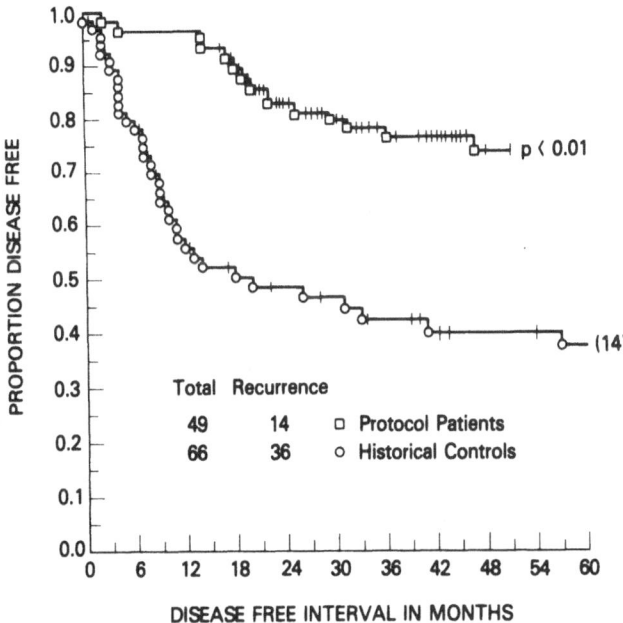

Fig. 3. Disease-free interval in soft tissue sarcoma
    protocol.

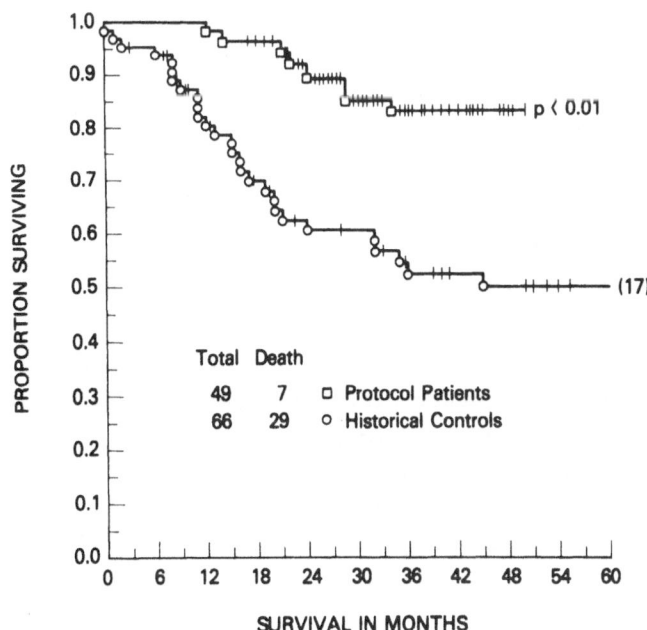

Fig. 4. Survival in soft tissue sarcoma protocol.

DISCUSSION

Soft tissue sarcomas have carried an overall poor prognosis, with most reported series citing five-year survival rates of 50% or below (1,2,3). Traditional treatment has been wide surgical excision, but even with radical extirpative surgery local recurrence rates have been high (1,2,3). Recently, therapeutic efficacy against sarcomas of modalities other than surgery has been demonstrated. Such modalities include radiotherapy (4), chemotherapy (5,6), and immunotherapy (7). The National Cancer Institute initiated a prospective investigation of the efficacy of adjuvant multimodality therapy in soft tissue sarcomas, attempting to assess whether limited surgery with radiotherapy could achieve satisfactory local control and whether adjuvant chemotherapy and immunotherapy were of any benefit in prolonging disease free survival.

A group of 66 patients with soft tissue sarcomas treated at the National Cancer Institute prior to 1975 served as historical controls for the present randomized study. The five-year survival of the historical control group was 49%, similar to the survival curves of the ten institution task force on soft tissue sarcomas of the American Joint Committee for Cancer Staging and End Results (8).

Protocol patients with extremity sarcomas receiving limb-sparing conservative surgery all had operations designed to remove all gross tumor and to achieve as wide a margin as possible while maintaining a functional extremity. Frequently such limb-sparing operations were extensive procedures, involving muscle group excisions or considerable soft tissue manipulations. Functional results of the conservative operations were generally satisfactory, with preservation of a useful extremity. However, many patients required braces or other prosthetic devices, particularly on lower extremities, in order to maximize their functional potential. Patients randomized to amputation generally tolerated surgery well. Adaptation to their disability and the use of prosthetic limbs was accomplished by most patients. With a planned program of physical therapy and occupational rehabilitation an intrinsic part of the postoperative care of all patients, most protocol patients were able to return to employment and a productive existence.

In the protocol for extremity sarcomas, the group of ten patients treated by radical surgery had no local recurrences, while the group of 16 patients receiving limb-sparing operations with radiotherapy had only two local recurrences. This result suggests limited resections followed by radiation therapy may be comparable to amputative procedures for controlling local disease. It is noteworthy, however, that several patients have experienced significant complications of radiation therapy, including three patients with chronic ulceration, one with flexion contractures, and one with sciatic neuropathy. The most severe complications of radiotherapy appears to occur in fields covering the proximal lower extremity. The precise role of radiotherapy for the control of soft tissue sarcomas will require continued evaluation, both for maintenance of local tumor control and for possible long term effects or complications of radiotherapy.

Protocol patients with sarcomas of the head-neck and trunk all received surgical excisions with radiotherapy to the tumor bed. Type of excision performed was related to the location and characteristics of the tumor for each individual, but surgical procedures uniformly were designed to remove all gross tumor and to obtain as wide margins as possible consistent with maintenance of function and reasonable morbidity. Operations were frequently extensive, particularly in retroperitoneal sarcomas where portions of viscera and vascular structures were frequently involved. Radiotherapy was given to all patients, with as high a dose as tolerated given to the tumor bed. Frequently, toxicity to normal tissues limited the total radiation dose to under 5000 rads. Radiotherapy complications did develop, chiefly local reactions, ulcerations, and gastrointestinal toxicity. One patient developed severe chronic radiation enteritis with malabsorption and functional intestinal obstruction. The patient died with no tumor at autopsy following surgery attempting to correct the intestinal disease.

410

Immunotherapy had no influence on disease free interval or survival when compared to the protocol patient groups that did not receive immunotherapy. Corynebacterium parvum therapy uniformly caused febrile reactions in patients and frequently resulted in minor skin ulcers or sterile abscesses. Experience among the present protocol patients suggests that this immunotherapy has no present role in the adjuvant treatment of soft tissue sarcomas.

The role of adjuvant chemotherapy appears to have importance in prolonging survival of sarcoma patients. Examination of all protocol patients, all of whom received chemotherapy, shows significantly improved disease free interval and survival as compared to historical control patients. This difference suggests that adjuvant chemotherapy delays or prevents dissemination of soft tissue sarcomas. However, the conclusion that chemotherapy is of benefit is based on comparison with remote historical control groups. Although the historical control patients were selected to match the characteristics of the protocol patients, absolute equivalence of the groups is not possible. Certain differences between protocol and control groups could exist, such as differing sizes of primary tumors, with smaller lesions in the control group; or differing

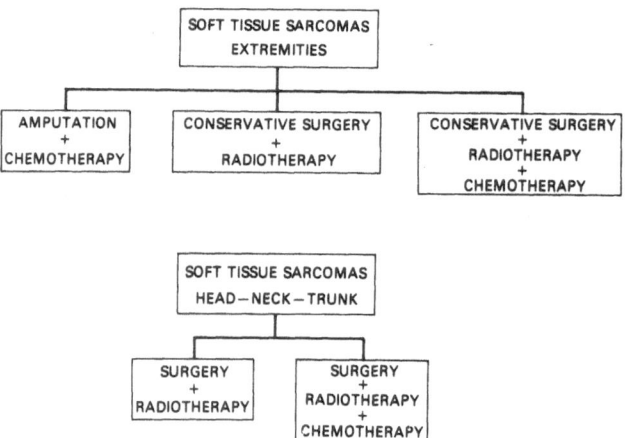

Fig. 5. Current soft tissue sarcoma protocols at National Cancer Institute.

times between diagnosis and treatment of the lesions, with early treatment for protocol patients or changing referral patterns resulting in more clinically favorable patients being admitted to the National Cancer Institute. All such differences could bias survival data in favor of protocol patients and against the historical group. In order to unequivocally establish the role of adjuvant chemotherapy in sarcoma treatment, the National Cancer Institute has instituted a sarcoma treatment protocol which currently randomizes patients with extremity tumors to receive amputation with chemotherapy, limb-sparing surgery with radiotherapy and chemotherapy, or limb-sparing surgery with radiotherapy alone. Head-neck and truncal sarcoma patients are randomized to receive surgery with radiation therapy or to receive surgery with both radiation and chemotherapy. Schema of current protocol is given in Figure 5.

REFERENCES

(1) Rosenberg, S.A., Kent, H., Costa, J., et al. Prospective randomized evaluation of the role of limb-sparing surgery, radiation therapy, and adjuvant chemoimmunotherapy in the treatment of adult soft-tissue sarcomas. Surgery 84:62-69, 1978.

(2) Shieber, W., Graham, P. An experience with sarcomas of the soft tissues in adults. Surgery 52:295-298, 1962.

(3) Cantin, J., McNeer, G.P., Chu, F.C., et al. The problem of local recurrence after treatment of soft tissue sarcoma. Ann. Surg. 168:47-53, 1968.

(4) Suit, H.D., Russell, W.O., Martin, R.G. Management of patients with sarcoma of soft tissue in an extremity. Cancer 31:1247-1255, 1973.

(5) Jacobs, E.M. Combination chemotherapy of metastatic testicular germinal cell tumors and soft part sarcomas. Cancer 25:324-332, 1970.

(6) Pinedo, H.M., Kenis, Y. Chemotherapy of advanced soft-tissue sarcomas in adults. Cancer Treat. Rev. 4:6786, 1977.

412

(7) Israel, L., Edelstein, R., Depierre, A., et al. Daily
intravenous infusions of Corynebacterium parvum in
twenty patients with disseminated cancer: A preliminary report of clinical and biologic findings. J.
Natl. Cancer Inst. 55:29-33, 1975.

(8) Russell, W.O., Cohen, J., Enzinger, F., et al. A clinical and pathological staging system for soft tissue
sarcomas. Cancer 40:1562-1570, 1977.

Acknowledgement

Results reported in the present study represent a cooper-
ative effort by many individuals in various branches and
divisions of the National Cancer Institute. In particular,
efforts of the following were important in the completion
of the study: Surgery Branch -- A.R. Baker, M.F. Brennan,
P.B. Chretien, M.H. Cohen, E.V. deMoss, M.W. Flye, H.F.
Sears, C. Seipp, P.H. Sugarbaker; Radiation Oncology
Branch -- E. Glatstein, H. Kent; Medicine Branch -- R.C.
Young; Clinical Pharmacology Branch -- B.A. Chabner;
Laboratory of Pathology -- J. Costa, B.L; Webber; Biometric
Research Branch -- R.M. Simon.

31 SOFT TISSUE SARCOMA: TREATMENT OF ADVANCED DISEASE IN THE ROYAL MARSDEN HOSPITAL

E. Wiltshaw, C. L. Harmer and J. A. McKinna

INTRODUCTION

Our interest in treating soft tissue sarcoma with chemotherapy began in 1960 when one of us (EW) found that even small doses of orally administered methotrexate could produce dramatic and sometimes worthwhile regressions. However, because of the rarity of these tumours, collection of cases was very slow and by 1967 only 32 could be reported (2).

In 1972 we felt that a concerted effort was needed to concentrate these unusual tumours under the care of one group within the hospital so that we could improve our expertise in managing sarcoma patients, while later we hoped to attract more referrals from outside. As a result, we formed the multidisciplinary Sarcoma Unit embracing surgery, radiotherapy and medicine. We held a weekly clinic and six-monthly open meetings. Patient accrual to this clinic is shown in Figure 1. Until this year, the rise in the number of new patients seen was dramatic, showing clearly that many doctors feel the need for advice and help when dealing with sarcomas. This year there has been a definite drop in referrals and we believe this is due to the lack of useful therapy which we can offer to the majority of patients. Better management programmes are clearly needed.

We report here a review of our total experience with chemotherapy. Table 1 shows the total number of cases seen at the clinic and those given chemotherapy. In all, 157 patients can be assessed for chemotherapeutic response.

A.T. van Oosterom et al. (eds.), Therapeutic Progress in Ovarian Cancer, Testicular Cancer and the Sarcomas, pp. 413-424. All rights reserved.
Copyright 1980 by Martinus Nijhoff Publishers, The Hague/Boston/London.

414

Table 1:   RMH Sarcoma Unit 1973-1979

No cases seen at the Clinic	375
No given chemotherapy	194
No therapeutically assessable	157

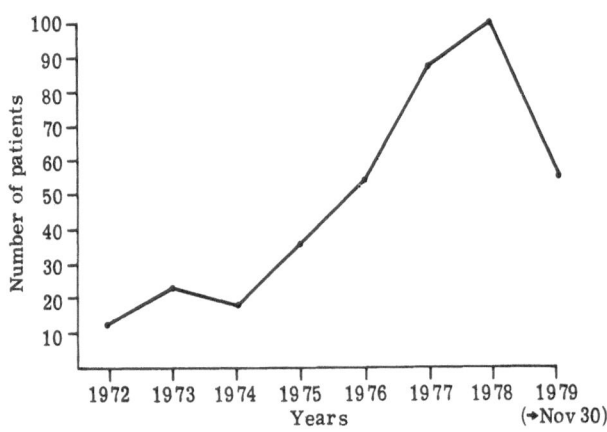

Number of new patients attending joint sarcoma clinic, 1972-1979

Table 2:   RMH Sarcoma Unit 1973-1979

Rejected Cases		
a.	Died within 1 month	17
b.	Less than 2 courses	5
c.	Lost to follow-up	9
d.	Adjuvant treatment	16
	Total	47

Forty-seven patients could not be assessed for the following
reasons: It was considered necessary that at least two
courses of drugs should be administered before considering
therapeutic benefit and 22 patients failed to meet this
requirement. Sixteen patients were given adjuvant treatment and are not considered further here, while a further
9 patients were lost to follow-up. All other cases were
assessable for tumour regression (measurable disease), had
a pathology review at the Royal Marsden Hospital, and 90%
had never been exposed to any cytotoxic drug

TREATMENT REGIMENS AND RESPONSES

From 1960 to 1979 sarcoma cases were treated by single agent
methotrexate or combination chemotherapy (MDS, STS I-IV).
The choice of regimen depended upon the year of entry.

1960-1970   oral or intra-arterial methotrexate
1970-1972   i.v. methotrexate infusions
1972-1973   MDS
1973-1975   STS I
1975-1977   STS II
1978-1979   STS III and STS IV.

Details of the treatment regimens are given in the appendix.
STS II was discontinued because of a low remission rate and
STS III has been stopped because of unacceptable toxicity.
Both myelosuppression and mucosal ulceration were serious
problems following STS III. STS IV is only used as second-
line chemotherapy. The one drug common to all treatment
schemes is methotrexate.

Table 3 shows the total number responding to each chemotherapy regimen, together with the percentage having a complete or partial regression. With all regimens, partial remissions were generally short-lived (up to 6 months) and
were of little benefit to patients. However, the occasional
case responded for more than a year and the longest partial
remission is continuing after 18 months.

Table 3: Sarcomas - Response and Regimen

Regimen	PR%	CR%	No Responding/ No Assessed
Mtx	13.5	11.5	13/52
MDS	7	21	4/14
STS I	26	21.7	11/23
STS II	22	5	11/40
STS III	26	9	4/11
STS IV	12	0	2/17

Bearing in mind the small number of cases in each treatment group, we cannot recommend one regimen over any other. It is likely that in order to say which one is the best, more than 100 cases would need to be randomised in each arm of a comparative trial. In fact, bearing in mind the very variable histology and natural history of these tumours, 100 patients in each grouping is almost certainly an underestimate.

Complete remissions (CR) occurred in relatively few cases, 5-21% depending on the schedule. The fact that, so far, no CR cases have occurred in the STS IV series may well be due to the fact that only patients failing to respond to one of the other regimens have been given this combination. A complete remission rate of around 10% is commonly seen in all reported series of sarcomas treated with chemotherapy, despite a considerable variation (5-80%) in overall remission rate. This point was well illustrated by the randomised studies reviewed by Pinedo et al (1). In this review there were studies where overall remissions and complete remissions were recorded. The overall remission rates varied from 13% to 57% and the CR rates from 0% to 19%. The most complete study with the largest number of patients compares CYVADIC and CYVADACT with 221 and 225 patients evaluable in each arm. The total response rates were 50% for CYVADIC and 39% for CYVADACT but the complete responses were 14% and 12% respectively. Our CR rate is in line with these larger series.

CHARACTERISTICS OF COMPLETE REMITTERS

Unfortunately, papers reporting on chemotherapy of sarcoma rarely give long-term follow-up results and even more rarely discuss which cases are most likely to benefit from treatment. This is unfortunate since for every 100 patients exposed to highly toxic and unpleasant therapy only about 5-15 will notice any benefit. Despite the fact that we have only 17 patients showing complete regression, we thought it worthwhile to look at these more closely. Leiomyosarcoma was our most common tumour (56 cases) but CR was seen in only 12.4%. Fibrosarcoma including cases classified as fibrous histiocytoma and those with neural elements (42 cases) rarely responded well. Only 4.7% achieved CR. Surprisingly, only 14 patients with liposarcoma were treated but the CR rate was 21.5%. If this figure was confirmed with a larger series, then these patients might well benefit from adjuvant treatment. Other histological subdivisions were too small to draw conclusions but one rather striking feature was seen in mixed mesodermal tumours. There was one CR in 5 cases treated, but there were also two partial remissions suggesting that this particular tumour may be particularly sensitive to cytotoxic drugs.

Despite these differences according to the histology, other features were far more important. In a total population of 157, 92 were females (58%), yet 16 out of 17 complete responders were female. Similarly, the primary tumour which responded most frequently arose in the pelvis (uterine, ovarian or pelvic retro-peritoneal tissues). Lastly, although embryonal sarcomas were not included in the study, we did include young patients (under 20 years of age) if the tumour histology was of adult type. The complete regressions were seen more frequently in the younger age groups. One last point is that locally recurrent or primary tumours responded more frequently than metastases. Twelve out of 17 CR cases had local tumour only when chemotherapy was started.

Table 4:   Characteristics of CR Cases
(Total 17)

Sex	Female 16	Male 1
Age	up to 30 years	24% CR
	31-60 years	11.7% CR
	>60 years	2.7% CR
Primary Site	Uterus/Pelvis	10/17 (58%)

We have stated that complete regressions are often worthwhile as opposed to partial remissions and Table 5 gives the length of response in each case. The median length of remission is 29 months and 5 continue in CR after more than 52 months. Two of the long-term survivors have died - one had a recurrence of a breast fibrosarcoma after 60 months and the other died at 92 months of radiation damage to the bladder and pelvic tissues. At autopsy there was no evidence of residual leiomyosarcoma which had originated in her uterus.

Table 5: Character of the Complete Responders

Length of Remissions
   8, 11, 13, 14, 15, 16, 19, 26, 29, 30, 34,
   52+, 56+, 60, 92, 104+, 110+
Median: 29 m
Treatment for Primary Tumour: 3 cases
   Remissions: 13, 104+, 110+
Remissions longer than 5 years 0/3 Recurrences

We were able to treat three primary tumours with chemo-therapy only. One was an undifferentiated sarcoma through-out the abdominal cavity, one was a retro-peritoneal leio-myosarcoma in the pelvis and the last was a lymphangio-sarcoma of the arm resulting from surgery and radiotherapy for a breast carcinoma. All three had a complete regression and the first two are continuing 104 and 110 months after chemotherapy. No other therapy has been given to these patients; surgical excision was not possible in either of them.

CONCLUSIONS

The formation of a multidisciplinary group to manage and advise on sarcoma cases is needed in the larger oncology centres and concentrating on these rare tumours rapidly leads to considerable expertise. Nevertheless, present treatment does not offer much benefit to the majority of cases. This is due mainly to the lack of effective chemotherapy.

    More effective use should also be made of present case material. We feel that large randomised trials of sarcomas of all kinds have failed to guide clinicians in judging which drugs to use. We advocate the concentration of sarcoma cases to a few centres and the use of one chemo-therapy regimen or at most two so that a large number of cases can be assessed and the characteristics of those likely to respond be better defined.

From our own studies it would appear that sarcomas arising in the uterus, ovary and retro-peritoneal tissues may be the most likely to benefit from present day chemo-therapy. In our experience complete remissions are virtually never seen in male cases. If confirmed by other studies, this unusual finding should be investigated further.

So far, there is little evidence that more complete remissions can be achieved by increasing the number of drugs used and we believe that the occasional practitioner of chemotherapy for sarcoma should give the simplest and safest regimen with which he is familiar. So far, no patient whose tumour has failed to respond to one combina-tion has later produced a complete regression on another combination, but the occasional case responds several times. One such case is illustrated in Table 6.

Local recurrence of liposarcoma was treated by the STS I regimen in December 1973 with complete remission for 34 months when she had a further local recurrence. Partial regression followed methotrexate infusions and response was assisted by surgery and radiotherapy. Recurrence occurred again, however, 26 months later and a further response is now being seen. It is possible that in this particular case radiotherapy should have been applied after CR had been achieved in 1973-74. We have noted that treat-ment for locally recurrent tumour is more successful than for metastatic disease, although many partial regressions were seen. Quite frequently, one or two metastatic lesions seem to be very resistant to therapy. Table 7 shows an example of this problem.

Table 6: Mrs P.F. - 42 years

Mass 1967

Diagnosis 11/73 - Myxoid Liposarcoma Thigh
                  and Broad Ligament

Treatment   - mass excised

12/73 Local Recurrence. STS I→CR

 6/75 STS I completed.

12/75 Cardiac Myopathy

10/76 Local Recurrence. Mtx 200 mg over
       36 hours q. 28 days.

 3/77 PR. Excision residual tumour thigh
       and pelvis.
       Radiotherapy to tumour bed 4,400 r.
       Mtx continued.

 6/78 Chemotherapy completed

12/78 Local Recurrence. Mtx 450 mg over
       36 hrs q. 28 days.

 9/79 PR.

Table 7: Mrs P.B. - 61 years

 2/75 Bleeding p.v.

 5/75 BSO and TH. Leiomyosarcoma of Uterus

 6/75 Radiotherapy 5,000 r. pelvis

 1/77 Local Recurrence + Lung Metastases

 2/77 STS II→CR

 6/78 Thoracotomy. Residual Tumour excised
       from R Lung

12/78 Recurrence Pelvis and Lung and Pericardium
       STS IV

 4/79 R Lung Lesions gone
       L Apical Lesion Slow Growth

11/79 One Lesion in Lung (L) remains

Complete response of local recurrence and lung metastases
apparently occurred following STS II but thoracotomy was
performed because we felt cure was unlikely. At thoracotomy
residual disease was seen and excised from the right lung.
Only 6 months later further recurrence developed in both
right and left lungs, in the pericardium and the pelvis.
STS IV was started and all but one left apical lesion has
disappeared. The proper management of this remaining lesion
would seem debatable. Surgical removal would almost certainly show more tumour on the left side and radiotherapy would
need to be given in very high doses to a relatively large
lesion, since 5,000 rads to the pelvis failed to prevent
recurrence in that area. Some surgeons in the United States
advocate surgery for apparent solitary metastases but long-
term results of this type of surgery after partially successful chemotherapy are sorely needed.

The two cases reported above show that even with good
responses to chemotherapy there are still very difficult
problems to resolve. We need to define much more clearly
the place of the three major treatment modalities under
these unusual circumstances.

APPENDIX: SARCOMA REGIMENS

Sarcoma Regimens

1) <u>Methotrexate</u>

    Oral: 2.5 mg - 10 mg daily for 2-15 days
                      (commonly 10 mg daily for 5 days
                      repeated every 2 weeks)

    Intravenous: a.   50-100 mg repeated every 2-3 weeks
                      b.   50-100 mg infusion over 18-36 hours
                          every 4 weeks.

    Intra-arterial: 50 mg in 24 hours for 4 days.

2) <u>MDS</u>

Cyclophosphamide	600 mg/m^2	(maximum 1 g)
5-Fluorouracil	500 mg/m^2	(maximum 1 g)
Vincristine	1 mg/m^2	(maximum 2 mg)
Actinomycin D	0.6 mg/m^2	(maximum 1 mg)
Methotrexate	200 mg i.v. infusion over 24 hours, followed by folinic acid 9 mg i.m. 6-hourly x4	

Course repeated every 28 days for 18 months

3) <u>STS I</u>

Adriamycin	60 mg/m^2	i.v. day 1
TIC Mustard	250 mg/m^2	i.v. days 1 and 2
Methotrexate	50 mg/m^2	i.v. infusion over 12-24 hours on day 1 with folinic acid rescue (as for MDS)

Course repeated every 21 days.
Adriamycin stopped after 10th injection.
Total duration 18 months.

4) <u>STS II</u>

Vincristine	1.4 mg/m^2 i.v. (maximum 2 mg)	⎫
Actinomycin D	1.4 mg/m^2 i.v. (maximum 2 mg)	⎬ day 1
Cyclophosphamide	600 mg/m^2 i.v. (maximum 1 g)	⎭
Adriamycin	60 mg/m^2 i.v.	⎫ day 21
Methotrexate	50 mg/m^2 i.v. infusion over 24h followed by folinic acid 15 mg 6-hourly for 36 hours.	⎭

Repeat cycle after further 21 days. Total 9 cycles.

5) <u>STS III</u>

Cyclophosphamide 600 mg/m^2 i.v. stat $\left.\begin{array}{l} \\ \\ \end{array}\right\}$

Vincristine 1.4 mg/m^2 i.v. (maximum 2 mg) day 1

Adriamycin 60 mg/m^2 i.v. stat

Methotrexate 5 mg/m^2 orally daily days 2-7

Cyclophosphamide 600 mg/m^2 i.v. stat $\left.\begin{array}{l} \\ \end{array}\right\}$ day 8

Vincristine 1.4 mg/m^2 i.v. (maximum 2 mg)

Repeat 3-4 weekly.

6) <u>STS IV</u>

BCNU 80 mg/m^2 i,v, stat $\left.\begin{array}{l} \\ \\ \end{array}\right\}$

Mitomycin C 0.04 mg/kg body weight i.v. stat day 1

VP-16 100 mg/m^2 i.v. stat

VP-16 100 mg/m^2 i.v. stat days 2&3

Repeat 3-6 weekly.

REFERENCES

1. PINEDO, HM, CHABNER, BA, NIEUWENHUIS, MG, and ROSENBERG, SA (1978) Soft tissue sarcoma in adults. Randomized Trials in Cancer: A Critical Review by Sites. Edited by Maurice J Staquet, Raven Press, New York 1978, p. 359-375

2. WILTSHAW, E (1967) Methotrexate in treatment of sarcomata. Brit Med J, 15 April 1967, 2:142-145

32 TREATMENT OF ADVANCED SOFT-TISSUE SARCOMAS IN ADULTS: PAST, PRESENT, AND FUTURE

H. M. Pinedo and A. T. van Oosterom

Although combination chemotherapy has had a major impact on the prognosis of children with rhabdomyosarcomas (1), chemotherapy has not yet acquired an important role in the management of this disease in the adult (2). Drugs which have proven to be highly effective in advanced childhood sarcoma have been incorporated into the programs for treatment of the primary tumor in this young age-group, whereas adjuvant chemotherapy in the adult is still experimental (3-5). These developments reflect the difference in sensitivity to chemotherapy between the sarcomas of adults and children, the latter being much more responsive (6).

The few reported data on response rates of single-agent treatment with Vincristine, Cyclophosphamide, or Actinomycin-D in children and adults with sarcoma, are shown in the first table.

Table 1.

SINGLE-AGENT TREATMENT IN CHILDREN AND ADULTS WITH SARCOMA (6)

AGENT	CHILDREN		ADULTS	
	No. of cases	Remission rate (%)	No. of cases	Remission rate (%)
Vincristine	20	50	10	0
Cyclophosphamide	42	62	14	14
Actinomycin-D	38	27	6	3/6[x]
DTIC	-	-	60	15
Adriamycin	-	-	357	27

x no definition of response

The duration of response in adults usually varies between
one and four months. A response lasting more than a year
is exceptional.

The combination of Vincristine, Actinomycin-D and Cyclophosphamide (VAC) had proven to be quite active in childhood
rhabdomyosarcoma. In contrast, Jacobs observed only 5/14
(29%) responses in adults with soft-tissue sarcomas treated with this combination (7). This same combination yielded only an 8% response rate in a randomized study performed at the Mayo Clinic (8), although the very low response
rate in this study can be atributed to the long interval
of 5 weeks between successive cycles.

In 1969 and 1970 the Southwestern Oncology Group (SWOG)
studied the activity of DTIC in 60 adults with sarcoma.
If patients with osteosarcoma and mesothelioma are excluded, the response rate in this study drops to only 15% (6,9).
The evolution of chemotherapy in adult soft-tissue sarcomas during the period between 1970 and 1980, has been cen-
tered around the anthracycline antibiotic Adriamycin, and
viewed retrospectively must be considered somewhat disappointing. Furthermore, few of the studies have been
randomized (10).

Significant advances were initially reported for combination regimens including Adriamycin (9), but it is now becoming more and more evident that these advances have been
of limited extent. It is clear that we have actually reached a dead end with the combination of Adriamycin, DTIC,
Cyclophosphamide and Vincristine.

Adriamycin is without doubt the most effective drug in our
present therapeutic armament for this tumor group (11,12).
Response rates with single-agent Adriamycin have ranged
from 9 to 70% (6). These differences can be partially explained by the different schedules and doses applied by
various investigators. Patients treated with a dose of
60-75 mg/m^2 tend to respond better than those treated with
lower doses, and response rates tend to be higher (25-40%)
in studies in which the drug was given in one bolus every
3 weeks (11+13), compared with those in which the drug was

given daily for 3 days (q 3 weeks) (14). The 3-weekly one
day schedule of administration has been applied in both the
non-randomized (12) and randomized (15) studies done by
the SWOG and in a randomized study of the Eastern Cooperative Oncology Group (ECOG) (13).

The 3-day regimen repeated at 3-week intervals had been
used in a previous study performed by the ECOG to compare
Adriamycin randomly with Cycloleucine (14). Response rates
of both drugs were below 20% with the schedules applied.
From the available data it may be concluded that when administered as a single-agent, Adriamycin should be given
in a dose of at least 70 mg/m^2 q 3 weeks. In most of the
studies there appears to be no difference in the response
of the various histological subtypes, although the number
of patients in each subtype group is often small (6). The
median duration of response to Adriamycin was 4-5 months,
and the duration of survival was 15 months for responders
as compared with 8 months for non-responders in the ECOG
study (13).

Studies performed in the early Seventies at the Southern
Research Institute in rodents bearing sarcoma 180, B 16 melanoma, or C3H breast carcinoma showed that the toxicity
of Adriamycin and DTIC given in combination was not additi-
ve, and almost full doses of each drug could be used (16).
Because both drugs had shown activity in soft-tissue sarcoma in man, Gottlieb et al. initiated in 1971 a non-randomized clinical study (SWOG-445) with these agents in
combination (12,16), which they called the ADIC regimen.
They selected the following schedule: Adriamycin 60 mg/m^2
on day 1 and DTIC 250 mg/m^2 on days 1 through 5. The cycles were repeated every 3 weeks. Doses were increased by
increments of 15 mg/m^2 for Adriamycin and 50 mg/m^2/ day
x5 for DTIC if the white blood cell count of the individual patient had not dropped below 3000/mm^3. Many of the patients could tolerate a dose of 75 mg/m^2 Adriamycin and
300 mg/m^2/day x5 of DTIC. An increased remission rate up
to 47% was observed with this regimen (6,12). Responders
tended to be younger and have had less prior chemotherapy.

There was, again, no difference in response between the various histological subtypes (Table 2).

Table 2.

RESPONSE TO THE COMBINATION OF ADRIAMYCIN AND DTIC, ACCORDING TO HISTOLOGICAL SUBTYPE

Histological type	No. of evaluable patients	Response rate (%)
Undifferentiated	26	58
Fibrosarcoma	31	42
Leiomyosarcoma	39	51
Liposarcoma	20	45
Rhabdomyosarcoma	20	40
Synovial cell sarcoma	11	45
Angiosarcoma	9	33
Neurofibrosarcoma	27	48
Total	183	47

Besides the increased remission rate, a slight increase in the duration of response was observed for ADIC as compared with both single-agent Adriamycin and single-agent DTIC treatment. The duration of survival increased with ADIC as compared with the duration obtained with Adriamycin alone.

A subsequent SWOG study with VADIC (Vincristine added to Adriamycin and DTIC) was performed in 1972-1973 (12). The addition of Vincristine gave a minimal advantage consisting of a reduction in the number of patients with progressive disease. Certainly the negligible toxicity of Vincristine was a dubious reason for maintaining this drug in subsequent regimens studied by many groups.

The next SWOG study (73-02) added Cyclophosphamide in a dose of 500 mg/m^2, administered on day 1 of each cycle, which gave the CYVADIC regimen (Table 3), (12).

Table 3.

CYVADIC REGIMENS[X] STUDIED BY THE SOUTHWESTERN ONCOLOGY
GROUP

Drugs	SWOG 73-02	SWOG 74-02
Cyclophosphamide	500 mg/m^2, day 1 i.v.	500 mg/m^2, day 1 i.v.
Vincristine	1,5 mg/m^2, day 1	1,5 mg/m^2, day 1[xx]
Adriamycin	50 mg/m^2, day 1	50 mg/m^2, day 2
DTIC	250 mg/m^2, days 1-5	250 mg/m^2, days 1-5

[X]q 3 weeks, [xx] weekly for 7 weeks

The original 73-02 study yielded a response rate of 59% in
soft-tissue sarcomas (6), whereas the slightly modified
CYVADIC regimen, studied in a randomized trial (SWOG 74-02),
resulted in a remission rate of 50% and a complete response rate of 15% (15). Thus, the complete plus partial
response rate achieved with CYVADIC was only slightly better than the rate obtained with the ADIC regimen (47%).
The toxicity reported for the CYVADIC regimen clearly indicates that introduction of other myelosuppressive drugs
into this combination will not be feasible (Table 4).

Table 4.

HAEMATOLOGIC TOXICITY ASSOCIATED WITH CYVADIC (EXPRESSED
IN PERCENTAGE OF 136 PATIENTS)

Nadir granulocyte count[x]			Nadir platelet count[xx]		
⟩1000	500-1000	⟨500	⟩100	50-100	⟨50
44%	29%	27%	79%	16%	5%

[x]cells/mm^3 ; [xx]cells x 10^3/mm^3

Toxicity was increased particularly by the addition of
Cyclophosphamide to VADIC.

Replacement of DTIC by Actinomycin-D (CYVADACT) yielded
a response rate of only 40% (15), which might indicate an
antagonism between Adriamycin and Actinomycin-D, a minimal
effect of Actinomycin-D in sarcomas, or a more frequent

reduction of the Adriamycin dose because of a more severe
toxic reaction to Actinomyin-D than to DTIC.

It is also of interest to mention a recent randomized
study performed in 27 patients by Rodriquez et al. at the
M.D. Anderson Hospital, in which an intensified CYVADIC
scheme was introduced. Three intensive courses were administered with or without the use of a protected environment
and prophylactic antibiotics (19). The starting dose of
Adriamycin and Cyclophosphamide were 60 mg/m^2 and 600 mg/m^2,
respectively. These doses were escalated at each cycle if
no infection occurred in the previous course. Only one infection episode occurred in the protected environment as
against six infections in the control group. The beneficial
effect on the response rate might well have been accounted
for by the Adriamycin by itself. There was, however, no
beneficial effect on the duration of response.

Clearly, it is not feasible to add any myelosuppressive
agent to the CYVADIC regimen without being forced to reduce
the dose of the other drugs, including that of Adriamycin.
Hence, one might observe a reduced effect of such a combination as compared to that of ADIC or even single-agent
Adriamycin. At present, one should consider the ADIC regimen as the standard regimen for adults with advanced soft-
tissue sarcoma.

Recently, the EORTC Soft-Tissue and Bone Sarcoma Group
performed a randomized study (62761) in patients with advanced sarcomas (20) to compare the standard CYVADIC regimen with a cyclic regimen in which Adriamycin plus DTIC
was alternated with Vincristine plus Cyclophosphamide.

Table 5.

CYVADIC REGIMENS STUDIED BY THE EORTC SOFT-TISSUE AND
BONE SARCOMA GROUP (PROTOCOL 62761)

Drugs	$S_1{}^x$	$S_2{}^{xx}$
Cyclophosphamide	500 mg/m^2, day 1 i.v.	1200 mg/m^2, day 29 i.v.
Vincristine	1,4 mg/m^2, day 1	1,4 mg/m^2, day 29
Adriamycin	50 mg/m^2, day 1	50 mg/m^2, day 1
DTIC	250 mg/m^2, days 1-5	250 mg/m^2, day 1-5

[x] q 4 weeks; [xx] q 8 weeks.

The only divergence from the original CYVADIC regimen was
the duration of the interval between the cycles (4 weeks
instead of 3 weeks). The aim of this study was to reevaluate
the CYVADIC regimen and to find out whether alternation would
result in prolongation of the duration of response. In both
arms the dosages of Adriamycin, Cyclophosphamide, and DTIC
were reduced by 33% for patients aged 60-75 years. Preliminary results have been reported recently (21). To date,
the results in 140 evaluable patients show a response rate
of 38.3% for the full-dose CYVADIC regimen; when the dosages were reduced the response rate dropped to 22.2% (Table 6).

Table 6.
EORTC TRIAL 62761: BEST OVERALL RESPONSE TO TREATMENT,
ACCORDING TO AGE-GROUP

Age-groups (yr)	CR (%)	PR (%)	NC (%)	Prog (%)	Total
15-59	15 (13,3)	17 (15.0)	41 (36.3)	40 (35.4)	113
60-75	1 (3.7)	5 (18.5)	6 (22.2)	15 (55.6)	27
Total	16 (11.4)	22 (15.7)	47 (33.6)	55 (39.3)	140

With respect to the dose-response relationship previously
observed for Adriamycin, the reduced response rate -compa-
red even to that obtained with ADIC - could be accounted
for by the reduction of the Adriamycin dose per cycle.
The longer interval between each cycle may explain the
lower response rate observed with the full-dose regimen
compared with the results obtained with the CYVADIC regimen studied in SWOG 74-03 (13). The cyclic regimen resulted in a response rate of only 15.9%, whereas the percentage for the CYVADIC regimen was 36.4. These data are
shown in Table 7, which includes the elderly group given
the adjusted dosage. These findings confirm the conclusion
that Vincristine and Cyclophosphamide are poor drugs for
the treatment of soft-tissue sarcoma, and are often unable
to maintain an effect achieved with the ADIC combination
administered 4 weeks earlier.

Table 7.

EORTC TRIAL 62761: BEST OVERALL RESPONSE TO TREATMENT

Regimen	CR (%)	PR (%)	NC (%)	Prog (%)	Total
4-drug	13 (16.9)	15 (19.5)	28 (36.3)	21 (27.3)	77
Cyclic	3 (4.8)	7 (11.1)	27 (42.8)	26 (41.3)	63
Total	16 (11.4)	22 (15.7)	55 (39.3)	47 (33.6)	140

Vincristine and Cyclophosphamide should therefore be excluded in new regimens to be studied. The data obtained in
the EORTC study also show that one should not evaluate
treatment only at 8 weeks, because remissions may be achieved even after 6 to 8 cycles of treatment. The duration of
response in the limited number of patients responding to
the cyclic S_2 regimen, appeared to be similar to that of
patients responding to the S_1 regimen. It is too early to
give data on survival, but there are clear indications that
the differences in response rates between the two regimens
and between the high- and low-dosage groups, will be reflected in the survival curves. The differences between the
survival curves of complete responders, partial responders,
patients with no change of disease, and patients with progressive disease are significant and independent of treatment.
When the many non-randomized studies performed during the
past decade are reviewed, the percentage of non-pre-
treated patients, the extent of disease, and the patients'
general condition should be taken into consideration.
Pre-treatment with other drugs probably reduces the remission rate significantly. The number of pre-treated patients has in all probability dropped sharply in studies
performed after reports on the responses observed in the
initial studies with single-agent Adriamycin therapy.
This factor might have even influenced the response rate
in the ADIC area compared with the preceding studies with
Adriamycin as a single-agent.
A response rate of 36% for Methotrexate has recently been
reported in a group of patients with soft-tissue sarcomas,

many of them not pre-treated (22). Three different regimens, including various other drugs, were used, but it is difficult to determine from the report which regimen was most effective. More details on this experience in England are reported in the preceeding chapter. In addition, evidence supporting the effectivity of Methotrexate comes from two small series comprising a total of 24 patients treated with high-dose Methotrexate after showing progression on CYVADIC (23,24). A total of 8 responders (33%) were observed in these two studies. At present, there is certainly no evidence that supports the use of high doses of Methotrexate in soft-tissue sarcoma. A study on low doses of Methotrexate in non-pre-treated patients definitely seems warranted. Our main aid should be to find new active drugs. In Chapter 34 the results of many recent Phase-II studies are reported. In the future we should seriously consider performing Phase II studies in non-pre-treated patients or possibly after a trial with single-agent treatment with either Adriamycin or a new antracycline analog. The EORTC Soft-Tissue and Bone Sarcoma Group has recently adopted the latter procedure. New anthracycline derivatives are under study in an attempt to find an agent with less side effects for the heart and the bone marrow. If such an agent proved to maintain its antitumor effect, we might be able to exploit the antitumor effect better. In cases of progression on single-agent treatment with an anthracycline analog, other new agents can be given a fair chance in Phase II studies performed in these patients with limited pre-treatment. This approach might help us to find more effective agents which could subsequently be incorporated into combination regimens including an anthracycline derivative The latter policy has been adopted by the EORTC Soft-Tissue and Bone Sarcoma Group for the early Eighties.

The following conclusions can be drawn from this survey:

1) Adult soft-tissue sarcoma is less responsive to chemotherapy than childhood sarcoma.

2) Adriamycin is the most effective agent in advanced
   adult soft-tissue sarcoma and forms the backbone
   of all effective chemotherapy regimens.

3) The addition of DTIC, Vincristine, and Cyclophosphamide
   has only increased the therapeutic effectivity to a
   limited extent; at present, one may consider the ADIC
   regimen as the standard treatment for soft-tissue sarcoma.

4) The dose-response relationship found for Adriamycin may
   explain the lower response rate in the older age-group
   in the EORTC study, whose doses had been adjusted.

5) The EORTC cyclic regimen gives a lower response rate
   than the 4-drug regimen.

6) Response to chemotherapy may occur slowly, and may not
   become apparent until administration of 6-8 cycles.

7) Phase II studies are extremely important to overcome
   the present deadlock in the treatment of sarcoma.

8) Phase II studies should be performed in either non-
   pre-treated patients or patients treated only with an
   anthracycline.

9) The development of an effective post-surgery adjuvant
   chemotherapy regimen may help us to circumvent the
   problem of drug resistance in advanced sarcoma.

REFERENCES

1. Pinedo, H.M., Võute, P.A.
   Combination chemotherapy in soft-tissue sarcoma.
   Recent advance in cancer treatment. p. 301,1977
   Ed. Tagnon, H.J., Staquet, M.J. Raven Press, New York.

2. Bramwell, V.H.C., Pinedo, H.M.
   Bone and soft-tissue sarcomas
   Cancer chemotherapy. The EORTC cancer chemotherapy
   Annual., chapter 20, p. 424, 1979
   Ed. Pinedo, H.M;, Excerpta Medica, Amsterdam.

3. Pinedo, H.M., Vendrik, C.P.J., Bramwell, V.H.C.,
   van Slooten, E., Deaking, D.P., van Unnik, J.A.M.,

Staquet, M., Sylvester, R., Bonadonna, G.
Evaluation of Adjuvant Therapy in Soft-Tissue sarcoma.
A collaborative Multidisciplinary Approach
EORTC protocol 62771. Eur. J. Cancer 15, 811, 1979.

4. Rosenberg, S.A., Kent, H., Costa, J., Weber, B.L.,
   Young, R., Chabner, B., Baker, A.R., Brennan, M.F.,
   Chretien, P.B., Cohen, M.H., Demoss, E.V., Sears, H.F.,
   Seiff, C., Simon, R.
   Prospective randomized evaluation of the role of limb
   sparing surgery, radiation therapy and adjuvant chemo-
   therapy in the treatment of adult soft tissue sarcomas
   Surgery, 84,62, 1978.

5. Bramwell, V.H.C., Võute, P.A., Rosenberg, S.A.,
   Pinedo, H.M.
   Adjuvant chemotherapy in soft-tissue sarcoma.
   Recent Results in Cancer Research vol. 68, p. 60-74
   1979.
   Ed. Bonadonna, G., Mathé, G., Salmon, S.E.
   Springer Verlag, Berlin-Heidelberg-New York.

6. Pinedo, H.M., Kenis, Y.
   Chemotherapy of adjuvant soft-tissue sarcoma in adults.
   Cancer Treatment rev. 4, 67, 1977.

7. Jacobs, E.M.
   Combination chemotherapy of metastatic testicular ger-
   minal cell tumors and soft part sarcomas.
   Cancer 25, 324, 1970.

8. Creagan, E.T., Hahn, R.G., Ahmann, D.L., Edmundson,
   J.H., Bisel, H.F., Eagan, R.T.
   A comparative clinical trial evaluating the combination
   of Adriamycin (NSC-123127), imidazole carboxamide (NSC-
   45388), Vincristine (NSC-67574), the combination
   Actinomycin-D. (NSC-3053), Cyclophosphamide (NSC-
   26271), Vincristine and a single-agent, Methyl-CCNU

(NSC-95441) in advanced sarcomas.
Cancer Treat. Rep. 60, 1385, 1976.

9. Gottlieb, J.A., Benjamin, R.S., Baker, L.H., O'Brien,
   R.M., Sinkovics, J.G., Hoogstraten, B., Quagliana, J.M.,
   Rivkin, S.E., Bodey, G.P., Rodriquez, V., Blumenschein,
   G.R., Saiki, J.H., Coltman, C., Brugess, M.A., Sullivan,
   P., Thigpin, T., Bottomley, R., Balcerzak, S., Moon,
   T.E.
   Role of DTIC (NSC-45388) in the chemotherapy of sarco-
   mas.
   Cancer Treatment Rep. 60, 199,1976.

10. Pinedo, H.M., Chabner, B.A., Nieuwenhuis, M.G.,
    Rosenberg, S.A.
    Soft-Tissue Sarcoma in adults.
    Randomized Trials in cancer.
    A critical review by Sites.
    The EORTC monograph series p. 359, 1978.
    Ed. Staquet, M., Raven Press, New York.

11. Benjamin, R.S., Wiernik, P.H., Bachur, N.R.
    Adriamycin: a new effective agent in the therapy of
    disseminated sarcomas.
    Medical and Pediatric Oncology 1, 63, 1975.

12. Gottlieb, J.A., Baker, L.H., O'Brien, R.M., Sinkovics,
    J.G., Hoogstraten, B., Quagliana, J.M., Rivkin, S.E.,
    Bodey, G.P., Rodriquez, V.T., Blumenschein, G.R.,
    Jaiki, J.H., Coltman, C., Burgess, M.A., Sullivan, P.,
    Thigpen, T., Bottomley, R., Balcerzak, S., Moon, T.E.
    Adriamycin (NSC-123127) used alone and in combination
    for soft tissue and bone sarcomas.
    Cancer Chemoth. Rep. 6, 271, 1975.

13. Rosenbaum, C., Schoenfeld, D.
    Treatment of advanced soft tissue sarcoma.
    Proc. Amer. Soc. Clin. Oncol. 18, 287, 1977.

14. Savlov, E.D., Knight, E., Costello, W.
    Study of Adriamycin versus cycloleucine in the treat-
    ment of sarcomas.
    Proc. Am. Assoc. Cancer Res. 15, 138, 1974.

15. Benjamin, R.S., Gottlieb, J.A., Baker, L.H., Sinkovics,
    J.C.
    Cyvadic vs. Cyvadact: a randomized trial of Cyclophos-
    phamide, Vincristine and Adriamycin + DTIC or Actino-
    mycin D in metastatic sarcomas.
    Proc. Amer. Ass. Cancer Res. 17, 256, 1976.

16. Griswold, D.F., Laster, W.R., Schabel, F.M.
    Therapeutic potentiation of Adriamycin and DTIC against
    B 16 melanoma, C3H breast carcinoma, Lewis Lung carci-
    noma and Leukemia L1210.
    Proc. Amer. Ass. Cancer Res. 14, 15, 1973.

17. Gottlieb, J.A., Baker, L.H., Quagliana, J.M.
    Chemotherapy of sarcomas with a combination of Adria-
    mycin and dimethyl triazeno imidazole carboxamide.
    Cancer 30, 1632, 1972.

18. Gottlieb, J.A.
    Ergebnisse der Adriamycintherapie.
    Adriamycine Symposium, Frankfurt am Main, p. 95, 1974.
    Ed. Ghione, M., Fetzer, J.B., Maier, E.,
    Springer Verlag, Heidelberg, Germany.

19. Rodriguez, V., Bodey, G.P., Freireich, E.J.
    Increased remission rate and prolongation of survival
    in patients with soft tissue sarcomas treated with
    intensive chemotherapy on a protected environment-
    prophylactic antibiotic programme (PEPA).
    Proc. Amer. Soc. Clin. Oncol. 18, 320, 1977.

20. Pinedo, H.M., Vendrik, C.P.J., Staquet, M., Kenis, Y., Sylvester, R.,
    EORTC randomized trial for metastatic soft-tissue sarcoma.
    Protocol 62761. March 1977. Eur. J. Cancer 13, 765, 1978.

21. Pinedo, H.M., Vendrik, C.P.J., Bramwell, V.H.C., Mouridsen, H.T., Somers, R., van Oosterom, A.T., Wagener, T., Lewis, B.J., de Pauw, R., Sylvester, R., Bonadonna, G.
    Re-evaluation of the Cyvadic regimen for metastatic soft-tissue sarcomas.
    Proc. Amer. Soc. Clin. Oncol. 20, 346, 1979.

22. Subramanian, S., Wiltshaw, E.
    Chemotherapy of sarcomas
    Lancet 1, 683, 1978.

23. Karakousis, C.
    High dose Methotrexate in metastatic sarcomas.
    Proc. Amer. Clin. Oncol. 19, 401, 1978.

24. Isacoff, W.H., Eilber, F., Tabbarah, H., Klein, P., Dollinger, M., Lemkin, S., Sheehy, P., Cone, L., Rosenbloom, B., Sieger, L., Block, J.H.
    Phase II clinical trial with high dose Methotrexate therapy and Citrovorum factor rescue.
    Cancer Treatm. Rep. 62, 1295, 1978.

33 TREATMENT OF CHILDHOOD SOFT TISSUE SARCOMAS

C. B. Pratt, H. Omar Hustu, A. P. Mahesh Kumar and S. L. George

Rhabdomyosarcoma (RMS) accounts for approximately 10% of the malignant solid tumors which occur in children. Because it is the most frequent soft tissue sarcoma (STS) of children, treatment of RMS has evolved since the early 1960s to utilize the combined modalities of surgery, radiation therapy and chemotherapy (1-24). In comparison to RMS, the other STS of children occur only rarely. Planned treatment of these latter tumor types is presently developing from the experience gained from the treatment of children with RMS as well as the results of treatment of adults with these tumors.

Since aggressive surgical attacks on RMS and many of the other STS have failed to produce a high percentage of cures (1,2,5-9,11-15,17,19,20,23,24), many patients have received radiation therapy and chemotherapy following surgery. The early spread of RMS and the incomplete resectability for more than two-thirds of these tumors has led to the investigation of these latter two modalities (4,8-20,23,24).

Supported in part by U.S. Public Health Service (CORE) Grant CA 21765 and by ALSAC.

RHABDOMYOSARCOMA

Staging and Treatments

At St. Jude Children's Research Hospital, stage-related treatment for RMS has been provided for 128 children treated by 3 multidisciplinary protocols since 1968. A staging scheme which considered localized, regional and generalized RMS was proposed for consideration of the treatment of patients with surgery, radiation therapy and chemotherapy according to the extent of disease (2).

Details of the surgical management including biopsies, exploration, resection and surgical reevaluation have been presented previously (24).

Chemotherapy with 3 or 4 agents - vincristine, cyclophosphamide and dactinomycin (Protocol I) with or without adriamycin (Protocols II, III) has been delivered to all patients; details have been previously reported (24). Patients with localized, completely resected disease or regional completely resected disease received these agents for a period of 6 or 12 months (Protocol I). Patients treated since 1973 (Protocols II, III) received 4 agents for a period of 1½ years, or until evidence of recurrent or progressive disease. Cyclophosphamide-adriamycin was alternated with vincristine-dactinomycin given weekly (Protocols II, III), intensively during the first 2 weeks and then alternating at weekly intervals. In the second protocol study, between 1973 and 1977, adriamycin was discontinued after a total dosage of 300 mg/m^2 had been delivered. In the more recent third protocol utilizing the same four agents, adriamycin was delivered in pulses during the first, seventh and thirteenth month of treatment. All agents were delivered to biological and clinical tolerance.

Radiation therapy was delivered concurrently with the initiation of chemotherapy for patients treated between 1968 and 1973. For patients treated since 1973, radiation therapy has been initiated approximately 6 weeks following beginning of chemotherapy, and after an evaluation of the patient's response to intensive chemotherapy. By protocol design, patients with localized or regional completely resected RMS did not receive radiation therapy. For patients with generalized tumor, radiation therapy was delivered to residual tumor following biopsy or indication of partial or complete response with chemotherapy.

RESULTS OF PROTOCOL TREATMENTS   (Table 1)

Seventeen patients were found to have localized or regional completely resected disease; 3 patients developed local recurrences, 2 developed distant metastases and 12 patients are continuously free of disease for up to 11 years.

Table 1.   Rhabdomyosarcoma I-III Protocols - Outcome for 128 Total Patients, by Stage

Stage I-IIA	17 Patients	12 NED
	3 Local Recurrences	
	2 Distant Metastases	
Stage IIB	73 Patients	40 NED
	13 Never Achieved CR	
	10 Local Recurrence	
	5 Distant Metastases	
	5 Died of Complications	
Stage IIIA	22 Patients	4 NED
	13 Never Achieved CR	
	3 Local Recurrence	
	2 Distant Metastases	
Stage IIIB	16 Patients	0 NED
	4 Never Achieved CR	
	12 Distant Metastases	

Seventy-three patients were found to have regional completely resected disease. Thirteen patients never achieved a complete response, 10 developed local recurrence of tumor, 5 developed distant metastases, 5 died of complications of treatment and 40 patients remain continuously free of disease activity from 3 months to 11 years. The deaths from complications resulted from intestinal obstruction [3], from generalized histoplasmosis [1] and from pneumonia [1] which was incidently associated with the presence of Pneumocystis carinii organisms.

Twenty-two patients had generalized tumor including distant metastases with normal bone marrow. Thirteen of these patients never achieved complete response, 3 developed local recurrence, and 2 developed additional distant metastatic spread; 4 patients remain continuously free of disease for periods up to 4 years from diagnosis.

Sixteen patients had generalized tumor associated with bone marrow infiltration by tumor cells. Four of these patients never achieved complete response, 12 developed distant metastases and none of the patients remains continuously free of disease.

Among these 128 patients admitted to the three prospective protocols, 30 patients never achieved a complete response. Twenty-eight patients developed recurrent disease during the first year following diagnosis, 6 developed recurrent disease within the second year following diagnosis, 1 developed recurrent disease during the third year following diagnosis and 1 patient developed generalized metastatic disease 5 years 1 month from initiation of treatment. Fifty-six patients remained continuously disease free from 3+ months to 11+ years.

Survival as Related to Protocol Treatment

By the RMS I protocol 14 of 34 patients survive without evidence of disease from 6 to 11 years. By the RMS II protocol 19 of 56 patients are continuously disease free for more than 3 years (33%). Following treatment

with the RMS III protocol 26 of 38 patients remain continuously disease free from 3 months to nearly 3 years; 3
patients are living with disease and an additional patient
died of complications related to treatment.

Overall disease free survival for patients admitted
to these protocols is shown in Figure 1.

FIGURE I. RHABDOMYOSARCOMA I-III PROTOCOLS

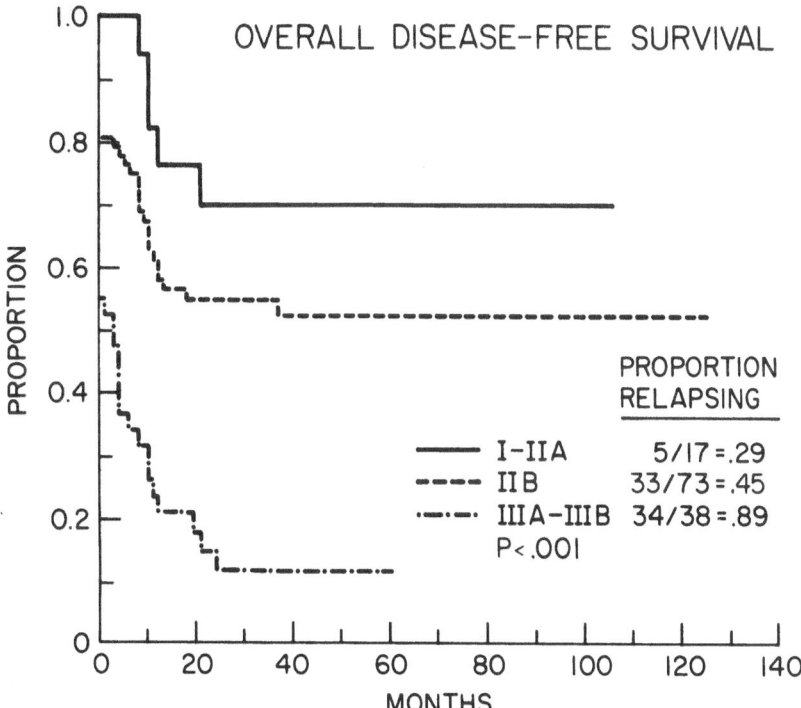

Extent of disease present at the time of diagnosis exerted
a significant effect on the disease free survival for
these patients (P <.001). However, survival for patients
with regional disease was similar to that of patients with
localized disease, provided that complete responses were
obtained.

There is as yet no statistical evidence of improvement of survival rates with the addition of adriamycin to

the other 3 agents. This may in part be related to the results of the second protocol in which the toxicity and morbidity were excessive, and associated with the deaths of 4 children as a result of complications as previously mentioned. There was 1 additional death of complications of a patient treated by the third protocol. Three of these deaths from complications were related to intestinal obstruction which followed laparotomy, combination chemotherapy, followed by abdominal or paraaortic nodal radiation therapy. An additional factor which may have complicated the survival of patients treated by the second protocol was that 21 of 56 patients had widely disseminated disease at the time of admission to protocol treatment; this incidence of advanced stage of disease was not encountered in patients admitted to the first and third protocols.

Response to Chemotherapy as Related to Histology and Extent of Tumor at Diagnosis

For patients with measurable indicators of disease activity an evaluation was performed for the response to combination chemotherapy which included vincristine, cyclophosphamide and dactinomycin, with or without adriamycin (Table 2).

Table 2. Response to Vincristine-Cyclophosphamide-Dactinomycin ± Adriamycin in Relation to Histologic Subtype. Rhabdomyosarcoma I-III Protocols (Measurable disease only)

Histology	Number Patients	CR	PR	MR	NR
Embryonal	54	13	30	3	8
Alveolar	12	6	4	1	1
Mixed	4	2	2	0	0
Sarcoma botryoides	2	0	2	0	0
Total	72	21	38	4	9
Proportion	1.00	0.29	0.53	0.06	0.12

Complete data was evaluable for 72 patients, of which 54 had the embryonal histologic variant. Among these 54 patients, 13 patients developed complete responses, 30 developed partial responses, 3 developed mixed responses and 8 patients failed to respond. Among 12 patients with the alveolar histologic subtype, 6 developed complete responses, 4 developed partial responses, and 1 developed a mixed response. There was no statistically significant difference in response rates among patients with embryonal and alveolar histologies (x^2 = 3.24, 2 d.f., P = 0.20). Two patients with sarcoma botryoides were evaluable for the effects of chemotherapy alone; both developed partial responses prior to treatment with radiotherapy. For 4 patients with the mixed histologic categorization, 2 patients developed complete responses and 2 had partial responses. Considering complete, partial and mixed responses, 66 of 72 patients, or 87%, developed response with these agents as delivered for measurable regional unresected or generalized disease.

Response to chemotherapy was also examined in relation to stage of disease at onset of treatment, and considered only patients with measurable indicators of disease activity (Table 3). In general, partial responses

Table 3. Childhood Rhabdomyosarcoma
Response to Chemotherapy with Vincristine-
Cyclophosphamide -Dactinomycin ± Adriamycin By
Extent of Tumor

Stage	Number Patients	CR	PR	MR	NR
IIB	35	8	25	1	1
IIIA-B	37	13	13	3	8
Total	72	21	38	4	9
Proportion	1.0	0.29	0.53	0.6	0.12

Table 4. Other Soft Tissue Sarcomas

Type	Number Surviving/Total	Male:Female	Age Range (Median) Years, Months
Liposarcoma	6/11	3:8	0.3 – 16.9 (6.6)
Synovial Sarcoma	7/11	9:2	4.6 – 20.10 (14.11)
Malignant Fibrous Histiocytoma	5/8	6:2	2.3 – 16.5 (9.3)
Fibrosarcoma	2/6	3:3	0.7 – 15.10 (7.6)
Schwannoma	1/5	2:3	9.0 – 16.0 (14.5)
Undifferentiated	1/4	3:1	1.4 – 17.6 (6.9)
Alveolar Soft Part	4/4	2:2	2.9 – 10.0 (6.9)
Hemangiopericytoma	1/4	2:2	0.6 – 17.1 (7.3)
Neurofibrosarcoma	1/4	1:3	9.11 – 13.5 (10.2)
Mesenchymoma	0/2	2:0	4.9, 10.7
Angiosarcoma	1/2	1:1	6.4, 13.1
	29/61	34:27	

were obtained more frequently than complete responses for patients with regional disease. The incidence of non-response was, as expected, higher in patients with disseminated disease (x^2 = 8.97, 2 d.f., P = 0.01).

Other Soft Tissue Sarcomas

Table 4 indicates the numbers of patients with the various STS other than RMS. The sex ratio and age range of patients with other soft tissue sarcomas are mentioned additionally. Liposarcoma and synovial sarcoma, among the most frequently encountered soft tissue sarcomas of adults, were the most frequent of the sarcomas other than RMS in children. The staging of our patients was consistent with that previously presented for children with RMS.

The chemotherapy and radiation therapy provided for patients with liposarcoma was similar with that used at the time of diagnosis for the treatment of children with RMS. Six of 11 patients survive; patients who died had regional unresectable or generalized tumor at diagnosis.

At diagnosis 7 of 11 children with synovial sarcoma had localized disease, whereas 3 had regional disease and only 1 had disseminated disease. Seven of 11 children are surviving, of which 6 are continuously free of disease from 2 to more than 9 years from diagnosis. Ten of 11 patients had primary tumor sites involving the upper or lower extremity. Seven patients with localized or completely resected synovial sarcoma received adjuvant vincristine-cyclophosphamide chemotherapy for 1 year following amputation or complete resection. Two patients developed metastatic disease at 1 year and 2½ years from initiation of chemotherapy.

Malignant fibrous histiocytoma, an unusual diagnosis among pediatric subjects, has been referred with increasing frequency in recent years. Because most of these patients had metastatic disease or unresected primary disease, an attempt has been made to evaluate single agents for this disease which has been reported to be resistant to the effects of chemotherapeutic agents.

Adriamycin produced a partial response in 1 of 5 patients treated with this agent. No responses have been observed in patients who have received cyclophosphamide, dactino-mycin, cis-Platinum-diamminedichloride, or high-dose methotrexate.

Although 4 of 6 patients with fibrosarcoma died, only 2 were evaluable for the effects of multiple agent chemo-therapy. The tumors of these patients failed to respond.

Four of the 5 patients with Schwannoma have expired. Each of these patients had evidence of neurofibromatosis and each of the patients who died of disease had either unresectable or metastatic disease at diagnosis. Each patient failed to respond to multiple agent combined chemotherapy.

Patients with undifferentiated sarcoma have also received treatment as delivered to patients with RMS during the period of time of their accession. One of 4 children is surviving at 1 year from diagnosis.

Each of the 4 patients with alveolar soft part sar-coma survives. One patient who received both radiation and multiple agent chemotherapy had no evidence of viable tumor with re-resection of the primary site. Another patient with primary tumor of the ethmoid region failed to respond to vincristine-cyclophosphamide-adriamycin-dactinomycin therapy. The additional 2 patients received surgical treatment alone.

Responses were obtained in both the patients with malignant mesenchymoma, the primary sites of which were the liver, following treatment with combined chemotherapy and radiation therapy. Both patients later died of pro-gressive disease.

The patients with hemangiopericytoma had either far advanced or unresectable regional disease at the time of diagnosis. Three of these patients were evaluable for the effect of chemotherapeutic agents generally used for the treatment of sarcomas. Measurable response of consider-able lengths of time were obtained following the use of

combined chemotherapy including vincristine, cyclophosphamide and dactinomycin, and in one instance adriamycin.

DISCUSSION

There has been significant improvement in the survival of patients who have received combined modality therapy for rhabdomyosarcoma in recent years. These improvements have been extended to patients with localized or
regional disease, but not to patients with evidence of
widespread metastatic disease at diagnosis. With combined
modality therapy, there has been an increase in the morbidity associated with the use of chemotherapy and radiation therapy. For patients failing to respond to combined
modality therapy or developing recurrent disease following
treatment, few additional agents of benefit are available.

Definitive statements cannot be made regarding the
responsiveness of STS of children other than RMS to either
single agent or combination chemotherapy. It is suggested
that, because of the rarity of these tumors, conventional
single agents be evaluated when possible in order to add
additional information to the paucity of information that
presently exists regarding the responsiveness of these
tumors to chemotherapeutic agents. While it is recognized
that the reports of CYVADIC chemotherapy (25) as advocated
by the Southwest Oncology Group and as used by the EORTC
(26) have provided meaningful data regarding adults with
these diseases, no such information presently exists
regarding response of these unusual tumors with the pediatric age group.

The successes as well as failures of the past must be
carefully evaluated to provide treatment for future patients with RMS and other STS according to site of primary
tumor and extent of tumor, with considerations for the age
of the patient. Surgery, radiotherapy and chemotherapy
must be applied with the aims of increasing response rates

as well as quality and duration of response, and decreasing the morbidity associated with combined modality therapy.

REFERENCES

1. Pinkel D, Pickren J: Rhabdomyosarcoma in children. JAMA 175:293-298, 1961.

2. Pratt CB: Response of childhood rhabdomyosarcoma to combination chemotherapy. J Pediatr 74:791-794, 1969.

3. Sagerman RH, Tretter P, Ellsworth RM: The treatment of orbital rhabdomyosarcoma of children with primary radiation therapy. Am J Roentgenol Radium Ther Nucl Med 114:31-34, 1972.

4. Pratt CB, Hustu HO, Fleming ID, Pinkel D: Coordinated treatment of childhood rhabdomyosarcoma with surgery, radiotherapy and combination chemotherapy. Cancer Res 32:606-610, 1972.

5. Kilman JW, Clatworthy W Jr, Newton WA Jr, Grosfeld JI: Reasonable surgery for rhabdomyosarcoma. A study of 67 cases. Ann Surg 178:346-351, 1973.

6. Donaldson SS, Castro JR, Wilbur JR, Jesse RH: Rhabdomyosarcoma of head and neck in children. Cancer 31: 26-35, 1973.

7. Ghavimi F, Exelby PR, D'Angio GJ, et al: Combination therapy of urogenital embryonal rhabdomyosarcoma in children. Cancer 32:1178-1185, 1973.

8. Jaffe N, Filler RM, Farber S, et al: Rhabdomyosarcoma in children. Improved outlook with a multidisciplinary approach. Am J Surg 125:482-487, 1973.

9. Tefft M, Jaffe N: Sarcoma of the bladder and prostate in children. Rationale for the role of radiation therapy based on a review of the literature and a report of fourteen additional patients. Cancer 32:1161-1177, 1973.

10. Holton CP, Chapman KE, Lackey RW, et al: Extended combination therapy of childhood rhabdomyosarcoma. Cancer 32:1310-1317, 1973.

11. Heyn RM, Holland R, Newton WA, et al: The role of combined chemotherapy in the treatment of rhabdomyosarcoma in children. Cancer 34:2128-2141, 1974.

12. Wilbur JR: Combination chemotherapy of embryonal rhabdomyosarcoma. Cancer Chemother Rep 58:281-284, 1974.

13. Ghavimi F, Exelby PR, D'Angio GJ, et al: Multidisciplinary treatment of embryonal rhabdomyosarcoma in children. Cancer 35:677-686, 1975.

14. Fernandez CH, Sutow WW, Merino OR, George SL: Childhood rhabdomyosarcoma: Analysis of coordinated therapy and results. Am J Roentgenol Radium Ther Nucl Med 123:588-597, 1975.

15. Ortega JA, Rivard GE, Issacs H, et al: The influence of chemotherapy on the prognosis of rhabdomyosarcoma. Med Pediatr Oncol 1:227-234, 1975.

16. Pullen DJ, Dyment PG, Humphrey GB, et al: Combined chemotherapy in childhood rhabdomyosarcoma. Cancer Chemother Rep 59:359-365, 1975.

17. Jereb B, Cham W, Lattin P, et al: Local control of embryonal rhabdomyosarcoma in children by radiation therapy when combined with concomitant chemotherapy. Int J Radiat Oncol Biol Phys 1:217-225, 1976.

18. Kumar APM, Wrenn EL Jr, Fleming ID, et al: Combined therapy to prevent pelvic exenteration for sarcoma botryoides of vagina and uterus. Cancer 37:118-122, 1976.

19. Maurer HM, Moon T, Donaldson M, et al: The Intergroup Rhabdomyosarcoma Study. A Preliminary Report. Cancer 40:2015-2026, 1977.

20. Hays EM, Sutow WW, Lawrence W Jr, et al: Rhabdomyosarcoma: Surgical therapy in extremity lesions in children. Orthop Clin North Am 8:883-901, 1977.

21. Tefft M, Fernandez CH, Moon TE: Rhabdomyosarcoma: Response with chemotherapy prior to radiation in patients with gross measurable disease. Cancer 39:665-670, 1977.

22. Kumar APM, Green AA, Smith JW, Pratt CB: Combined therapy for malignant tumors of the chest wall in Children. J Pediatr Surg 12:991-999, 1977.

23. Green DM, Jaffe N: Progess and controversy in the treatment of childhood rhabdomyosarcoma. Cancer Treat Rev 5:7-27, 1978.

24. Pratt CB, Hustu HO, Kumar APM, et al: Results of treatment of childhood rhabdomyosarcoma at St. Jude Children's Research Hospital 1962-1978. J Natl Cancer Inst (In press).

25. Gottleib JA, Baker LH, O'Bryan RM, et al: Adriamycin (NSC-123127) used alone and in combination for soft tissue and bony sarcomas. Cancer Chemother Rep (Part 3) 6:271-282, 1975.

26. Pinedo HM, Vendrik CK, Staquet M, et al: E.O.R.T.C. protocol for the therapy of metastatic soft tissue sarcoma, a randomized trial. Eur. J. Cancer 13: 765-771, 1977.

34 NEW DRUGS FOR THE TREATMENT OF SOFT TISSUE SARCOMAS

D. J. Stewart, R. S. Benjamin, L. H. Baker, B. S. Yap and G. P. Bodey

Adriamycin remains the most effective drug in the treatment of soft tissue sarcomas (1). Although a number of other agents, including DTIC, cyclophosphamide, vincristine, actinomycin-D, chlorambucil, mitomycin-C, and dibromodulcitol, are reported to have activity in these diseases (2), none has a reproducible response rate of more than 20% in adults with soft tissue sarcomas. While Adriamycin-containing combinations such as CYVADIC (cyclophosphamide, vincristine, Adriamycin, and DTIC) induce responses in more than 50% of patients (3), the duration of Adriamycin therapy is limited by cumulative cardiotoxicity and relapse frequently occurs following discontinuation of Adriamycin (4). Hence, new therapeutic modalities are greatly needed for soft tissue sarcomas. Currently, investigations are underway, both to define new drugs with activity against these tumors, as well as to determine methods of enhancing the therapeutic index of older drugs. Below is a discussion of new drugs unrelated to Adriamycin that have been used in the treatment of soft tissue sarcomas, followed by a discussion of experience with newer anthracyclines and with new methods of administering Adriamycin.

NEW DRUGS

Antibiotics   (Table I)

Azotomycin is an antitumor antibiotic isolated from the bacterium Streptomyces ambofaciens, and is a diazo analog of L-glutamine (5). In a broad phase II trial published 11 years ago, 4 of 16 patients with soft tissue sarcomas experienced partial remissions (6). Technical problems in the manufacture of the drug delayed further testing until recently when a second phase II trial was conducted in which none of 8 fully evaluable patients with soft tissue sarcomas responded (5).

An additional case report documents a patient with a uterine hemangio-pericytoma who achieved a prolonged complete remission on second-line therapy with azotomycin (7). This is a relatively toxic drug, producing nausea and vomiting severe enough to frequently result in prerenal azotemia (5), and drug-related deaths have been noted, both from granulocytopenia-associated sepsis and from emesis-induced hypovolemic shock and aspiration pneumonia (5).

Neocarzinostatin is an acidic single chain polypeptide isolated from Streptomyces carzinostaticus (8). In phase I-II trials 1 of 14 sarcoma patients experienced a partial remission (8, 9, 10, 11). It was not stated whether this patient had a soft tissue sarcoma or a bone sarcoma. The major toxicity of neocarzinostatin consists of myelosuppression, nausea and vomiting, fever, and allergic reactions. In addition, renal and hepatic dysfunction, hypophosphatemia, and hyponatremia are not uncommon (8).

Piperazinedione, a piperazine derivative obtained from the fermentation products of a strain of Streptomyces (12), produced no responses in 3 patients with unspecified types of sarcomas in 1 phase I-II trial (12), but produced one partial remission in 19 patients with uterine sarcomas treated in a phase II trial (13). The major toxic effect of this drug was myelosuppression (12).

Pyrazofurin, a C-ribonucleoside antibiotic isolated from the fermentation broths of Streptomyces candidus, induced only 1 minor response in 6 patients with unspecified types of sarcomas in a phase I trial (14) and no responses in 20 evaluable patients with soft tissue sarcomas in a phase II trial (15).

In view of activity demonstrated in phase I and early phase II trials, further studies may be warranted with azotomycin and neocarzinostatin, but sufficient patients have been treated with piperazinedione and pyrazofurin to conclude that they probably only have limited activity in soft tissue sarcomas.

Antimetabolites

Antimetabolites that have recently undergone clinical investigations in patients with soft tissue sarcomas are listed in table 2. During phase I trials of L-Alanosine, 3 patients with soft tissue sarcomas were treated. None responded (16). 5-Azacytidine, a pyrimidine antagonist, has undergone 2 broad phase II studies in patients with

Table 1: Antibiotics in Sarcomas

Drug	Type of Study	No. Evaluable Patients	No. with ≥50% Regression	No. with Improvement <50%	Reference No.
Azotomycin	Phase II	25	5(20%)	0	5, 6, 7
Neocarzinostatin	Phase I & II	14*	1*(7%)	0	8*, 9, 10*, 11*
Piperazinedione	Phase I & II	22*	1(5%)	0	12*, 13
Pyrazofurin	Phase I & II	26*	0	1(4%)	14*, 15

* Not stated in all cases whether patients had soft tissue sarcoma or other types of sarcoma.

solid tumors. In one study 3 evaluable patients with soft tissue sarcomas progressed on treatment (17). In a second study, a single patient with an unspecified type of sarcoma achieved a partial remission (18). Toxic effects of 5-azacytidine include myelosuppression and severe nausea and vomiting (17, 18).

Baker's antifol, a triazene that inhibits dihydrofolate reductase, was ineffective in 4 patients with unspecified types of sarcomas when used in high doses with citrovorum factor rescue (19). At conventional doses a patient with a synovial cell sarcoma experienced a remission during a phase I trial (20), but none of 28 patients with a variety of soft tissue sarcomas responded during a subsequent phase II trial (21).

In a phase I study of N^6-benzyladenosine-5'-monophosphate, the riboside of N^6-benzyladenosine, no sarcoma patients responded, although the actual number of patients with soft tissue sarcomas is not specified (22). Four children with rhabdomyosarcoma (23) and 2 adults with unspecified soft tissue sarcomas (24), showed no response to cyclocytidine, the anhydrous form of cytosine arabinoside. A single patient with a leiomyosarcoma treated with the uridine analogue 3-deazauridine during a phase I trial also did not respond (25).

Fifteen patients with soft tissue sarcomas were included in a phase II trial of diamino-dichlorophenyl-methylpyrimidine (DDMP) administered at doses of 50 mg/m^2 per week or 90 mg/m^2 every 3 weeks with citrovorum factor rescue (26). This dihydrofolate reductase inhibitor induced a partial remission in one patient and stabilized disease progression in 2 additional patients. Toxicity included myelosuppression, rash, stomatitis, anorexia, and headache.

N-Phosphonacetyl-L-aspartate (PALA) has recently undergone phase I testing in a number of centers. Of 8 patients with unspecified types of sarcomas, 1 achieved a partial remission and 2 had minor responses (27, 28, 29). Toxic effects consisted of nausea and vomiting, rash, mucositis, paresthesias, diarrhea, phlebitis, fever and myelosuppression (27, 29).

High dose methotrexate followed by citrovorum factor rescue has produced 12 remissions in 57 evaluable soft tissue sarcoma patients (30, 31, 32, 33), including 5 responses in 10 patients with rhabdomyosarcoma (30, 31). Some patients received vincristine along with the methotrexate. It remains to be determined whether high dose methotrexate offers any therapeutic advantage over optimally administered

Table 2: Antimetabolites in Sarcomas

Drug	Type of Study	No. Evaluable Patients	No. with ≥50% Regression	No. with Improvement <50%	Reference No.
L-Alanosine	Phase I	3	0	0	16
5-Azacytidine	Phase II	4*	1*(25%)	0	17, 18*
Baker's Antifol	Phase I & II	33	1(3%)	0	19*, 20, 21
N⁶-Benzyladenosine-5'-monophosphate	Phase I	?	0	0	22*
Cyclocytidine	Phase I & II	6	0	0	23, 24
3-Deazauridine	Phase I	1	0	0	25
DDMP	Phase II	15	1(7%)	0	26
PALA	Phase I	8*	1*(13%)	2*(25%)	27*, 28*, 29*
Methotrexate (high dose) & Citrovorum factor	Phase II	57	12(21%)	0	30, 31, 32, 33

* Not stated in all cases whether patients had soft tissue sarcoma or other types of sarcoma.

regular dose methotrexate in this disease. The addition of moderately high doses of methotrexate with citrovorum factor to the CYVADIC regimen has produced no augmentation of response rate over that seen with CYVADIC alone (34), and methotrexate without citrovorum factor administered by a variety of doses and schedules has given a 37% response rate in soft tissue sarcomas (35). In this latter study, a small proportion of the patients received their methotrexate intraarterially.

Of the antimetabolites discussed above, PALA definitely warrants further investigation in view of its apparent activity in phase I trials and 5-azacytidine and DDMP are of some interest. Inadequate information is available to make any judgment on cyclocytidine, 3-deazauridine, and N^6-benzyladenosine-5'-monophosphate. Baker's antifol has modest activity at best and high dose methotrexate with citrovorum factor rescue may have no advantage over regular dose methotrexate.

Metal-based Compounds (Table 3)

Cis-Diammine dichloroplatinum-II (CDDP) has produced remissions in 4 of 26 children with soft tissue sarcomas (36, 37, 38, 39) and 3 of 49 adults (40, 41). Hence, the response rate in soft tissue sarcomas appears to be lower than that seen in osteosarcoma (42). Six patients with soft tissue sarcomas have been treated with intraarterial CDDP without therapeutic benefit (43).

Gallium nitrate was administered to 22 patients with unspecified types of sarcoma in phase I trails (44, 45). A partial remission was seen in a patient with a fibrosarcoma and a minor response was seen in a leiomyosarcoma. These results are encouraging for a phase I trial , and a phase II trial is currently being undertaken by the Southwest Oncology Group.

Table 3: Metal-Based Compounds in Sarcomas

Drug	Type of Study	No. Evaluable Patients	No. with ≥50% Regression	No. with Improvement <50%	Reference No.
Cis-diammine-dichloro-platinum-II	Phase II	75	6(8%)	1(1%)	36, 37, 38, 39, 40, 41
Galium nitrate	Phase I	22*	1(5%)	1(5%)	44*, 45*

* Not stated whether patients had soft tissue or other types of sarcoma.

Alkylating Agents

As indicated in table 4, generally negative results in soft tissue sarcomas were obtained with a variety of alkylating agents. Aniline mustard (N,N-β-dichloroethylaniline, NSC 18429) was ineffective in both of 2 patients with myxoliposarcomas treated in a broad phase II trial (46). In a phase II study conducted by the Southwest Oncology Group, the alkylating agent dianhydrogalactitol did not result in any responses in 27 patients with a variety of soft tissue sarcomas (47). Likewise, hexamethylmelamine is relatively inactive. Out of 38 patients with soft tissue sarcomas and 43 with unspecified types of sarcoma treated with hexamethylmelamine, only 4 (2%) have responded (48, 49).

Peptichemio, a mixture of 6 synthetic oligopeptides, each of which contains an m-(di (2-choroethly) amino)-L-phenylalanine residue, did exhibit some activity, in that a single child with a rhabdomyosarcoma treated with this drug responded (50). However, 5 adults with unspecified types of sarcoma failed to respond (51). Major toxic effects were nausea and vomiting (mild), phlebitis, alopecia, skin rash, urticaria, fever, and cumulative myelosuppression (51).

Yoshi 864 (1-propanol, 3, 3'-imminodi-dimethane sulfonate (ester) hydrochloride) an alkylating agent effective in murine mechlorethamine-resistant tumors, did not produce any objective responses in 11 patients with unspecified types of sarcoma and one patient with a hemangiopericytoma, but did produce disease stability in 7 (52). Although results with this drug have not been encouraging, further studies would be necessary before it could be concluded that it is inactive in sarcomas.

Cyclophosphamide is an active drug in childhood sarcomas (2), although its activity in adult soft tissue sarcomas is marginal. In a recent study in children with a variety of malignancies, cyclophosphamide was given with i.v. hydration at a dose of 750 mg/m^2 every second day for 5 treatments (53). Two courses were given 3 weeks apart. These high doses of cyclophosphamide produced complete remissions in 2 out of 3 children with rhabdomyosarcoma and a partial remission in a single patient with a synovial cell sarcoma. Major toxicity included myelosuppression, nausea and vomiting, and hemorrhagic cystitis. This approach deserves further exploration in the treatment of soft tissue sarcomas.

Table 4: Alkylating Agents in Sarcomas

Drug	Type of Study	No. Evaluable Patients	No. with ≥50% Regression	No. with Improvement <50%	Reference No.
Aniline Mustard	Phase II	2	0	0	46
Dianhydrogalactitol	Phase II	27	0	0	47
Hexamethylmelamine	Phase II	81*	4*(2%)	0	48, 49*
Peptichemio	Phase II	6*	1(17%)	0	50, 51*
Yoshi 864	Phase II	12*	0	0	52*
High dose Cyclophosphamide	Phase II	4	3(75%)	0	53

* Not stated in all cases whether patients had soft tissue or other types of sarcoma.

Nitrosoureas   (Table 5)

The nitrosuoreas BCNU, CCNU, MECCNU and streptozotocin have previously been noted to have modest activity in sarcomas (2, 54), although in some cases not enough patients have been treated to give an accurate assessment of the response rate. In a recent phase II study of ACNU (1-(4-amino-2-methyl-5-pyrimidinyl)methyl-3-(2-chloroethyl)-3-nitrosourea) 1 patient with a fibrosarcoma experienced a complete remission while single patients with liposarcoma and leimyosarcoma failed to respond (55). Toxicity included myelosuppression, nausea and vomiting, and lassitude (55).

Chlorozotocin, a water-soluble nitrosourea, produced no responses in 6 soft tissue sarcoma patients during phase I studies (56, 57). However, during a subsequent phase II study, 3 responses were seen among 21 patients (58). Toxic effects consisted of cumulative myelosuppression and renal toxicity, and mild hepatic toxicity (56, 57).

Phase I studies have just recently been completed with a new nitrosourea, PCNU (1-(2-chlorothyl)-3-(2,6-dioxo-3-piperidyl)-1-nitrosourea) (59). The only patient with a soft tissue sarcoma continues to show stability of a previously slowly growing synovial cell sarcoma 52 weeks after starting on treatment.

All of these drugs are of considerable interest and deserve further investigation.

Plant Products

A variety of plant products have had limited trials in patients with soft tissue sarcomas (Table 6). Bruceantin, a plant-derived simarouboulide, failed to produce any responses in 5 patients with sarcoma treated during phase I trials (60, 61). Maytansine, a naturally occurring ansa macrolide, has been ineffective in 6 patients with unspecified types of sarcoma during phase I trials and 20 patients with soft tissue sarcomas during phase II trials (62, 63, 64).

The semi-synthetic vinca alkaloid vindesine likewise produced no responses in 5 patients in early trials (65, 66). However, because of evidence that continuous infusion may be a more effective treatment schedule than rapid infusion for vinca alkaloids (67), we are currently conducting a phase II trial of continuous infusion of vindesine and vinblastine in patients with soft tissue sarcomas (68). To date, 6 patients have been treated with each drug and none have responded.

Table 5: Nitrosoureas in Sarcomas

Drug	Type of Study	No. Evaluable Patients	No. with ≥50% Regression	No. with Improvement <50%	Reference No.
ACNU	Phase II	3	1(33%)	0	55
Chlorozotocin	Phase I & II	27	3(11%)	0	56, 57, 58
PCNU	Phase I	1	0	0	59

Table 6: Plant Products in Sarcomas

Drug	Type of Study	No. Evaluable Patients	No. with ≥50% Regression	No. with Improvement <50%	Reference No.
Bruceantin	Phase I	5*	0	0	60*, 61
Maytansine	Phase I & II	26*	0	0	62, 63*, 64
Vindesine	Phase I & II	11	0	0	65*, 66, 68*
Vinblastine continuous infusion	Phase II	6*	0	0	68*
VM-26	Phase II	33	1(3%)	0	69, 70
VP-16213	Phase II	41*	3(7%)	0	69, 71*

* Not stated in all cases whether patients had soft tissue or other types of sarcoma.

VM-26 and VP-16213 are semisynthetic podophyllotoxins. VM-26 induced only 1 response in 33 patients with soft tissue sarcomas treated in phase II studies (69, 70) and VP-16213 has resulted in only 3 responses out of 41 patients (69, 71).

Hence, further information is necessary before judging the efficacy of bruceantin, vindesine and vinblastine in soft tissue sarcomas. Maytansine, VM-26 and VP-16213 appear to have little activity in this disease. Miscellaneous (Table 7)

AMSA (4'-(9-acrindylamino)-methanesulfon-m-anisidide) is an acridine dye that binds to DNA both by intercalation and external binding (72). In 4 phase I studies, a combined total of 9 patients with sarcomas were treated with this drug and 1 achieved a remission (72, 73, 74, 75). In an ongoing phase II study, 1 of 22 patients with soft tissue sarcomas has responded (68). Toxicity consists mainly of myelosuppression, mild nausea and vomiting, and phlebitis (72).

Anguidine (diacetoxyscirpenol)is the principal phytotoxic metabolic product of the fungus Fusarium equiseti. Five patients with sarcomas were included in phase I studies, and 1 patient responded (76, 77). Toxic effects included nausea and vomiting, hypotension, central nervous system toxicity, diarrhea, chills and fever, erythema, stomatitis, dyspnea and myelosuppression (76). Both myelosuppression and antitumor efficacy may have been enhanced by administering the drug by continuous infusion over 4 days (77).

One patient with a soft tissue sarcoma has achieved a partial remission and 1 has had a minor response on cytembena (sodium cis-β-4-methoxybenzoyl-β-bromoacrylate) (78, 79). Overall, 24 soft tissue sarcoma patients were included in phase I and II trials.

In a recent phase I study with IMPY (imidazolopyrazole) neither of 2 patients with soft tissue sarcomas responded (68).

Two patients with soft tissue sarcomas have been treated with interferon (80). Neither responded. The interferon inducer poly ICLC (polyriboinosinic-polyribocytidylic acid) has also recently undergone phase I testing (81). Six patients with unspecified types of sarcoma failed to respond.

Razoxane (ICRF 159) did not produce any responses in 11 patients with soft tissue sarcomas treated in a phase II trial (82). However, this agent is known to be a radiosensitizer, and 41 of 53 patients treated with a combination of razoxane and irradiation achieved remission. Many of these were complete remissions (83, 84). Only 3 of 18 patients with unspecified types of sarcoma receiving a combination of razoxane and Adriamycin responded (85).

Table 7: Miscellaneous Drugs in Sarcoma

Drug	Type of Study	No. Evaluable Patients	No. with ≥50% Regression	No. with Improvement <50%	Reference No.
AMSA	Phase I & II	31*	2(6%)	0	68, 72, 73* 74*, 75
Anguidine	Phase I	5*	1(20%)	0	76, 77*
Cytembena	Phase I & II	25	1(4%)	1(4%)	78, 79
Impy	Phase I	2	0	0	68
Interferon	Phase II	2	0	0	80
Poly ICLC	Phase I	6*	0	0	81*
Razoxane a) alone	Phase II	11	0	0	82
b) radiation	Phase II	53	41(77%)	0	83, 84
Hyperthermia a) alone	Phase II	1	0	0	86
b) radiation	Phase II	2	1(50%)	0	87

* Not stated in all cases whether patients had soft tissue or other types of sarcoma.

Localized hyperthermia with or without concommitant irradiation has also been used in 3 patients with soft tissue sarcomas (86, 87). One response was seen. In addition, in a study that included patients with Kaposi's sarcoma, the combination of heat plus irradiation resulted in more prolonged remissions than radiation alone (88).

In summary, among the miscellaneous agents tested, cytembena appears to have limited activity in soft-tissue sarcomas. AMSA, anguidine, IMPY, interferon, razoxane and hyperthermia have not yet been adequately evaluated, although anguidine is of interest in view of the fact that 1 of 5 patients achieved remission during phase I trials, and razoxane in combination with irradiation appears to be highly active.

New Anthracycline Antibiotics

Because of the activity of Adriamycin, there is a great deal of interest in related anthracyclines. A number of these have undergone phase I and early phase II trials as outlined in Table 8. It is hoped that one can be developed that lacks cardiotoxicity. The most thoroughly studied is carminomycin, an anthracycline developed in the USSR. In 48 patients with soft tissue sarcomas treated with this drug, 27% had partial remissions with a median duration of 9 months, and 19% had minor responses, lasting for a median of 3.5 months (89). Diagnoses included synovial cell sarcoma, rhabdomyosarcoma, stromal sarcoma of the uterus, liposarcoma, fibrosarcoma, and angiosarcoma. Partial remissions were seen in each cell type. The majority of patients had not had prior chemotherapy. Toxicity consisted primarily of leukopenia and nausea and vomiting, although thrombocytopenia was also seen occasionally. Minor side effects consisted of headache, weakness, anorexia, alopecia, stomatitis, and rarely, diarrhea. No cardiac toxicity, other than occasional minor electrocardiographic changes was noted. Carminomycin has been reported to be less cardiotoxic than Adriamycin in a rat model (90), but further observation will be necessary to confirm this clinically. Carminomycin has also been used in combination with vincristine and cyclophosphamide in children with sarcomas with a reported objective improvement rate of 100%. Some patients had irradiation and surgery in addition to the drug combination.

Experience with the other anthracyclines is still too limited to permit accurate assessment of their activity in soft tissue sarcoma. However, early results with detorubicin (14-diethoxacetoxy-daunorubicin)

Table 8: Anthracycline Antibiotics in Sarcomas

Drug	Type of Study	No. Evaluable Patients	No. with ≥50% Regression	No. with Improvement <50%	Reference No.
Aclacinomycin A	Phase I	3	0	0	94
AD-32	Phase I	1	0	0	95
4'-epi-adriamycin	Phase I	1	1(100%)	0	93
Carminomycin	Phase I & II	48	13(27%)	9(19%)	89
Detorubicin	Phase II	2	2(100%)	0	92
Quelamycin	Phase I	2	0	0	96, 97
Rubidazone	Phase II	2	0	0	98

are encouraging. This drug, currently under investigation in France, produced a complete remission in 1 child with rhabdomyosarcoma and a partial remission in another patient with an abdominal liposarcoma (92). Toxicity included nausea and vomiting, alopecia, and myelosuppression. Congestive heart failure has been observed in a single patient treated with this drug. 4'-epi-adriamycin induced a partial remission in a single patient with a Kaposi's sarcoma (93). Aclacinomycin A, AD-32, quelamycin, and rubidazone have so far produced no responses in a small number of patients with soft tissue sarcomas treated with these agents (94, 95, 96, 97, 98).

New Methods of Administering Adriamycin

A variety of mechanisms have been explored in an attempt to improve the therapeutic index of Adriamycin (table 9). Adriamycin has been complexed with DNA in the hope that the molecule would be too large to be taken up by cardiac cells, thereby decreasing the cumulative cardiotoxicity of Adriamycin. In recent studies, 1 patient with a liposarcoma treated with this drug in combination with DTIC responded (99). Unfortunately, cardiac toxicity did not appear to have been altered (99).

Because of suggestive evidence that high peak levels of Adriamycin may be important in the development of Adriamycin-induced cardiomyopathy, it was felt that continuous infusion of Adriamycin over 24-96 hours might be less cardiotoxic than rapid high dose infusions. To date, 21 sarcoma patients have been treated with continuous infusion Adriamycin plus DTIC, along with rapidly infused cyclophosphamide (100). There have been 3 (14%) complete remissions, 9 (43%) partial remission, 2 minor responses, and 6 patients have had stable disease. Patients are being monitored by serial endomyocardial biopsies, and early results strongly suggest that this method of administering Adriamycin may indeed be less cardiotoxic than is rapid infusion (101). Other toxicity is comparable to that seen with standard CYVADIC regimens (3), although stomatitis is somewhat more prevalent. Thus, continuous infusion Adriamycin appears to be at least as effective in the treatment of sarcomas as is rapid infusion and a reduction in cumulative cardiac toxicity may enable more prolonged maintenance of treatment in responding patients. This may be important since relapse very frequently occurs following discontinuation of Adriamycin (4).

Table 9: New Methods of Administering Adriamycin

Method	No. Evaluable Patients	No. with ≥50% Regression	No. with Improvement <50%	Reference No.
Adriamycin – DNA**	1	1	0	99
Continuous Infusion**	21*	12*(57%)	2*(10%)	100*
Intraarterial	8	5(63%)	0	101
Protective Enviroment**	24*	17*(71%)	0	103*
Amphotericin – B**	2	0	0	104
High dose adriamycin, cyclophosphamide, total body irradiation, and autologous bone marrow rescue	1	1(100%)	0	106

* Not stated in all cases whether patients had soft tissue or other types of sarcoma.

** Given in combination with DTIC ± cyclophosphamide and vincristine.

In an attempt to achieve high local concentrations of drug, Adriamycin has been given by intraarterial infusion. Five out of 8 patients
with soft tissue sarcomas treated by this approach achieved partial
remissions (102). In another study, pre-operative intraarterial Adriamycin and local irradiation made limb salvage possible in 16 of 17
patients with soft tissue sarcoma, and none had relapsed by 4-34 months
after surgery (103).

Of 15 patients treated in protective environments with high doses
of drugs on the CYVADIC regimen (cyclophosphamide 500-800 mg/m^2, Adriamycin 50-80 mg/m^2, DTIC 250-400 mg/m^2/day x 5 days), 4 (27%) achieved
complete remission and 7 (47%) achieved partial remissions (104). Thus,
increasing doses of drugs appears to result in increased efficacy.

Amphotericin-B has been used in combination with Adriamycin-containing regimens in 2 Adriamycin-resistant patients with soft tissue
sarcoma (105). Neither patient responded. It is postulated that amphotericin-B may enhace uptake of some chemotheraputic drugs into cells.
A single soft tissue sarcoma patient treated with the combination of
amphotericin-B and a nitrosourea also failed to respond (106). Insuf-
ficient patients with sarcoma have been treated with this approach to
permit assessment of its efficacy.

A single child with a rhabdomyosarcoma responded to treatment with
high doses of adriamycin and cyclophosphamide, total body irradiation
and autologous bone marrow rescue (107). This approach deserves further
investigation.

In conclusion, Adriamycin-containing regimens such as CYVADIC remain
the most active form of treatment for soft tissue sarcomas. It is hoped
that by altering the method of administration the response rate can be
even further enhanced and the duration of remission prolonged. A number
of new agents outlined in Table 10 have shown sufficient activity in
phase I and early phase II trials to be of further interest. A number of
other agents had little evidence of activity, but many of these have
been studied in only a small number of patients.

*Table 10: Summary of Activity of
New Drugs in Sarcoma*

Possible Activity	Inconclusive	Low Activity (<10% in Phase II trials)
4'-epi-adriamycin	Aclacinomycin	Piperazinedione
Carminomycin	AD-32	Pyrazofurin
Detorubicin	Quelamycin	Baker's Antifol
Azotomycin	Rubidazone	CDDP
Neocarzinostatin	L-Alanosine	Dianhydrogalactitol
5-Azacytidine	Cyclocytidine	Hexamethylmelamine
DDMP	3-Deazauridine	Maytansine
PALA	N^6-Benzyladenosine-5'-monophosphate	VM-26
Gallium nitrate	Aniline Mustard	VP-16213
Peptichemio	Yoshi 864	Cytembena
ACNU	Bruceantin	
Chlorozotocin	Vindesine	
AMSA	Vinblastine	
Anguidine	Interferon	
High dose Methotrexate	Poly ICLC	
High dose Cyclophosphamide	Razoxane	
Razoxane plus irradiation	Impy	
	PCNU	

472

REFERENCES

1. Benjamin, R.S., Wiernik, P.H. and Bachur, N.R.: Adriamycin:
    A New Effective Agent in the Therapy of Disseminated Sarcomas.
    Med. and Pediat. Oncol. 1:63-76, 1975.

2. Wasserman, T.H., Comis, R.L., Goldsmith, M., et al: Tabular
    Analysis of the Clinical Chemotherapy of Solid Tumors. Cancer
    Chemother. Rep. 6:399-419, 1975.

3. Benjamin, R.S., Baker, L.H., Rodriguez, V. et al: The Chemo-
    therapy of Soft Tissue Sarcomas in Adults. IN: Management of
    Primary Bone and Soft Tissue Tumors. (Univ. Texas System Cancer
    Center, M.D. Anderson Hospital & Tumor Institute) 21st Annual
    Clinical Conf. on Cancer (Chicago, ILL.) Yearbook Med. Pub.,
    Inc., 1977, p. 309-315.

4. Yap, B.S., Sinkovics, J.G., Benjamin, R.S., et al: Survival and
    Relapse Patterns of Complete Responders in Adults with Advanced
    Soft Tissue Sarcomas. Proc. Am. Assoc. Cancer Res.
    20:352, 1979.

5. Chang, P. and Wiernik, P.H.: Phase II Study of Azotomycin in
    Sarcomas. Cancer Treat. Rep. 61:1719, 1977.

6. Weiss, A.J., Ramirez, G., Grage, T., et al: Phase II Study of
    Azotomycin (NSC-56654). Cancer Chemother. Rep. 52:611-614, 1968.

7. Sooriyaarachchi, G.S., Ramirez, G., Roley, E.L., et al: Heman-
    giopericytoma of the Uterus. J. Surg. Oncol. 10:399-406, 1978.

8. McKelvey, E.M., Burgess, M.A., McCredie, K.B., et al: Neo-
    carzinostatin: A Phase I Clinical Trial with Five-day Inter-
    mittent and Continuous Infusions. Cancer 44:1182-1188, 1979.

9. Rivera, G., Howarth, C., Aur, R.J.A., and Pratt, C.B.: Phase I
    Study of Neocarzinostatin in Children with Cancer. Cancer Treat.
    Rep. 62:2105-2107, 1978.

10. Ohnuma, T., Christopher, N., Cuttner, J. and Holland, J.F.:
    Phase I Study with Neocarzinostatin Tolerance to Two Hour
    Infusion and Continuous Infusion. Cancer 42:1670-1679, 1978.

11. Griffin, T.W., Comis, R.L., Lokich, J.J., et al: Phase I and
    Preliminary Phase II Study of Neocarzinostatin. Cancer Treat.
    Rep. 62:2019-2025, 1978.

12. Benjamin, R.S., Keating, M.J., Valdivieso, M., et al: Phase I-II
    Study of Piperazinedione in Adults with Solid Tumors and Acute
    Leukemia. Cancer Treat. Rep. 63:939-943, 1979.

13. La Gasse, L., Thigpen, T., and Morrison, F.: Phase II Trial of
    Piperazinedione in Treatment of Advanced Endometrial Carcinoma,
    Uterine Sarcoma and Vulvar Carcinoma. Proc. Am. Assoc. Cancer
    Res. 20:388, 1979.

14. Salem, P.A., Bodey, G.P., Burgess, M.A., et al: A Phase I
    Study of Pyrazofurin. Cancer 40:2806-2809, 1977.

15. Gralla, R.J., Sordillo, P.P., and Magill, G.B.: Phase II Evaluation of Pyrazofurin in Patients with Metastatic Sarcoma. Cancer Treat. Rep. 62:1573, 1978.

16. Stewart, D.J.: Unpublished Data.

17. Velez-Garcia, E., Vogler, W.R., Bartolucci, A.A., and Arkun, S.N.: Twice Weekly 5-Azacytidine Infusion in Disseminated Metastatic Cancer: A Phase II Study. Cancer Treat. Rep. 61:16 75-1677, 1977.

18. Weiss, A.J., Metter, G.E., Nealon, T.F., et al: Phase II Study of 5-Azacytidine in Solid Tumors. Cancer Treat. Rep. 61:55-58, 1977.

19. Benjamin, R.S.: Unpublished Data.

20. Rodriquez, V., Gottlieb, J., Burgess, M.A., et al: Phase I Studies with Baker's Antifol (BAF)(NSC 139105). Cancer 38:690-694, 1976.

21. Thigpen, J.T., O'Bryan, R.M., Benjamin, R.S., and Coltman, C.A., Jr.: Phase II Trial of Baker's Antifol in Metastatic Sarcoma. Cancer Treat. Rep. 61:1485-1487, 1977.

22. Catane, R., Kaufman, J.H., Nime, F.A., et al: Phase I Study of N^6-Benzyladenosine-5'monophosphate . Cancer Treat. Rep. 62:1371 1373, 1978

23. Finklestein, J.Z., Higgins, G., Krivit, W., and Hammond D.: Evaluation of Cyclocytidine in Children with Advanced Acute Leukemia and Solid Tumors. Cancer Treat. Rep. 63:1331-1333, 1979.

24. Burgess, M.A., Bodey, G.P., Minow, R.A., and Gottlieb, J.A.: Phase I-II Evaluation of Cyclocytidine. Cancer Treat. Rep. 61: 437-443, 1977.

25. Stewart, D.J.: Unpublished Data.

26. Alberto, P., DeJager, R.L., Brugarolas, A., et al: Phase II Study of Diamino-Dichlorophenyl-Methylpyrimidine with Folinic Acid Protection and Rescue. Proc. Am. Assoc. Cancer Res. 20:323, 1979.

27. Valdivieso, M., Moore, E.C., Loo, T.L. et al: Phase I Clinical Study of N-(Phosphonacetyl)-L-Aspartate (PALA, NSC 224131). Proc. Am. Assoc. Cancer Res. 20:187, 1979.

28. Ervin, J.J., Blum, R.H., and Canellos, G.P.: N-Phosphonacetyl-L-Aspartate (PALA), Phase I Trial. Proc. Am. Assoc. Cancer Res. 20:200, 1979.

29. Ohnuma, T., Hart, R., Roboz, J., et al: Clinical and Pharmacological Studies with Phosphonacetyl-L-Aspartate (PALA). Proc. Am. Assoc. Cancer Res. 20:344, 1979.

30. Von Hoff, D.D., Rozencweig, M., Louie, A.C., et al: "Single"-Agent Activity of High-Dose Methotrexate With Citrovorum Factor Rescue. Cancer Treat. Rep. 62:233-235, 1978.

474

31. Isacoff, W.H., Eilber, F., Tabbarah, H., et al: Phase II Clinical Trial with High-Dose Methotrexate Therapy and Citrovorum Factor Rescue. Cancer Treat. Rep. 62:1295-1304, 1978.

32. Vaughn, C., and Baker, L.: Personal Communication.

33. Ambinder, E.P., Perloff, M., Ohnuma, T., et al: High-Dose Methotrexate Followed by Citrovorum Factor Reversal in Patients with Advanced Cancer. Cancer 43:1177-1182, 1979.

34. Lynch, G., Magill, G.B., Golbey, R.B., et al: Combination Chemotherapy of Soft Part Sarcomas with Cyomad (S-7) Proc. Am. Assoc. Cancer Res. 20:116, 1979.

35. Subramanian, S., and Wiltshaw, E.: Chemotherapy of Sarcoma. The Lancet. 1:683, 1978.

36. Gaynon, P., Baum, E., Greenberg, L., et al: A Phase II Trial of Cis-Platinum Diammine Dichloride (NSC 119825) in Refractory Childhood Tumors. Proc. Am. Assoc. Cancer Res. 20:394, 1979.

37. Nitschke, R., Fagundo, R., Berry, D.H.: Weekly Administration of Cis-Dichlorodiammineplatinum (II) in Childhood Solid Tumors: A Southwest Oncology Group Study. Cancer Treat. Rep. 63:497-499, 1979.

38. Kamalakar, P., Freeman, A.I., Higby, D.J., et al: Clinical Response and Toxicity with Cis-Dichlorodiammineplatinum (II) in Children. Cancer Treat. Rep. 61,835-839, 1977.

39. Leventhal, B., and Freeman, A.: Cis-Diammine Dichloro Platinum. A Phase II Study in Pediatric Malignancies. Proc. Am. Assoc. Cancer Res. 20:197, 1979.

40. Hayes, D.M., Cvitkovic, E., Golbey, R.B., et al: High Dose Cis-Platinum Diammine Dichloride. Cancer 39:1372-1381, 1977.

41. Samson, M.K., Baker, L.H., Benjamin, R.S., Lane, M.: Cis-Diammine Dichloroplatinum(II) (NSC-119875, DDP) in Advanced Soft Tissue and Bony Sarcomas; a Southwest Oncology Group Study. (Submitted for Publication).

42. Ochs, J.J., Freeman, A.I., Douglass, H.O., et al: Cis-Dichlorodiammineplatinum(II) in Advanced Osteogenic Sarcoma. Cancer Treat. Rep. 62:239-245, 1978.

43. Calvo, D.B.III: Personal Communication.

44. Samson, M.K., and Baker, L.: Personal Communication.

45. Bedikian, A.Y., Valdivieso, M., Bodey, G.P., et al: Phase I Clinical Studies with Gallium Nitrate. Cancer Treat. Rep. 62: 1449-1453, 1978.

46. Young, C.W., Yagoda, A., Bittar, E.S.: Therapeutic Trial of Aniline Mustard in Patients With Advanced Cancer. Cancer 38: 1887-1895, 1976.

47. Kimball, J.C., and Cangir A.: Phase II Trial of Dianhydrogal-actitol in Advanced Soft Tissue and Bony Sarcomas: A Southwest Oncology Group Study. Cancer Treat. Rep. 63:553-554, 1979.

48. Borden, E.C., Larson, P., Ansfield, F.J., et al: Hexamethyl-melamine Treatment of Sarcomas and Lymphomas. Med. and Ped. Onc. 3:401-406, 1977.

49. Blum, R.H., Livingston, R.B., Carter, S.K.: Hexamethyl-melamine a new drug with activity in solid tumors. Eur.J. Cancer 9:195-202, 1973.

50. Otten, J. and Maurus, R.: Clinical Trial of Peptichemio in Solid Tumors of Childhood. Cancer Treat. Rep. 62:1015-1019, 1978.

51. Grose, W.E., Burgess, M.A. and Bodey, G.P.: Clinical Evaluation of Peptichemio. Cancer Treat. Rep. 63:385-389, 1979.

52. Altman, S.J., Metter, G.E., Nealon, T.F., et al: Yoshi 864 (1-Propanol, 3,3'-Iminodi-, Dimethanesulfonate Ester, Hydro-chloride): A Phase II Study in Solid Tumors. Cancer Treat. Rep. 62:389-395, 1978.

53. Kende, G., de Castro, L.A., Freeman, A.I. and Bjornsson, A.: High-Dose Cyclophosphamide in Childhood Cancer. Proc. Am. Assoc. Cancer Res. 19: 387, 1978.

54. Slavik, M.: Clinical Studies with Nitrosoureas in Various Solid Tumors. Cancer Treat. Rep. 60:795-800, 1976.

55. Saijo, N., Nishiwaki, Y., Kawase, I., et al: Effect of ACNU on Primary Lung Cancer, Mesothelioma, and Metastatic Pulmonary Tumors. Cancer Treat. Rep. 62: 139-141, 1978.

56. Kovach, J.S., Moertel, C.G., Schutt, A.J.: A Phase I Study of Chlorozotocin (NSC 178248). Cancer 43:2189-2196, 1979.

57. Gralla, R.J., Tan, C.T.C. and Young, C.W.: Phase I Trial of Chlorozotocin. Cancer Treat. Rep. 63:17-20, 1979.

58. Kelley, R.W., Samson, M.K., Brownlee, R.W., et al: Phase II Evaluation of Chlorozotocin in Advanced Human Cancers. Submitted for Publication.

59. Stewart, D.J.: Unpublished Data.

60. Garnick, M.B., Blum, R.H., Canellos, et al: A Phase I Study of Bruceantin (NSC 165563). Proc. Am. Assoc. Cancer Res. 20:326, 1979.

61. Bedikian, A. Personal Communication.

62. Eagan, R.T., Ingle, J.N., Rubin, J., et al: Early Clinical Study of an Intermittent Schedule for Maytansine (NSC-153858): Brief Communication. J. Natl. Cancer Inst. 60:93-96, 1978.

63. Blum, R.H. and Kahlert, T.: Maytansine: A Phase I Study of an Ansa Macrolide with Antitumor Activity. Cancer Treat. Rep. 62:435-438, 1978.

64. Wasserman, P. and Baker, L.: Personal Communication.

65. Currie, V.E., Wong, P.P., Krakoff, I.H. and Young, C.W.: Phase I Trial of Vindesine in Patients with Advanced Cancer. Cancer Treat. Rep. 62:1333-1336, 1978.

66. Rossof, A.H., Chandra, G., Walter, J., and Showel, J.: Phase II Trial of Vindesine (Desacetyl Vinblastine Amide Sulfate) in Advanced Metastatic Cancer. Proc. Am. Assoc. Cancer Res. 20: 146, 1979.

67. Yap, H.Y, Blumenschein, G.R., Hortobagyi, G.N., et al: Continous 5-day Infusion Vinblastine in the Treatment of Refractory Advanced Breast Cancer. Proc. Am. Assoc. Cancer Res. 20:334, 1979.

68. Yap, B.S.: Unpublished Data.

69. Radice, P.A., Bunn, P.A., Jr., and Ihde, D.C.: Therapeutic Trials with VP-16-213 and VM-26: Active Agents in Small Cell Lung Cancer, Non-Hodgkin's Lymphomas, and Other Malignancies. Cancer Treat. Rep. 63:1231-1239, 1979.

70. Bleyer, W.A., Krivit, W., Chard, R.L., Jr., and Hammond, D.: Phase II Study of VM-26 in Acute Leukemia, Neuroblastoma, and Other Refractory Childhood Malignancies: A Report from the Children's Cancer Study Group. Cancer Treat. Rep. 63:977-981, 1979.

71. Bleyer, W.A., Chard, R.L.; Krivit, W. and Hammond, D.: Epipodophyllotoxin Therapy of Childhood Neoplasia: A Comparative Phase II Analysis of VM-26 and VP 16-213. Proc. Am. Assoc. Cancer Res. 19:373, 1978.

72. Legha, S.S., Gutterman, J.U., Hall, S.W., et al: Phase I Clinical Investigation of 4'-(9-Acridinylamino)methanesulfon-m-anisidide (NSC 249992), a New Acridine Derivative. Cancer Res. 38:3712-3716, 1978.

73. Von Hoff, D.D., Howser, D., Gormley, P., et al: Phase I Study of Methanesulfonamide, N-[4-(9-acridinylamino)-3-methoxyphenyl]-(m-AMSA) Using a Single-Dose Schedule. Cancer Treat. Rep. 62:1421-1426, 1978.

74. DeJager, R., Bodey, J.J., Dupont, D., et al: Phase I Study of Oral 4'-(9-acridinylamino)-methanesulfon-m-anisidide (NSC-249992). Proc. Am. Assoc. Cancer Res. 20:429, 1979.

75. Schneider, R., Sklanoff, R. and Ochoa, M.: Phase I Trial of AMSA (4'-[acrindylamino]-methanesulfon-m-anisidide). Proc. Am. Assoc. Cancer Res. 20:114, 1979.

76. Murphy, W.K., Burgess, M.A., Valdivieso, M., et al: Phase I Clinical Evaluation of Anguidine. Cancer Treat. Rep. 62:1497-1502, 1978.

77. Adler, S., Lowenbraun, S., Jarrell, R., et al: Study of Anguidine (NSC 141537) by Continuous Infusion for Treatment of Solid Tumors. Proc. Am. Assoc. Cancer Res. 20: 306, 1979.

78. Baker, L.H., Samson, M.K. and Izbicki, R.M.: Phase I and II Evaluation of Cytembena in Disseminated Epithelial Ovarian Cancer and Sarcomas. Cancer Treat. Rep. 60:1389-1391, 1976.

79. Matejovsky, Z. Effects of Cytembena in the Treatment of Malignant Musculoskeletal Tumors. Neoplasma 18:473-480, 1971.

80. Christopherson, I.S., Jordal, R. Osther, K., et al: Interferon Therapy in Neoplastic Disease. Acta Med. Scand. 204:471-476, 1978.

81. Levine, A.S., Sivulich, M., Wiernik, P.H. and Levy, H.B.: Initial Clinical Trials in Cancer Patients of Polyriboinosinic-Polyribocytidylic Acid Stabilized with Poly-L-lysine, in Carboxymethylcellulose [Poly(ICLC)],a Highly Effective Interferon Inducer. Cancer Res. 39:1645-1650, 1979.

82. Dyment, P.G., Starling, K.A., Land, V.J., et al: ICRF-159 (Razoxane) in the Treatment of Pediatric Solid Tumors: A Southwest Oncology Group Study. Cancer Treat. Rep. 63:1397-1398, 1979.

83. Hellmann, K., Ryall, R.D.H., MacDonald, E., et al: Comparison of Radiotherapy with and without Razoxane (ICRF 159) in the Treatment of Soft Tissue Sarcomas. Cancer 41:100-107, 1978.

84. Rhomberg, W.J.: Radiotherapy Combined with ICRF-159 (NSC 129943). Int. J. Radiat. Oncology Biol. Phys. 4:121-126, 1978.

85. Chlebowski, R., Pugh, R., McCracker, J. et al: A Phase I-II Trial of Combination Therapy with Adriamycin and ICRF. Proc. Am. Assoc. Cancer Res. 20:167, 1979.

86. Marmor, J.B., Pounds, D., Postic, T.B., and Hahn, G.M.: Treatment of Superficial Human Neoplasms by Local Hyperthermia Induced by Ultrasound. Cancer 43:188-197, 1979.

87. Hornback, N.B., Shupe, R.E., Shidnia, H. et al: Preliminary Clinical Results of Combined 433 Megahertz Microwave Therapy and Radiation Therapy on Patients with Advanced Cancer. Cancer 40:2854-2863, 1977.

88. Kim, J.H., Hahn, E.W., Tokita, N., and Nisce, L.Z.: Local Tumor Hyperthermia in Combination with Radiation Therapy. 1. Malignant Cutaneous Lesions. Cancer 40:161-169, 1977.

89. Perevodchikova, N.I., Lichinitser, M.R. and Gorbunova, V.A.: Phase I Clinical Study of Carminomycin: Its Activity Against Soft Tissue Sarcomas. Cancer Treat. Rep. 61:1705-1707, 1977.

90. Zbinden, G. and Brandle, E.: Toxicologic Screening of Daunorubicin (NSC-82151), Adriamycin (NSC-123127), and their Derivatives in Rats. Cancer Chemother. Rep. 59:707-715, 1975.

91. Gusev, L.: Chemotherapy of Angiogenic Sarcomas in Children. Pediatrii (Mosk.) 7:73-76, 1978.

92. Jacquillat, Cl., Auclerc, M.F., Weil, M., et al: Clinical Activity of Detorubicin: A New Anthracycline Derivative.

478

Cancer Treat. Tep. 63:889-893. 1979.

93. Villani, F., Bonadonna, G., and Veronesi, U.: Phase I Study of
     4'-Epi-Adriamycin. Proc. Am. Assoc. Cancer Res. 20:172, 1979.

94. Ogawa, M., Inagaki, J., Horikoshi, N. et al: Clinical Study of
     Aclacinomycin A. Cancer Treat. Rep. 63:931-934, 1979.

95. Blum, R.H., Garnick, M.B., Israel, M., et al: Initial Clinical
     Evaluation of N-Trifluoroacethyladriamycin-14-valerate (AD-32),
     an Adriamycin Analog. Cancer Treat. Rep. 63:919-923, 1979.

96. Brugarolas, A., Pachon, N., Gosalvez, M., et al: Phase I Clinical
     Study of Quelamycin. Cancer Treat. Rep. 62:1527-1534, 1978.

97. Cortes-Funes, H., Gosalvez, M., Moyano, A., et al: Early Clinical
     Trial with Quelamycin. Cancer Treat. Rep. 63:903-907, 1979.

98. Skovsgaard, T., Hansen, H.H., Mouridsen, H.T., et al: Clinical
     Trial of Rubidazone in Solid Tumors and Malignant Lymphomas.
     Cancer Treat. Rep. 62:1053-1058, 1978.

99. Benjamin, R.S.: Unpublished Data.

100. Benjamin, R.S.: Unpublished Data.

101. Benjamin, R.S., Ewer, M.S., Mackay, B., et al: An Endomyocardial
     Biopsy Study of Anthracycline-Induced Cardiomyopathy--Detection,
     Reversibility and Potential Amelioration. Proc. Am. Assoc. Cancer
     Res. 20:372, 1979.

102. Shah, P., Baker, L.H., and Vaitkevicius, V.K.: Preliminary Exper-
     iences with Intra-Arterial Adriamycin. Cancer Treat. Rep. 61:1565-
     1567, 1977.

103. Morton, D.L., Eilber, F.R., Weisenbarger, T.H., et al: Limb
     Salvage Using Preoperative Intraarterial Adriamycin and Radiation
     Therapy for Extremity Soft Tissue Sarcomas. Aust. N.Z. J. Surg.
     48:56-59, 1978.

104. Rodriguez, V., Bodey, G.P., and Freireich, E.J.: Increased Remis-
     sion Rate and Prolongation of Survival in Patients with Soft Tis-
     sue Sarcomas Treated with Intensive Chemotherapy on Protected
     Environment Prophylactic Antibiotic Program (PEPA). Proc. Am.
     Assoc. Cancer Res. 17:320, 1976.

105. Krutchik, A.N., Buzdar, A.U., Blumenschein, G.R. and Sinkovics,
     J.G.: Amphotericin B and Combination Chemotherapy in the Treat-
     ment of Refractory Metastatic Breast Carcinoma and Sarcoma. Cancer
     Treat. Rep. 62:1565-1567, 1978.

106. Presant, C.A., Klahr, C., Olander, J., and Gatewood, D.: Ampho-

tericin B Plus 1,3-Bis(2-Chloroethyl)-1-Nitrosourea (BCNU-NSC-No. 409962) in Advanced Cancer. Phase I and Preliminary Phase II Results. Cancer 38:1917-1921, 1976.

107. Kaizer, H., Leventhal, B.G., Santos, G.W., et al: The Use of Cryopreserved Autologous Bone Marrow Following Marrow-Lethal Chemoradiotherapy in the Treatment of Selected Pediatric Malignancies. Proc. Am. Assoc. Cancer Res. 19:402, 1978.

35 CURRENT AND FUTURE MANAGEMENT OF SOFT TISSUE SARCOMAS
Panel Discussion, held on December 8th, 1979

Chairman: J. F. Holland (New York)
Panel members: D. Crowther (Manchester),
H. M. Pinedo (Amsterdam), Ch. B. Pratt (Memphis),
W. F. Sindelar (Bethesda), D. J. Stewart (Houston),
J. A. M. van Unnik (Utrecht) and E. Wiltshaw (London)

CHAIRMAN: Topics to be discussed are:
1) surgical management, 2) combination of radiotherapy and
chemotherapy, 3) radiotherapy, 4) chemotherapy, 5) new
approaches.

1. Surgical Management

Is there a place for frozen section, biopsy and diagnosis
in determining the extent of operation in adults and in
children ?

DR. VAN UNNIK : I suppose I have to give the same answer
as Professor Van Rijssel : it has to be done by an
experienced pathologist.

There must be a good understanding between the surgeon and
the pathologist. In soft-tissue pathology, it isn't always
possible to give a histological diagnosis, but you can
give some useful information. Sometimes you can recognize
a high grade malignancy in tumors by identifying cellularity
and mitosis. The exact diagnosis is often only possible on
paraffin slides.

For a definite diagnosis we need a large biopsy. An
illustrating example I heard some time ago concerned a
surgeon who did not trust his pathologist, so he divided the
biopsy into three parts and sent each one to three
different pathologists. The answer he got was that it was
a fibro-sarcoma, it was a metastasis of an adenocarcinoma,
it was a malignant biphasic synovio-sarcoma. Then the
surgeon said : "Now, I'm sure pathologists are good for

nothing". But, you really need a large-scale biopsy. This is what I want to stress.

DR. SINDELAR : We utilize frozen sections at our Institution basically for two purposes. Firstly not for definitive diagnosis but to determine whether or not we have, in the pathologist's opinion, an adequate amount of tissue for a subsequent histologic confirmation. Very frequently, these tumors are heterogeneous and a very small sampling does not suit the pathologist.
Secondly frozen sections are useful to determine margins.

DR. PINEDO : What about needle biopsy, which has been introduced and accepted in the adjuvant study of the Sarcoma group of the E.O.R.T.C. ?

DR. VAN UNNIK : I'm afraid I'll have to give nearly the same answer. For a definite diagnosis, we really need to have a large biopsy.

CHAIRMAN : Does it differ in children, Dr. Pratt ?

DR. PRATT : It's necessary to complete most of the staging procedures, prior to the decision about the first surgical procedure. The type of soft-tissue tumor is crucial in children.

CHAIRMAN : So that our general proposition would be : that definitive planning should not be based on a one-stage operation but based upon biopsy and better understanding of what the tumor is.

DR. SINDELAR : An important point to be made regarding biopsies, is that these are not trivial procedures. Biopsy incisions have to be placed so that they can be totally excised with the specimen. This is not often considered by surgeons and really needs to be stressed.

CHAIRMAN : The width of the margin that one takes with a neoplasm is another thing, it seems to me, you could speak to, Dr. Sindelar. Is it acceptable to take the muscle compartment in which the tumor is located ?

Or should you be beyond the muscle compartment in which it is located ?

DR. SINDELAR : You've hit upon an area of considerable controversy. The biologic behaviour of most sarcomas tends to respect fascial planes. So, in the case of extremity lesions, a complete excision of a fascial compartment should be a curative operation. However, there are relatively few other anatomic areas in the body where this can be done.

The biopsy or the operation itself often traverses various fascial planes, thereby opening those to potential contamination. The question of margins, of course, is : how much is enough ? Often, the location of the tumor determines what sort of margin you will get, and the closest margin, generally, is that which is on or nearest to a structure which cannot be surgically sacrificed.

DR. CROWTHER : A good case can be made out for centralizing the surgical service. We have referrals from all over a large region and each surgeon, who refers a case might deal with perhaps only a few cases a year. Certainly, we get a lot of our cases - or more than we want - referred in which the primary lesion itself has only been shelled out. Quite often the comment that we get is that it was easily shelled out. But of course this is a very false way of looking at it, because in nearly all those cases it's a false capsule - it can very easily be shelled out - but almost certainly tumor will be left behind.

DR. PINEDO : Dr. Sindelar, do you take a biopsy of the lymph nodes draining the tumor area of an extremity as a routine, even if not palpable.

DR. SINDELAR : No, we do not routinely sample lymph nodes, if they are not clinically suspect. Sarcomas rarely go to lymph nodes. In our surgical excisions, we do not routinely include the draining lymph nodes unless they are contiguous or a part of the structure which we feel is potentially contaminated.

CHAIRMAN : The statement has been made, that the proper operation for sarcoma of an extremity is amputation. What is the frequency with which you are seeing amputated patients, as a necessity for extremity sarcomas in Britain, for example, in Amsterdam, and Houston ? With what frequency do you see patients who require amputation ?

DR. CROWTHER : Eighty percent get local wide excision. So only 20 % are amputated.

DR. PINEDO : On the Continent, it's the same.

DR. STEWART : I can't give any firm figures, because we make an attempt to reduce the tumor size first by intra-arterial or systemic chemotherapy. We then make an attempt at local excision, if we can.
CHAIRMAN: What is the nature of your intra-arterial chemotherapy?
DR. STEWART: Right now, it's continuous-infusion adriamycin plus DTIC.
CHAIRMAN: Comments or questions from the floor related to this surgical aspect?

DR.MUGGIA: When you're dealing with the mediastinum or intra-abdominal tumor, do you rely on frozen sections.
DR. PRATT : When you're dealing with retroperitoneal disease. You have to consider the resectability of the lesion.

DR. SINDELAR : Frozen sections are useful to determine margins. In retroperitoneal sarcomas, surgery is limited by the proximity of non-sacrificable structures- liver, vena cava, aorta and so on. If you get a positive margin, you can't do anything about it. However, if you get a positive margin in, for example the renal fossae, where you have 2 more centimeters of fat that you can take out, then I think you might go ahead. It has to be individualized, depending on the location your're working in.

2. *Combination of radiotherapy and chemotherapy*

CHAIRMAN : Combinations of radiotherapy and chemotherapy
have been used in childhood sarcomas. Could we have a
discussion on similar approaches in adults ?

DR. PINEDO : There is certainly a place for the combination
in the treatment of the primary tumor in the adult.
Many radiotherapists and medical oncologists are afraid of
combining the radiation therapy and high-dose adriamycin
because of complications. In the adjuvant study of the
E.O.R.T.C., we have left the possibility to combine the
two at the same time. Radiation therapy is given according
to strict guidelines after the operation if indicated.
Concomittantly, chemotherapy (CYVADIC) may be started.
Most elect to wait until the radiation therapy has ended.

CHAIRMAN : That would be a very great variable in your
study if it's not randomly studied. There is controversy
in the United States concerning radiotherapy to the
operative site, as reported by Dr. Suit (Boston). It's an
uncontrolled observation. Is radiotherapy indicated after
low-grade sarcomas and is it effective after high-grade
sarcomas.

DR. PINEDO : The simultaneous use of radiation and
adriamycin is particularly dangerous in the head and neck
region.

CHAIRMAN : My question still is : which of these programs
of treatment has the greatest likelihood of eradicating the
tumor ? I'm not convinced that either chemotherapy or
radiotherapy are effective as an adjuvant.

DR. CROWTHER : I agree with that. There have been no properly
randomized studies conducted with large enough numbers of
patients to prove that radiotherapy is useful as an
adjuvant. If you treat locally recurrent disease with
radical radiotherapy, about a third of those may well
survive for 5 years without local recurrence. Half of the
patients relapse with lung metastases, so that, combined

treatment may be required. It's also true for adjuvant
chemotherapy : there have been no randomized controlled
studies. These are badly needed with stratifications for
site, grade, histological type, and adequacy of surgery.
The E.O.R.T.C. are just managing to get together now and I
hope that those studies will be successful in future.

DR. MUGGIA : I'd like to call attention to a preliminary
report in the International Journal of Radiation Oncology
Biology and Physics by the group at Sidney Farber Cancer
Institute, Dr. Blum and coworkers. They combined adriamycin
and radiation therapy with surgery in a very heterogeneous
group of patients with advanced locally invasive tumors.
They had good results with the combination, given
sequentially. The sequences differed according to the
extent and location of disease. They have had some
recurrences, but the preliminary experiences look quite
favorable.

DR. SINDELAR : I agree with all that's been said. It needs
to be pointed out that, in marginal surgical excisions with
positive microscopic margins radiotherapy can control local
disease. It probably cannot control gross residual disease
and that distinction should be made. I fully agree with the
previous comments that this needs to be looked at in some
systematic fashion.

CHAIRMAN : It should be pointed out that the principal drug
is adriamycin and we do not know the optimal way to use it
as an adjuvant. It's amazing how, as a collective body,
we've not yet done a proper study. Are there comments or
questions from the floor?

3. Radiotherapy

DR. CHASSAGNE (Villejuif) : I would like to comment about
some type of Curie-therapy which has not yet been mentioned.
We have an experience in about 50 children with
rhabdomyosarcomas in collaboration with Drs. Schweisgut and
Lemerle. We had very few local recurrences. We have
published a paper on vaginal sarcoma botryoides, with 12

cases and no failures. The children are managed with chemotherapy first, about two or three courses and then they
receive local treatment with Curie-therapy.
The Curie-therapy spares the bones, because it's a local
treatment. That is the main advantage. Also, it lasts only
for 5 to 6 days.

In adults, we do not have as extensive an experience as in
children. We do implantation at the time of surgery. I'm
sure in the States you have the same experience - at least
Dr. Delclos at MD. Anderson is doing it and also Dr. Henschke
has used it. Radium implants are placed via plastic tubes
during operation.

CHAIRMAN : Do you use frozen sections to determine the margins?

DR. CHASSAGNE (interrupting) : No, our pathologists find it
very difficult to interpret frozen sections, because of
fibrotic tissue coming from previous surgery. We put the
tube inside the surgical scar and wait for the definitive
pathological report, and then load the tube.

CHAIRMAN : How many rads do you then give ?

DR. CHASSAGNE : If it's localized disease, we have given
at least 7000 rads in adult sarcoma. For the childhood
rhabdomyosarcomas, we give a smaller dose.

DR. WILTSHAW : Intra-lesional Curie-type therapy for large
adult sarcomas was abandoned some time ago, in our hospital
and also probably in Manchester.

CHAIRMAN : That's in the large tumor. But my understanding
was that Dr. Chassagne was talking about the tumor bed
after the surgery.

DR. CHASSAGNE : I would not advise to do this in large
rhabdomyosarcomas.   If however,you have tumor close to
major arteries and nerves local Curie-therapy may play a
role.

DR. CROWTHER : The question of the Manchester therapy is

being raised. We don't use local implantation following surgical excision, nor have we done in the past. There is an interesting technique however, which is known as growth restraint, with just 100 rads a week given palliatively to bulky tumors. Some good responses to that type of approach, with five-year disease-free survivals have been seen.

DR. STEWART : One of the potential treatments for the future for localized unresectable disease is hyperthermia. Some centers implant thermistors in large unresectable tumors, heat them up to roughly 43° C and get fairly extensive necrosis around the termistors. It's possible that it could gain some application in treating a tumor bed.

CHAIRMAN : There is a great deal of technicological advance in this particular area with different kinds of hyperthermia producing methods.

DR. SINDELAR : Just to make one further comment on radio-therapy, which is obviously a difficult area. The Japanese have had considerable experience with intra-operative radiation, where vital structures in the abdomen, following tumor section, are moved out of the way and, one dose radiation is given to the tumor bed. This is beginning to be explored in the United States and may well offer some hope for therapy in difficult areas, such as the retroperitoneal sarcomas.

DR. VAN OOSTEROM : It's highly surprising that none of you has commented on the data of razoxane (ICRF - 159) plus radiotherapy reporting 77 % responses in Dr. Stewart's presentation.

DR. STEWART : That sounds good for local disease control or pre-operative use. I don't have any personal experience with it, so I can't comment further.

DR. CROWTHER : There have been a number of radiotherapy series with similar response rates. For example, McNeer reported on 58 patients, 72 % response and in 38% no recurrences in a period over 5 years. The Windyer Report with

14 out of 22 complete remitters, using 6000 plus rads, 8
did not recur in a period longer than 5 years. Radiotherapy
alone can control local disease quite well.

4. Chemotherapy

CHAIRMAN : Let's move on then to chemotherapy and immunotherapy. We've established that there is no standard drug
other than adriamycin. Combinations involving adriamycin
are still controversial and under study. Is it ethical to
study a drug in previously untreated patients with
metastatic sarcoma ?

DR. STEWART : It depends on which patient population you
study. One might be able to identify patients at high-risk
of not responding to conventional drugs. The stem cell
assay could also provide some guidance.

CHAIRMAN : There is no question that the whole in vitro
sensitivity testing is very attractive. Since that is still
on the horizon it is reasonable to test new drugs in
untreated patients with metastatic sarcoma. The EORTC
Sarcoma Group will study anthracycline analogs such as
4-Epi Adriamycin, Carminomycin and Aclacinomycin A. I find
this not only ethical, but imperative.

DR. CROWTHER : I would have a proviso, that patients with
simple local recurrence be excluded.

DR. PINEDO : After seeing the data of Dr. Wiltshaw with
methotrexate this agent should also be included in Phase II
studies in untreated advanced cases.

DR. WILTSHAW : In fact, my patients were not pre-treated.
The addition of adriamycin and all other drugs to
methotrexate did not increase our complete remission rate,
the partial remission rate was quite variable.
I have wondered whether there are some responsive sarcomas,
which will respond to almost anything you give. That is
why, we get 10 % complete responses in all our series.

Perhaps methotrexate is as good as any other agent at getting complete remissions. I certainly would think high dose methotrexate should be tried.

DR. MUGGIA : However, in your combination studies, you always used the rescue technique with methotrexate and you may have negated the anti-tumor effect from methotrexate. In your earlier experience where you used it as a single agent it was more effective. I would have doubts whether the high-dose methotrexate can fare all that well. There is some information on high-dose methotrexate and the response rate was not as good as your single-agent low-dose methotrexate, especially for complete remissions.

DR. WILTSHAW : The numbers involved are so small that I really don't think one could comment on that.

DR. PINEDO : But at present there is no reason at all to give high-dose methotrexate to soft-tissue sarcomas. Do you agree ?

DR. WILTSHAW : Yes.

DR. PINEDO : There have been two studies with high-dose methotrexate. Isacoff observed 5 responses in 11 patients and Karakusis 3 responses in 13 patients, which is actually more or less what you have been seeing with your low-dose methotrexate studies.

In the EORTC we have just completed a study of methotrexate given as 80 milligrams per m^2 per week in patients pre-treated with CYVADIC. The response rate in this population is only one in 13. But the lead from London should be pursued in previously untreated patients.

CHAIRMAN : This is one of the studies, that the National Cancer Insitute and Dr. Muggia in particular have been trying to merchandize for some time : a good critical comparison between high-dose methotrexate and low-dose methotrexate, because it does have a fundamental biologic question. You recall that Dr. Rosen was absolutely unambiguous in having ten anecdotes of his own, where a higher dose methotrexate in the macro range made a difference. And yet we raise the concept that low-dose unrescued methotrexate would be preferable in soft-tissue sarcoma.

DR. MUGGIA : That was my major point. In the combinations employing methotrexate, Dr. Wiltshaw has always used citrovorum factor rescue. This may not be equivalent to testing methotrexate itself in the combination.

5. New approaches

CHAIRMAN : Immunotherapy ? Would anyone like to speak for or against immunotherapeutic procedures in soft-tissue sarcoma ?

DR. SINDELAR : I guess I'm the only one here who talked on immunotherapy. It showed absolutely no effect in our patients, and particularly the corynebacterium parvum was badly tolerated. These data do not support a role for this type of immunotherapy in the treatment of sarcomas.

CHAIRMAN : Is it worth investigating ?

DR. SINDELAR : I think that depends on your predisposition I personally think not. Others may.

CHAIRMAN : These tumors are among the classical RNA-virus induced tumors in birds and animals. Is there any use for anti-viral medications or interferon ?

DR. CROWTHER : Interferon certainly is a very expensive drug and difficult to get. The first area in which it's going to be used is probably not in soft-tissue sarcomas. As to immunotherapy, there have been some uncontrolled studies of immunotherapy. Townsend reported on 18 patients, locally resected and treated with BCG and tumor-cell vaccines who had a 61 % disease-free survival, and compared them with 15 control patients who were locally resected and had a 33 % disease-free survival. This was one of the studies which suggested that perhaps a control study should be set up. But, of course, as we've heard from Dr. Sindelar, his with C-parvum was negative.

CHAIRMAN : BCG and C-parfum are different materials. Certainly one could be active and the other not. I don't think that they are mutually exclusive. Has the extensive study of BCG in Texas led at one time or another through soft-tissue sarcoma land?

DR. STEWART : I am not familiar with those studies at MD Anderson. I wanted to get back to interferon. It must be studied in this disease, since osteogenic sarcoma is one tumor in which evidence for activity in the adjuvant situation has been reported. In limited experience on patients with metastatic tumors of various origins, interferon - just as any other drug - seems to do best in patients with only very small tumors. There have been responses in breast carcinoma, lymphoma and multiple myeloma. It definitely deserves a trial.

DR. CLETON : In this country, many people are concerned about the role of interferon. How good is the evidence of Strander in osteosarcoma? How good is the evidence in myeloma and in non-Hodgkin lymphomas? Dr. Rosen, on the panel on osteosarcoma said : If I had enough interferon, I would treat half of my patients with interferon. I don't think there is all that much evidence that interferon has done anything in humans yet, but you may have more recent information.

CHAIRMAN : I think that statement couldn't stand as such, Dr. Cleton. The American Cancer Society did buy a considerable amount of interferon from Helsinki and it's currently under study in about ten American institutions, in four diseases : breast, lymphoma, myeloma and melanoma. And there are responses in each of those tumor types among the institutions. The data particularly from Gutterman at the MD Anderson Hospital, where he has seen responses in each of those tumor types. The data of Strander are persuasive to those who've seen them first hand, and relate to biochemical markers. It is my proposition that it is an active compound; it is surely not a panacea. I have seen people who have failed on it, but I've seen tumor regression. It is important to recognize that it is a natural substance, and being a natural substance opens up a whole proposition of how the regressions are brought about and what role it may play in natural defense against tumors. I have looked at Strander's data and they are equal to adriamycin in the adjuvant treatment of osteosarcoma.

DR. CLETON : This was again with historical controls !

CHAIRMAN : We cannot go back to discussing the questions of historical controls. But, as was pointed out, the only basis for saying that historical controls are different from a 20 % survival is one series of patients at the Mayo Clinic. It is a small series and if you added five patients with relatively benign tumors you would certainly get a better survival. Rather than say the whole world has always been wrong, it would be easier to have someone go look and see whether or not by chance a few relatively benign tumors got into the Mayo Clinic series.

DR. MUGGIA : I do accept the Mayo Clinic data. Their pathologists have thoroughly reviewed and published their data. Mayo has the foremost pathologists in this field

CHAIRMAN : Absolutely, no question about it. But I can assure you that the classification of osteosarcoma at the Mayo Clinic has changed.

DR. STEWART : However, we can all agree, that interferon would be a substance of great investigative interest. Nevertheless we shouldn't adopt it into the therapeutic armamentarium as if it worked, without a proof.

DR. MUGGIA : To change the subject, is there anybody who has experience with 5-fluorouracil ? In the very extensive review, Dr. Stewart, there was one agent that did not appear. In the old gynecologic literature, there are some responses to 5-fluorouracil in uterine sarcomas. It is of interest now that PALA is used in combination with 5-fluorouracil, and some responses are observed. This might be worth looking at.

DR. PINEDO : How many responses did you see with 5-FU plus PALA ?

DR. STEWART : The data was presented at the most recent Phase I meeting of the N.C.I. It was two out of five soft-tissue sarcoma patients who responded to this combination. One osteogenic sarcoma and one chondrosarcoma did not.

INDEX

498

DRUGS

Single agent

Combinations

BCD	bleomycin + cyclophosphamide + actinomycin D 331, 353, 358
BP	bleomycin + cisplatin 204
CAP	cyclophosphamide + adriamycin + cisplatin 7, 24, 130, 153
CHAD	cyclophosphamide + hexamethylmelamine + adriamycin + cisplatin 67, 70, 130
CHexUP	cyclophosphamide + hexamethylmelamine + 5-fluorouracil + cisplatin 130
COMPADRI II	332, 336
CONPADRI I	332, 336
CYVADACT	cyclophosphamide + vincristine + adrimaycin + actinomycin D 416
CYVACT	cyclophosphamide + vincristine + actinomycin D 332
CYVADIC	cyclophosphamide + vincristine + adriamycin + DTIC 331, 416, 426, 428, 429, 430, 431, 440, 449
HexaCAF	hexamethylmelamine + cyclophosphamide + methotrexate + 5-fluorouracil 7, 53, 56, 69, 129, 130, 152
HexaCAF L-PAM	hexamethylmelamine + cyclophosphamide + methotrexate + 5-fluorouracil - L-PAM 154
PVA	cisplatin + vincristine + actinomycin D 280
PVB	cisplatin + vinblastine + bleomycin 151, 161, 166, 185, 188, 196, 235, 247, 270, 274, 275, 278
PVBA	cisplatin + vinblastine + bleomycin + adriamycin 197
PVBACT	cisplatin + vinblastine + bleomycin + actinomycin D 222
PVBPACT	cisplatin + vinblastine + bleomycin + prednison + actinomycin D 221
PBVPA	cisplatin + bleomycin + VP16-213 + adriamycin 168
T7	actinomycin D + adriamycin + bleomycin + methotrexate, high dose + vincristine 336, 353, 354
VAB I	vinblastine + actinomycin D + bleomycin 204, 208, 235
VAB II	vinblastine + cisplatin + actinomycin D + bleomycin 204
VAB III-IV	vinblastine + cisplatin + actinomycin D + adriamycin 205, 206, 207
VAC	vincristine + actinomycin D + cyclophosphamide 426, 440
VADIC	vincristine + adriamycin + DTIC 331, 428
VA MTX	vincristine + adriamycin + methotrexate 333
VB	vinblastine + bleomycin 160, 186, 188, 196, 204, 235, 250
VBP+VP16	vinblastine + bleomycin + cisplatin + VP16-213 187
VP	vinblastine + cisplatin 275
VMMC-PAM	vincristine + mitomycin C + L-PAM 331